Exercise Physiology

LABORATORY MANUAL

D1364680

third edition

Exercise Physiology
LABORATORY MANUAL

Gene M. Adams

California State University
Fullerton

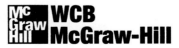

Boston, Massachusetts   Burr Ridge, Illinois   Dubuque, Iowa
Madison, Wisconsin   New York, New York   San Francisco, California   St. Louis, Missouri

WCB/McGraw-Hill

A Division of The **McGraw·Hill** Companies

EXERCISE PHYSIOLOGY LABORATORY MANUAL

Recycled paper

 This book is printed on recycled paper containing 10% postconsumer waste.

3 4 5 6 7 8 9 0 QPD/QPD 9 0 9 8

ISBN 0–697–29500–1

Publisher: *Ed Bartell*
Executive editor: *Vicki Malinee*
Developmental editor: *Shirley Oberbroeckling*
Marketing manager: *Pam Cooper*
Project manager: *Ann Fuerste*
Production supervisor: *Deb Donner*
Cover © Yoav Levy/Photo Take
Illustrations by Janet Inez Adams
Art editor: *Joyce Watters*
Compositor: *Shepherd, Inc.*
Typeface: *10/12 Times Roman*
Printer: *Quebecor Printing Book Group/Dubuque*

www.mhhe.com

Contents

Preface

The third edition of *Exercise Physiology Laboratory Manual* is faithful to its original objective which is to familiarize students with many of the basic laboratory procedures and tests in Exercise Physiology. It is designed to complement the typical Exercise Physiology lecture course. No single manual can ever be an exhaustive survey of all laboratory tests or experiments in exercise physiology. Thousands of different tests have been used by persons interested in exercise performance, ranging in sophistication from Ancient Greek "evaluators" visually inspecting Spartan athletes[1] to modern exercise scientists monitoring isotopic tracers.

The field and laboratory experiences suggested in this lab manual are designed not only to reinforce the basic principles learned in the lecture course but also to teach the basic principles and skills of measurement and evaluation in the field of exercise physiology. Although computerized methods facilitate testing, particularly calculations, they often do not provide students with an optimal understanding of the principles of testing. Too often the principles of measurement are lost when all that is required is pressing a "magic button" on an instrument. Thus, one of my purposes is not to teach students how to use all of the constantly evolving exercise instruments, but to help students understand what the instruments are attempting to measure and how they do it.

Chapter Format

The third edition retains the successful format of its predecessors. The topic of each chapter is introduced by presenting its significance, purpose, physiological rationale, and accuracy. The introductory material is followed by a Method section, which includes information about the test equipment, the technician and subject preparations, and the test procedures and calculations. The Method section is followed by a Results and Discussion section, which includes information regarding the interpretation of the tests, such as norms and standards.

New to this Edition

This edition has been enhanced by the addition of the following features:

- Boxes for the Accuracy sections and Calibration sections focus on these topics for particular chapters of special interest to students, instructors, and researchers. It allows one to skip easily over these sections if this information is not of immediate concern.
- In each Method section, a listing format of the procedural steps facilitates a "cook-book" style of administrating the field or laboratory tests.
- New illustrations have been added throughout the text to clarify concepts, equipment, and procedures.
- Updated norms have been added along with more user-friendly forms.
- I have retained the classical references while updating many others, thus providing students and instructors with the means to pursue further investigations into their research interests.

The Customized Option

My goal for this and previous editions has been to make the "Manual" as generic as possible, so that it is applicable to most Exercise Physiology Laboratories. This edition is even more flexible than the first two by giving instructors the exciting option of customizing the manual to meet their specific needs and interests. They can now choose to include only those chapters—in specially bound volumes—that fit their course and teaching methods. For those instructors who prefer the full twenty-five chapters, the complete version of the Manual is also available. For either option, the framework of the manual remains flexible enough for instructors to substitute their own tests and equipment, if they so desire, while assuring that the basic principles of laboratory procedures are followed.

The first three chapters of the "Manual" are required of both customized and complete versions. Chapter TE (Terminology) begins with the terms important for understanding and measuring exercise, such as those related to fitness, mass, force, work, velocity, power, and energy. The chapter continues with a discussion of meteorological terms, such as temperature and relative humidity. Also, the chapter presents some common statistical terms used in exercise physiology, such as variable, relationship, norms, and standards. Chapter TE also summarizes the types of tests often associated with fitness and exercise; these are categorized into three types: field, field/laboratory, and laboratory tests. Because accurate assessment is paramount to reliable and valid testing,

---

[1]Mechikoff, R., & Estes, S. (1993). *A history and philosophy of sport and physical education.* Dubuque, IA: Brown & Benchmark.

the terminology chapter also includes a brief discussion of calibration. The terminology chapter ends with a discussion of the major components of a research paper or abstract: introduction, purpose, method, results, discussion, and conclusion.

Chapter UN (Units of Measure) begins with a discussion of the International System of measurement. This logically leads to a discussion of the American and metric systems. The units of these two systems dealing with length, mass, volume, and other terms presented in the first chapter (TE) are discussed with respect to their conversions and precision. Chapter UN also includes a discussion of such basic data as name, date, and gender, that are usually required for data collection in all laboratory tests.

The third chapter—Dynamic Strength (DS)—is required because it incorporates many of the terms and units presented in the first two required chapters. Specifically, Chapter DS applies the terms and measuring units to three different free-weight strength tests.

The manual is arranged in a logical order according to the physical fitness continuum presented in the first chapter. Thus, the initial chapters present field and laboratory tests for strength and anaerobic fitness; the middle chapters present aerobic fitness tests, including cardiovascular and respiratory tests; the latter chapters present flexibility and kinanthropometry (body composition) tests. Regardless of the chapter sequence, each chapter may stand alone in order to accommodate flexible scheduling of laboratory sessions.

For more information concerning this new Custom Option, please contact your McGraw-Hill sales representative or refer to the custom order form included in this text.

My philosophical approach to learning laboratory procedures is consistent with the following quote:[2]

> "A learner does not act without thinking and feeling, or think without acting and feeling, or feel without acting or thinking."

In essence, this means that the student is encouraged to get involved in the topic by being *active* during the lab session and to *feel* what it is like to be tested. By *thinking* about these actions and feelings, the student then can truly *know* the topic.

This manual is a fruitful combination of the "knowing" I received from my former teachers and role models. My first teacher, Dr. Larry Morehouse, introduced me to Exercise Physiology and contributed to the framework by which to build my future knowledge in Exercise Physiology. My second teacher, Dr. Herbert deVries, contributed to my technical and research skills while enhancing my knowledge and encouraging my involvement in the profession. My role model, Dr. Fred Kasch, provided a model for applying what I knew to the general public and students. The three men contributed to my admiration for all pioneers of exercise physiology and to my excitement toward the field of Exercise Physiology. I am also grateful to my colleagues from all parts of the country who contributed their encouragement and ideas. I especially want to thank the following instructors who took time to offer their insightful opinions about this edition of the manual:

Cindy Abbott, California State University, Fullerton
Dakin E. Anderson, Winona State University
Walter D. Andzel, Kean College of New Jersey
Barry Beedle, Elon College
William Cockerham, Fresno Pacific College
Lori Dewald, Shippensburg University of Pennsylvania
Elizabeth Dowling, Old Dominion University
Richard Green, Gonzaga University
Ute Jannsen-Kerr, Santa Fe Community College
Gig Leadbetter, Mesa State College
John Liu, Bryan College
Bonita Marks, University of North Carolina, Chapel Hill
Greg Martel, University of Maryland
Jerry Mayhew, Truman State University
Steven Morrison, Pennsylvania State University
Vincent Paolone, Springfield College
Donald Rodd, University of Evansville
John P. Sanko, University of Scranton
Sheri Savoie, Louisiana State University
Mark Spencer, Norfolk State University
Mark Stanbrough, Emporia State University
Marilyn Strawbridge, Butler University
Mary Frances Visser, Mankato State University
Henry Williford, Auburn University at Montgomery

Gene Adams

---

[2]Barrow, H. M., & McGee, R. (1971). *A practical approach to measurement in physical education.* Philadelphia: Lea & Febiger, p. 145.

Exercise Physiology Laboratory Manual, Third Edition
by Gene Adams
Textbook Order Form

Option 1 - To order the standard *Exercise Physiology Laboratory Manual* textbook, make note of the ISBN number and contact your bookstore with this information. ISBN 0-697-29500-1

Option 2 - To order a Custom *Exercise Physiology Laboratory Manual* (minimum order is 50 custom manuals), please complete this form (**front and back**) .

Professor Name _____

School _____

Department _____ Course Name _____

Address _____

City _____ State _____ Zip _____

Phone/Fax _____ E-mail _____

Textbook Order Coordinator _____

Enrollment (Please be as accurate as possible for ordering purposes) _____

      Note: Minimum order is 50 custom manuals.

Please indicate which bookstores will be ordering the text, along with the phone numbers.

1. _____   2. _____   3. _____

Phone# _____   Phone#_____   Phone # _____

Option 3 - Determine what additional WCB/McGraw-Hill materials or your own materials you would like bound with the selections you indicated on the reverse Custom Order Form. Then contact our Primis Custom Publishing team at 1-800-228-0634 for order and pricing information.

Exercise Physiology Laboratory Manual
Custom Order Form

Step 1: **Make your selections. Place numbers in the column marked "presentation order" to indicate the order in which you would like your customized selections to appear in your textbook.**

Suggested Pricing: $13 for up to 7 labs, $1.30 per each lab thereafter.

Selections	Presentation Order	Selections	Presentation Order
TE Terminology		EB Exercise Blood Pressure	
UN Units of Measure		RE Resting Electrocardiogram	
DS Dynamic Strength		EE Exercise Electrocardiogram	
SS Static Strength		LV Lung Volumes	
IS Isokinetic Strength		ER Exercise Respiration	
SP Speed—40-, 50- and 60-Yard Sprints		FL Lower Trunk Flexibility	
VP Vertical Power		BM Body Mass Index	
NC Anaerobic Cycling (Wingate)		GR Girth	
NS Anaerobic Stepping		SF Skinfolds	
NT Anaerobic Treadmill Tests		HW Hydrostatic Weighing	
AR Aerobic Running and Walking		AP Appendixes	
AS Aerobic Stepping		Appendix A Cardiopulmonary Resuscitation	
AC Aerobic Cycling		Appendix B Reporting Units and Symbols	
OC Maximal Oxygen Consumption		Appendix C Metric-American Conversions	
RB Resting Blood Pressure		Appendix D Sample Problems and Solutions	

Step 2: **Complete the course information and school name for the cover and send this form to our Primis team (See below):**

Professor or course name to appear on cover: _____

School name to appear on cover: _____

Step 3: Don't forget to contact our Primis Custom Publishing team if you would like to add any additional materials to those indicated above. Call Primis Custom Publishing, mail or Fax to:

WCB/McGraw-Hill Publishers
Primis Custom Publishing
2460 Kerper Blvd.
Dubuque, IA 52001
Fax: (319) 589-4766 Phone: (800) 228-0634

Chapter TE   Terminology

Probably nothing is more motivating for exercise science students than to know that the field's professional organizations affirm the importance of an education in exercise science laboratories. For example, the Exercise Science Council of The National Association for Sport and Physical Education (NASPE) has stated that students of exercise science are expected to "demonstrate the use of (1) health and fitness field and laboratory instruments, (2) techniques, (3) procedures, and (4) equipment."[20] The committee asserts that in conjunction with this basic standard, students should be able to "evaluate and interpret exercise testing results." The logical first step in acquiring such abilities for the exercise physiology student is to master the scientific language of physiological testing.

The beginning student of Exercise Physiology is introduced to many new terms and often is exposed to unfamiliar measuring units. If these are not mastered early, the performance tests administered in a laboratory course of exercise physiology will have little meaning. It would be similar to studying a new subject written or taught in a foreign language. Two former editors of the highly respected journal *Medicine and Science in Sports and Exercise* emphasized the importance of standardizing terminology and measuring units in the field of exercise physiology.[13,30,31,32,33] The terms and units presented in *Exercise Physiology Laboratory Manual* are faithful to their recommendations of standardization.

Many of the terms used to orient the beginning student in a course of exercise physiology laboratory may be organized into the following six categories: (a) exercise, (b) meteorological, (c) statistical, (d) calibration, (e) types of tests, and (f) scientific writing terms.

Exercise Terms

Familiarization with exercise terms is essential to the understanding of the measurement of physical performance. To understand physical performance one needs to become familiar with fitness terms, especially those that are health-related and those related to a fitness continuum; the continuum being those physical fitness components that can be categorized according to time. After becoming familiar with the fitness terms, we will familiarize ourselves with some of the most common measurement terms in exercise physiology such as mass, force, work, velocity, power, and energy.

Fitness and Health Relationship

Fitness and health are not synonymous, especially when health is viewed traditionally as an absence of disease. However, *optimal* health implies that individuals have the potential to achieve their highest possible fitness level. Accordingly, a high physical fitness level promotes optimal exercise performance.

One modification of the World Health Organization's conceptual definition of physical fitness states that fitness is "the ability to carry out physical activities satisfactorily."[24] The five traditional fitness components listed in Table 1—(1) strength, (2) muscular endurance, (3) cardiorespiratory or cardiovascular endurance, (4) flexibility, and (5) body composition—may also be categorized as health-related fitness components.[1] These fitness components are not only directed at exercise performance but also at such hypo-active prone diseases or functional disabilities as heart disease, obesity, and muscle pain.[5] Muscular power, including speed of movement, is a **non**-health-related fitness component that is of primary concern to competitive exercise participants. Table 1 also gives examples of how each of these health-related fitness components are frequently measured in field (weight room, gym, track/field, etc.) or laboratory settings.

Except for flexibility and body composition, three of the other health-related fitness components—strength, muscular endurance, and cardiorespiratory endurance—may be classified according to their relationship to time, either in seconds (s) or minutes (min). The ranges of times selected for each component in Figure 1 are based on an optimally paced and all-out effort by the performer under normal conditions. This general time relationship is faithful to the typical tests that measure these three fitness components. For example, strength can usually be measured in less than 4 s, but is difficult to sustain longer than this; muscular endurance is often measured between 10 and 180 s, and cardiorespiratory endurance is measured in 3 min or more. In order to apply distances to this model, one must consider the specific fitness of each person. For muscle endurance, the time zone between 10 s and 180 s, represents a person's all-out effort to sustain optimal performance for the duration of any event in the 10–180-s time period. This period could represent running distances over 100 meters and less than 1200 meters (three laps of a 400-meter track). For example, if a male and female ran

Table 1 Health-Related Fitness and Measurement Examples

Fitness Terms	Measurement Examples	
	Field	Laboratory
Muscular Strength	Maximal Lift (e.g., 1-RM)	Isokinetic Dynamometry (e.g., Torque)
Muscular Endurance	Timed Repetitions (e.g., Situps)	Wingate Cycle (e.g., rpm)
Cardiorespiratory Endurance	Timed Distance (e.g., 1.5-Mile Run)	Maximal Oxygen Consumption (e.g., Graded Exercise Test)
Flexibility	Linear Range of Motion (e.g., Sit-and-Reach)	Degrees Range of Motion (e.g., Leighton Flexometry)
Body Composition	Height-Weight Relationship (e.g., Body Mass Index)	Lean-Fat Relationship (e.g., Hydrostatic Weighing)

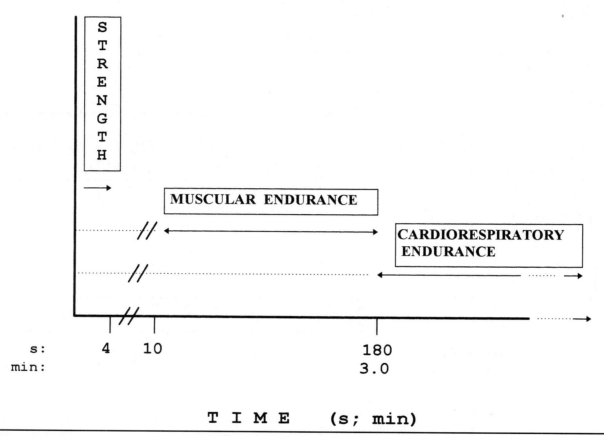

Figure 1 The relationship between three of the health-related fitness components and time.

800 meters in 100 s and 110 s, respectively, each would be deemed world class performers; whereas if a person ran about half this distance, 400 meters, in the same time—100 to 110 s—it would be fairly typical for the average young adult. Swimming distances, of course, would be shorter, and cycling distances would be greater for any given time periods.

One problem with relating these three fitness components to these general time periods is that there can be significant differences between the shorter and longer times within each designated time interval. Hence, by subdividing the time zones based on physiological factors, more specific terminology may be applied.

Fitness-Time Continuum

Using the term continuum to describe fitness allows us to identify some other fitness components that are important and that may require different testing and training procedures. A version of such a fitness-time continuum is shown in Table 2 and Figures 2 and 3. It is an approximate classification of exercise/fitness derived by combining the various analyses or reports of running events[27,46,50] and bioenergetic systems.[11,12,19,22,36,37,42,43,45,49,51,55] This continuum shows and labels transition periods and divisions between and within the three major time-related fitness components (strength, muscular endurance, and cardiorespiratory endurance).

Table 2 Traditional Fitness Categories Subdivided on the Basis of Bioenergetics and Time

Fitness Category	Bioenergetic Pathway	Time Period
Strength	Short-Anaerobic (SAn)	<4 s
	Phosphagenic (Stored ATP)	
Power (Strength and Speed)	Short-Anaerobic Phosphagenic (ATP + PC)	4–10 s
Muscular Endurance		10–180 s
Power-Endurance (Strength, Speed, and Muscle Endurance)	Short-Anaerobic Phosphagenic and Glycolytic	10–30 s
Mid Muscular-Endurance	Long-Anaerobic (LAn) Glycolytic	30–90 s 0.5–1.5 min
Mixed Endurance (Muscle and Cardiorespiratory Endurance)	Anaerobic and Aerobic Glycolytic and Oxidative	90–180 s 1.5–3.0 min
Cardiorespiratory Endurance	Aerobic	>180 s >3 min
Short-Aerobic (SA)	Oxidative	3–60 min = SA
Long-Aerobic (LA)	Oxidative + Hydration + Nutrition Factors	>60 min = LA

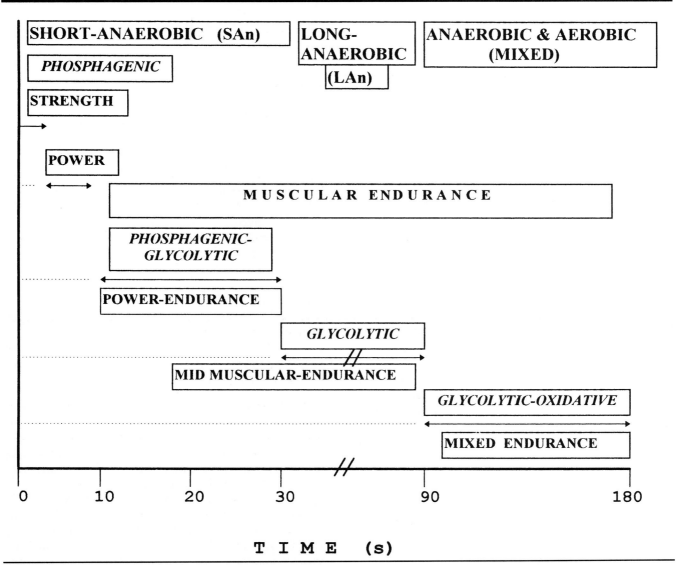

Figure 2 The fitness continuum representing the relationship between time and fitness based on significant contribution of the anaerobic (phosphagenic and glycolytic) bioenergetic pathway (italics).

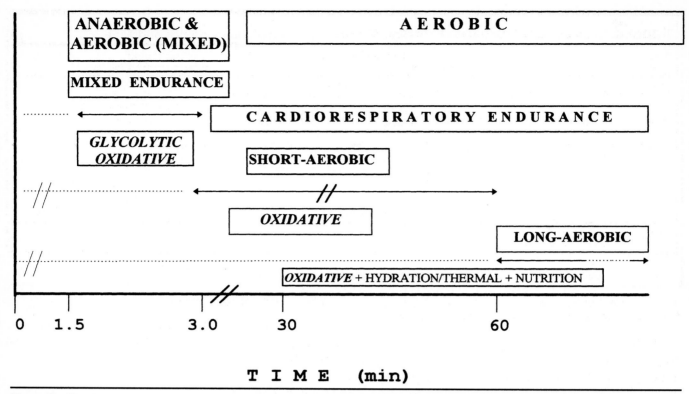

| | ANAEROBIC & AEROBIC (MIXED) | | | AEROBIC | | |

Figure 3 The fitness continuum representing the relationship between time and fitness based on significant contribution of the aerobic (oxidative) bioenergetic pathway.

From the biochemical point of view, exercise may be divided into at least five categories based on the predominant metabolic pathway or combination of two pathways (Table 2).

The bioenergetic pathways are metabolic paths that are responsible for providing the energy substance, adenosine triphosphate (ATP) for muscle action. As noted in Table 2 and Figures 2 and 3, the two major metabolic pathways—aerobic and anaerobic—produce this useable chemical energy—ATP—so that the muscles can transfer it to mechanical energy (movement). Both the anaerobic and aerobic pathways may be divided into short and long components.

Short-Anaerobic (SAn)

The short-anaerobic pathway is mainly a phosphagenic system, especially for movements requiring strength and power (strength combined with speed). The glycolytic pathway contributes to movements related to power-endurance. Strength is dependent upon the stored ATP in the muscle fibers, which is immediately available for muscle action. The maximal transfer of this chemical energy (ATP) to mechanical energy occurs during a maximal muscle contraction. This supply may last up to three[12] or four seconds[36] during a maximal contraction. An early 1900s leader of physical education proposed such a short test of strength to determine a student's health and progress.[38] Power actions receive their energy from both ATP and phosphocreatine

(PC); this supply may last for 10s when used at a maximal rate. Movements that are relatively less forceful and slower, but are able to persist up to 30 s, combine the slower ATP-producing glycogen system with that of the faster phosphagenic system. This short-anaerobic fitness component may be referred to as power-endurance, the beginning portion of muscular endurance.

Long-Anaerobic (LAn)

The 30–90 s midportion of muscular endurance, called mid muscular-endurance, is mainly dependent on the glycolytic pathway for its source of ATP. This is the system that causes performers of these events to accumulate high lactate values.

Mixed-Endurance

The third and final portion of muscular endurance is called mixed-endurance. For optimally sustained movements between 90 s (1.5 min) and 180 s (3 min), it relies on substantial contributions from both the aerobic and anaerobic pathways. Performances closer to the shorter end of this range, that is, closer to 1.5 min, will have a greater glycolytic contribution than those all-out performances nearing the 3-min time. Typical running events for this pathway could extend from 400 m to 800 m. These events also cause very high lactate values, attesting to the significant contribution of the glycolytic pathway;

Table 3 Fitness Tests Presented in This Lab Manual

Fitness Continuum Tests			
	Anaerobic		Aerobic
Strength	Short-Anaerobic	Long-Anaerobic	Short-Aerobic
Dynamic Free-Weights (Upper Body)	Sprints (40-50-60 yd)	Wingate Cycle (Power/Endurance)	1.0-Mile/9-min Run
			1.5-Mile/12-min Run
Static Dynamometry (Handgrip)	Vertical Jump	Anaerobic Step	Forestry Step
			Astrand Cycle
Isokinetic (Leg Extension and Flexion)	Wingate Cycle (Power)	Fast Treadmill and Slow Treadmill Runs	Power-170 Cycle
			Maximal $\dot{V}O_2$
			Exercise ECG
			Exercise Blood Pressure
			Exercise Respiration
Noncontinuum Tests			
Flexibility: Sit-and-Reach			
Body Composition: Stature-Weight Indexes; Girths; Skinfolds; Densitometry			

but successful performance is also dependent upon a significant contribution from the aerobic pathway.

Aerobic

The aerobic pathway is an oxidative pathway that predominates in optimally paced exercise of durations longer than 3 min. It too may be divided into two major portions, one called **short-aerobic (SA)** from about 3 min to 60 min, and another called **long-aerobic (LA)** for prolonged efforts greater than 60 min. In brief, long-aerobic tasks still depend on the oxidative pathway, but require more consideration of nutritional and hydrational factors for successful performance than do the short-aerobic tasks.

Summary of Fitness Terms

The anaerobic pathway is a high-power system producing ATP at high rates (high power) but producing small amounts (low capacity). The aerobic pathway is just the opposite—a low-power but high-capacity system. The mixed pathway, which involves significant contributions from both aerobic and anaerobic pathways, is moderate in power and capacity. **Flexibility,** a traditional fitness component, cannot be categorized meaningfully into the fitness-time continuum. Although **body composition** is a traditional fitness component, it is also not suited for the fitness-time continuum. However, it may be viewed as the expected *by-product* of these time-designated fitness components of the fitness continuum.

Many of the tests presented in this manual may be categorized according to the fitness continuum, that is, the predominant metabolic pathway being evaluated by the test; others are simply referred to as noncontinuum tests such as flexibility or body composition tests (Table 3). Skill-related performance, such as agility, balance, and sports skills, are not within the scope of this laboratory manual.

Measurement Terms

Some of the most common measurement terms in exercise physiology are mass, force, work, velocity, power, and energy.

Mass (M)

Mass is a basic physical quantity that is defined as the quantity of matter in an object. Under normal acceleration of gravity, mass is equivalent to weight. Two common units of measure for mass or weight are the gram and kilogram. Mass and force are two basic quantities that are similar under certain circumstances. In some instances mass is considered equal to the force lifting the mass, such as when lifting your own weight and/or the barbell against gravitational forces. However, in actuality, the muscles need to exert forces greater than the mass due to various factors (e.g., mechanical leverage).

Force (F)

Force is a derived term (mass × acceleration) and is defined as that which changes or tends to change the state of rest or motion in matter.[4] Thus muscular activity (exercise) generates force. Because torque is often associated with force measurements, it is mentioned here, but it could stand alone as a basic physical variable.[33] Torque consists of a rotational force applied to a lever. A person applying a maximal force to a resistance or load, whether it be against gravity or a lever, is displaying the fitness component of strength. Most muscular activity, however, uses forces that are submaximal.

Forces may be related to three of the major fitness components when using weight-lifting as the representative exercise mode. Each component can be associated with an estimated range for the percentage of a maximal contraction. By virtue of the definition of strength, this health-related fitness component requires a muscle action that is at, or at least very near, 100% of maximal. The forces necessary to perform activities associated with muscle endurance have a large range and are less than those required for strength. Based on the relationship between the number of maximal repetitions and one maximal repetition when weight-lifting (see Chapter DS) and the approximate amount of time it would take to perform such repetitions, muscular endurance actions may be estimated to require about 40% to 90% of maximal. The forces necessary to perform the number of lifts inherent to cardiorespiratory endurance are usually less than 40% of a maximal contraction.[14] This model should illustrate how forces can be related to fitness components for some activities, specifically, in this case, weight lifting.

Work (w)

Work is a derived term, meaning that it is comprised of more than one basic physical quantity. It is a product of two basic quantities—force and distance, but not time.

Often, work is thought of as the force applied upward *against* gravity for a given displacement or distance (D). This may be classified as positive work (^+w), or concentric exercise (Eq. 1). For example, the work or exercise performed while ascending steps or running on a sloped treadmill is calculated as positive work. Cycling on a cycle ergometer is also positive work. On the Monark® cycle ergometer the visibility of the vertical work can be appreciated by observing the lift of the weighted pendulum at the side of the ergometer. This force can also be read on the dial indicator at the top-front panel of the ergometer.

$$^+w = F \times D \qquad \text{Eq. 1}$$

The work calculated for step tests should consider the negative work (^-w) or eccentric component. Eccentric exercise represents the muscle action when descending the step. For step-test purposes, negative work is considered to be about one-third of the positive work[3,41] (Eq. 2).

$$^-w = \tfrac{1}{3} \times \,^+w; \text{ or } = \,^+w \div 3; \text{ or } = 0.33 \times \,^+w \qquad \text{Eq. 2}$$

The combined components of positive work and negative work comprise total work (w). This combination can be presented either as an addition equation (Eq. 3) or a multiplication equation (Eq. 4). The horizontal component (e.g., back and forth movements in stepping) of work usually is considered only when calculating the total energy cost in terms of oxygen consumption.

Addition: $\qquad\qquad w = \,^+w + \,^-w \qquad$ Eq. 3

Multiplication: $\qquad w = 1.33 \times \,^+w \qquad$ Eq. 4

Velocity (v)

Velocity is synonymous with speed. It is the quotient of distance divided by time (D/t). The fitness components can be related to speed based on approximate world-record times for various running events.[23,27] The obvious reference point for maximal velocity is the 100-m event, in which runners achieve maximal velocity within 4 to 5 or 6 s, or between 30 to 40 or 50 m,[18,55] and could maintain this up to the eleventh second.[54] The velocities for the other running events, and their associated fitness components, can be quantified as a percentage of the maximal velocity (Fig. 4). A static contraction exhibits zero velocity because there is no visible movement. The formula for velocity is presented in Equation 5.

$$v = D/t; \text{ or } D \div t \qquad \text{Eq. 5}$$

Power (P; ẇ)

Power is a derived quantity that is a function of work over time (w/t or ẇ), that is, the *rate* of work. It is the mathematical product of force and velocity. The formula for power is expressed in different ways in Equation 6.

$$P = w/t = w \cdot t^{-1} = F \times (D/t) = F \times (D \cdot t^{-1}) = F \times v \qquad \text{Eq. 6}$$

Notice that the format in two of the formulas multiplies by the negative power exponent (e.g., $^{-1}$); this is the recommended reporting style of the International System and of most scientific journals.

Contrary to what one might first think, maximal power is not achieved by either maximal velocity or maximal force. It is achieved by the optimal combination of velocity and force,[53] as depicted in Figure 5. Thus, to achieve maximal power a person must exert against a submaximal resistance, which also means that the movement will not reach the maximal velocity of unloaded limbs.

Power is also a term often used when referring to the rate of transforming metabolic energy to physical performance,[34] such as aerobic power and anaerobic power. However, instead of viewing this as a power term, as would a physicist, the exercise physiologist would probably view this more as an energy term.

Energy (E)

Energy is a derived term providing a description of the amount of metabolic energy released due to the combination of visible mechanical work and the heat of the body itself. It may be calculated from the total amount of work produced and the known or estimated efficiency of the exerciser, which is a major determinant of heat generation. The metabolic oxygen cost during exercise on a cycle ergometer is estimated from the power level plus the oxygen cost of "zero" power cycling and resting metabolism.[35]

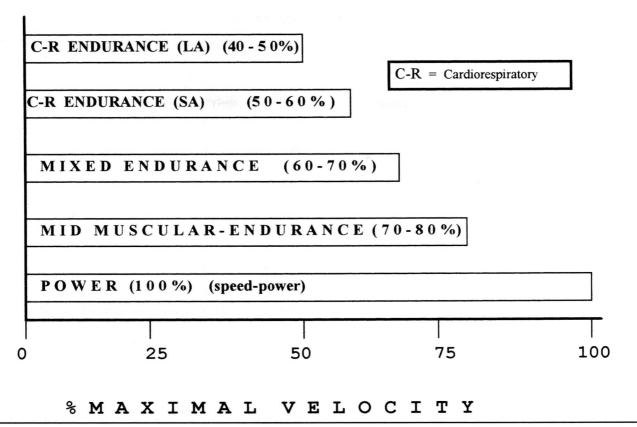

% M A X I M A L   V E L O C I T Y

Figure 4 The relationship between fitness components and maximal running speed (velocity).

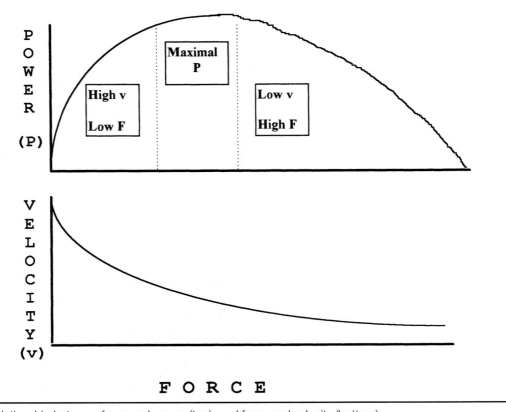

F O R C E

Figure 5 The relationship between force and power (top), and force and velocity (bottom).

Meteorological Terms

Meteorology is the study of the weather. The primary meteorological concerns of the exercise physiologist are temperature, relative humidity, and barometric pressure.

Temperature (T)

Temperature is one of the seven basic physical quantities, according to the International System of nomenclature.[56] Americans are familiar with the fahrenheit scale, but the two most common units for scientists are the celsius scale and the kelvin scale. The fahrenheit (F) scale is usually not printed in scientific research journals.

Celsius (C) Scale

This was formerly called the centigrade scale, but the preferred term is *celsius*.[6] The Swedish mathematician Anders Celsius arbitrarily chose to make the freezing and boiling points of water $0°$ and $100°$, respectively.

Kelvin (K) Scale

The basic thermal scale for the International System (SI) is the kelvin scale, named after the nineteenth century physicist. It has an absolute zero, meaning that the coldest temperature is truly $0°$ (no *minus* or *below zero*). For example, it is not possible to have a temperature colder than $0 °K$; a temperature of $0 °C$ or $32 °F$ is a temperature of $273 °K$.

Relative Humidity (RH)

Humidity, or air saturation, is a meteorological term indicating the relative amount of water in the air. If the RH is 100%, then the air contains the most amount of water it can possibly hold at that air temperature. Air can hold more water at higher temperatures than it can at lower temperatures. Typically, relative humidities at exercise are not apt to affect exercise if they are between 20% and 60%; RH levels below or above this range may be classified as *dry* or *wet*, respectively.

Barometric Pressure (P$_B$)

The term barometric pressure refers to the air pressure of the environment. Altitudes can be estimated from air pressures, and weather patterns can be dictated by changes in air pressures. At sea level, barometric pressure does not influence exercise performance. For exercise physiologists, barometric pressure is important in measuring certain physiological variables such as respiratory volumes.

Statistical Terms

The term *statistics* can have more than one meaning.[39] In a broad sense, it includes the method of organizing, describing, and analyzing quantitative (numbers) data, in addition to predicting outcomes or probabilities. The combined term *basic statistics* is sometimes used to describe group data with such statistics as the mean (average, *M*) and standard deviation (*SD*).

Some of the statistical terms commonly used in an exercise physiology laboratory are (a) **variables,** (b) **relationships,** (c) **norms,** and (d) **standards.**

Variable

A variable may be considered a characteristic. The characteristics or variables mentioned in this manual usually have quantitative values that vary among a sample or population. Some of the measured variables discussed in this manual are strength, run/walk time, oxygen consumption, heart rate, blood pressure, and percent body fat. A variable may be either independent or dependent.

Independent Variable

This variable is manipulated or changed (varied) in order to determine its relationship to the dependent variable.[52] Its measuring unit is usually placed on the horizontal (X) axis of a graph (e.g., time in minutes or seconds, power in watts). The experimenter (or technician) controls the independent variable.[29]

Dependent Variable

This variable is measured before and/or after manipulation of the independent variable; its measuring unit is usually placed on the vertical (Y) axis of a graph (e.g., heart rate in b · min^{-1}).

Relationships

There are several terms to consider under the relationship heading. Most of these terms use the unit of measure called the **correlation coefficient (*r*)** to express the extent of the relationship. The correlation coefficient may describe the accuracy of a test, such as its reliability, validity, and objectivity; or it may relate one variable to another, possibly estimating or predicting one variable from the other.

Certain visual relationships may be observed when one variable is plotted on a graph with another variable. When the graphic line (best fit) is straight and ascending, it is called a linear and **direct** (or positive) **relationship.** Thus, as one value of a variable increases, the value of the other variable increases proportionately. When the plotted points on the graph form a descending straight line, it is called a linear and **indirect** (negative) **relationship.** In this case, as one value of a variable increases, the other variable decreases.

Reliability

Reliability is a measure of the reproducibility or consistency of a test. Ideally, reliabilities of tests should be based on a sample of at least thirty subjects.[40] A reliable test gen-

Table 4 Some Criteria for Qualifying Reliability Correlations

Category	Correlation Criteria
High	.9+
Good	.80–.89
Fair	.70–.79
Poor	<.70

Note: Based on references 10,26,39,48.

erates high correlations when values from repeated trials of that test are compared. Table 4 lists some of the criteria for qualitatively categorizing correlations ranging from poor to high.[10,26,39,48] The criterion for an acceptable correlation may vary with the opinions of various investigators; a recommended minimum test-retest correlation can be as low as .70,[48] or, more stringently, as high as .85.[26] A perfect correlation is 1.0, but this would rarely occur.

The reliability of a test may be affected by the experimental and biological error (variability). Experimental variability is due to lab procedures, instrumentation, and environment; thus it represents the technological error in a test. Biological variability or error is due to the natural periodicity (hourly, daily, weekly, etc.) or inherent biological fluctuations of the human subject.[28]

Objectivity

Although similar to reliability, objectivity is distinct in that it represents the ability of a test to give similar results when administered by different administrators. It is sometimes referred to as the *inter-observer reliability*.

Validity

This is a measure of the test's ability to measure what it claims to measure. Again, a test with high validity has a good correlation between the criterion (actual or true) value and the test. The r need not be as high for validity as for reliability to establish a meaningful relationship.

Prediction

The relationship between one variable and one or more other variables allows transformation into an equation to estimate one of the variables. The line of best fit of the graphic plot of one variable to another is termed a **regression line;** when it is transformed into an equation it is called a **regression equation.** Sometimes regression equations are presented in the form of a **nomogram;** a nomogram is a series (two or more) of vertical or diagonal lines by which to predict one variable from one or more other variables.

The statistical term that describes the predictive error of a regression equation is the **standard error of estimate** (*SEE*). This is a type of standard deviation around the predicted scores from the regression line. For example, if the predicted lean weight is 40 kg, and the *SEE* is 5 kg, then 68% of the scores will be between 35 kg and 45 kg. Thus, the standard error of the estimate indicates the amount of error to be expected in a predictive score.[8] Using percent fat predictions as an example of *SEE* criteria, one authority[25] recommends that the *SEE* not be greater than 3.1% fat units for nonunderwater-weight determinations in women. Using aerobic fitness predictions as an example, another researcher[17] suggests an acceptability *SEE* criterion of less than 15%.

Norms

Norms and standards enhance the interpretation of test scores. **Norms** are values that relate an individual's score to those of the general population. Some authorities[7] suggest that the minimum number of subjects to establish norms be set at 100. If the population sample number is less than 100, or if the sample differs significantly in its characteristics from the one in which it is being compared, it is probably more appropriate to refer to its values as *comparative scores,* rather than norms. The derived percentiles (*%ile*) or standard deviations (*SD*) developed from norms are often described in accordance to such descriptive categories as poor, below average, average, above average, and excellent (Fig. 6). The Canadian Standardization Test uses percentile ranges from 81 to 100 as excellent, 61 to 80 as above average, 41 to 60 as average, 21 to 40 as below average, and 1 to 20 as poor.[21] Thus, if a person is categorized as excellent in a certain fitness component, then that person ranks better than 80% of the population.

Standards

Standard is a term often used synonymously with norms. However, it more appropriately is used to connote a desirable or recommended value or score.[2] The term *criterion-referenced standards (CRS)* is a professionally popular term.[16] It has the advantage over normative standards for fitness tests because CRS indicate the levels necessary for good health, regardless of the level of physical fitness of the reference group.[9,15,44,47] The CRS for fitness tests may be based on professional expertise and scientific research, in addition to normative data.[15] Thus, CRS are standards that represent recommended levels of performance. Because the CRS are absolute standards, they do not consider the number of persons who meet the standard. For example, a normative standard such as the mean or the 50th percentile may not meet the desirable level of performance. The CRS levels allow easy recognition of the adequacy or inadequacy of a person on that particular fitness/health variable. Also, as long as a person meets the CRS criterion, he or she has the same merit as someone who scores extremely high on the variable.

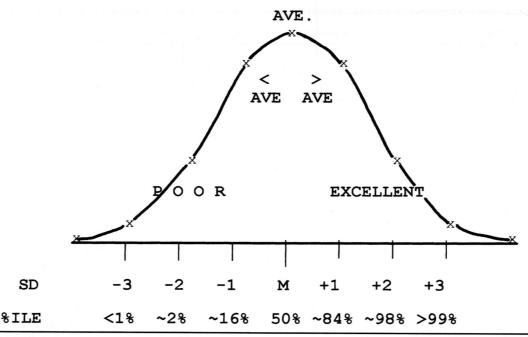

AVE.

< >
AVE AVE

POOR   EXCELLENT

SD	-3	-2	-1	M	+1	+2	+3
%ILE	<1%	~2%	~16%	50%	~84%	~98%	>99%

Figure 6 A typical normal curve and possible placement of qualitative categories (Canadian Test) based on a chosen multiple of the standard deviation and percentiles.

Because the criterion standards are based partially on human judgment, and because of testing errors or subject motivation, the cutoff scores may cause false merit or false nonmerit. Also, the merit levels do not indicate levels at which a person may need to be successful in recreational or competitive sports; they are concerned only with better health.

Thus, *norms* describe a person's position within a population, whereas *standards* describe the criteria suggested for appropriate health or fitness of a population. A test battery that provides both norms and standards is the AAHPERD Health-Related Test.

Calibration Terms

The term **calibration** refers to the fine tuning of the measuring instruments in order to enhance the reliability, validity, and objectivity of testing. Often an instrument is calibrated at three or more points along its measurement scale. These points usually include the lowest point (e.g., zero), an approximate midpoint, and the highest point. For example, a platform scale for measuring body weight may be calibrated at the zero point (0 kg), at the approximate midpoint (70 kg), and at the high point (136 kg). The midpoint and high-point calibrations are possible if calibrated weights are used. Calibrated (certified) weights are those that are certified by a highly accurate scale at a reputable weight dealer. Midpoint and high-point adjustments cannot be made on many instruments. Thus the experimenter may develop a correction factor based upon any discrepancy between the observed and known values at the high and midpoints, or the experimenter may adjust the zero to minimize or eliminate the discrepancy at the most critical interval of the particular measurement.

Types of Tests

Most of the tests described in this manual require measurements during exercise or postexercise conditions, not resting conditions. The value of performance testing of humans is analogous to that of testing cars; the best way to test the performance of the car is not solely by observing it as it sits there, but by observing it as it motors along the highway. Similarly, the best way to evaluate human performance is to observe (measure) the human during or immediately after exercise. The various tests used to measure physical performance may be based upon their predominant use on the field or in the lab or both; thus, the tests described in this book are designated as one of three types: (a) field, (b) field/lab, and (c) lab.

Field Tests

Field tests are common in physical education/kinesiology. Exercise physiologists need to be familiar with field tests because they often measure or estimate variables (e.g., physical fitness components) that are discussed in a course of exercise physiology. Field tests in physical education were developed at the turn of the twentieth century in order to test large groups of persons as accurately and economically as possible outside of a laboratory setting. Unless outside variables (e.g., weather, terrain, motivation, etc.) are strictly

Table 5 Categorization of Tests According to Field, Field/Lab, or Lab

Field	Field/Lab	Lab
Free-Weight Strength	Handgrip Dynamometry	Isokinetic Leg Strength
Sprints	Vertical Jump	Maximal Oxygen Consumption
40-yd	Anaerobic Step	Treadmill Anaerobic Power
50-yd	Wingate Cycle	Exercise Electrocardiogram
60-yd	Forestry Step	Vital Capacity
1.5-Mile/12-Min Run	Astrand Cycle	Forced Expiratory Volume
AAHPERD Run	P-170 Cycle	Lung Volumes
Stature-Weight	Blood Pressure	Max Voluntary Ventilation
Body Mass Index	Girths	Exercise Ventilation, Tidal Volume and Frequency
	Skinfolds	Densitometry (Underwater)
	Sit-Reach Flexibility	

controlled, field tests are not appreciated in research as are the more controlled laboratory tests. However, this does not mean that field tests cannot be as valid as some laboratory tests. In addition to their use in physical education classes, field tests are popular as screening and maintenance tests for military and safety/emergency personnel (e.g., firefighters, lifeguards, police, and rangers). Some familiar field tests are situps, pushups, and pullups. Two typical *aerobic* field tests are the 1.5-Mile Run Test and the AAHPERD 1.0-Mile Run Test.

Field/Lab Tests

Field/lab tests may be administered either under field or laboratory conditions. This usually means that minimal equipment is required, but that the test should be performed under conditions that approximate those in the laboratory setting. In other words, slightly more stringent controls are placed on field/lab tests compared to those placed on field tests. An example of a field/lab test is the Forestry Aerobic Step Test. A long step bench may easily be carried outside the laboratory facility, along with any accessory equipment such as a metronome and stopwatch. Stadium bleachers may substitute for the bench in the laboratory, allowing for simultaneous testing of a large group of subjects.

Lab Tests

Lab tests often require more sophisticated, expensive, and/or bulky equipment than the field or field/lab tests. In addition, more rigid controls are placed on some of the extraneous variables such as weather and motivation. These controls are made not only during the test but prior to the test. For example, a subject undergoing a true lab test should not be influenced by such factors as a heavy meal or a cup of coffee. Due to the more stringent controls and greater complexities in laboratory tests, technicians must be more knowledgeable and skilled in testing procedures and interpretation of testing. Laboratory tests do not lend themselves well to testing more than one person simultaneously,

and, therefore, require more time per subject. In general, compared to field tests, lab tests offset their less practical characteristics by virtue of their more precise and accurate characteristics.

A summary of the tests described in this book are listed in Table 5 under the test headings *Field, Field/Lab,* or *Lab.* Some of these may be placed in two or all three categories depending upon the sophistication applied by the investigator or technician. For instance, densitometry (hydrostatic weighing) may be performed in a swimming pool and without prior measurement of residual volume. Thus, depending upon the sophistication selected, it could be classified as either a field/lab test or a lab test.

Scientific Writing Terms

The parts of a research article in scientific journals have traditional terms or headings for each part. A research abstract contains all of these same parts as the full-length article, but is much shorter and acts as a summary of the study. Typically, the following parts are included in scientific articles and abstracts: (1) introduction/purpose, (2) method, (3) results/discussion, and (4) conclusion. An abstract of a research study is usually placed at the front of the written article. However, if it does not appear at the beginning, it may be presented as a summary at the end of the article.

Research articles often range in length from about three to six pages in many scientific journals and up to nearly one hundred pages in special journal supplements, master's theses, and doctoral dissertations. However, these articles may be reduced to merely 150–500 words in an abstract. For example, one journal in the field, *Research Quarterly for Exercise and Sport,* presently averages about 200 words per abstract, whereas another, *Medicine and Science in Sports and Exercise,* averages 300–350 words. Also, when researchers submit abstracts for consideration of presentation at conventions, they often are given special forms with an outlined "box" (about 5 × 5 in.; 14 × 14 cm) by which to limit the length of their abstract (see inserted box). There is abundant use of abbreviations in abstracts in

Title of Abstract

Name(s) of Investigator(s)

Introduction and Purpose:

Introduction: Importance, significance, and possibly a brief historical perspective of the topic.
Purpose: State of the problem; research question; hypotheses and their rationale.

Method: Description of participants, instrumentation (apparatus), procedures, experimental design and statistical methods.

Results and Discussion:

Results: Summary of major findings; statistical values.

Discussion: Explanations (rationale) and implications of the findings; interpretation; confounding variables; confirmation or refutation of prior studies; future studies.

Conclusion: A final statement related to your purpose; the answer to your research question.

Notes: The names and affiliations of the investigators are not included when submitting abstracts for blind review. The titled subheadings (e.g., "Method") usually are not printed.

order to squeeze as many words as possible into these boxes. Not every item discussed under each major part of a research paper needs to be covered in the abstract because of the abstract's brevity. However, each major section (Introduction/Purpose; Method; Results/Discussion; and Conclusion) must be addressed.

Abstract Introduction and Purpose

Introduction

An abstract should first catch the reader's attention by stating the *importance* or *significance* of the study. Perhaps the study settles some controversial issue or benefits a particular group such as educators, coaches, or scientists. Sometimes a brief historical perspective may be included. The importance/significance is usually no longer than one or two sentences.

Purpose

The purpose of the study is merely a statement concerning the problem that the study is trying to solve. It may be presented in the form of a research question, such as, "What is the aerobic fitness level of the students in our exercise physiology lab class?" or it may be stated definitively, such as, "The purpose of this study was to determine the level of fitness in the exercise physiology lab class." Sometimes there is more than one purpose to a study, or one of the purposes is secondary to another.

The purpose may include the hypothesis of the investigators. This is a statement regarding the expected outcome. For instance, the investigators might feel that physical educators will have higher fitness levels than that of the average person. A **physiological rationale,** which provides the basis for the study or for the type of test chosen to solve the problem, may be included. Thus, statements regarding the physiology, validity, and reliability of a test may be included here.

Method

The description of the method for solving the research problem follows the description of the purpose. Often this portion of the abstract is overdone; three or four statements should be sufficient for most method sections, unless the investigators are concerned with a research problem dealing with the type of methodology per se. The method portion of an abstract often includes the following: (1) general description of the instrumentation, procedures, and calculations; (2) description of participants (subjects); and (3) experimental design, statistical method, and sampling procedure.

Results and Discussion

The results usually summarize and evaluate the group data from a tabular form to a statistical form (e.g., mean, standard deviation, and range). The interpretation of the results may be best applied if norms and standards exist for the particular testing method of the study.

The discussion should include a physiological rationale (a reason) for the results, and may include any confounding variables affecting the results. It may mention whether the findings confirm or refute previous research. Also, the findings may have raised questions that may be answered by further research.

Conclusion

The conclusion should be very succinct, simply answering the research question that was proposed in the purpose of the study. It should be as obviously presented as the purpose. Thus, it often begins as follows: "The investigators conclude that . . ."; or it is the last sentence of the abstract.

Summary of Terminology

Many of the basic terms and units used in exercise physiology are summarized in Table 6. As with learning any new

Table 6 Common Terms and Units for Exercise, Meteorology, Statistics, Calibration, Tests, and Scientific Writing

Term	Unit
Exercise	
Force (F)	N; kg
Work (w)	J; kJ; N $\cdot$ m; kg $\cdot$ m
Velocity (v)	m $\cdot$ min^{-1}; m $\cdot$ s^{-1}; km $\cdot$ h^{-1} mph; rad $\cdot$ s^{-1}; $°$ $\cdot$ s^{-1}
Power (P)	W; J $\cdot$ s^{-1}; J $\cdot$ min.$^{-1}$; –kJ $\cdot$ s^{-1}; kJ $\cdot$ min^{-1}; N $\cdot$ m $\cdot$ s^{-1}; N $\cdot$ m $\cdot$ min^{-1}; kg $\cdot$ m $\cdot$ s^{-1}; kg $\cdot$ m $\cdot$ min^{-1}
Energy (E)	J; kJ; kcal; VO$_2$; L $\cdot$ min^{-1}; ml $\cdot$ min^{-1}; ml $\cdot$ kg^{-1} $\cdot$ min^{-1}; MET
Meteorology	
Celsius (C)	$°$C
Kelvin (K)	$°$K
Relative Humidity (RH)	% RH
Barometric Pressure (P$_B$)	torr
Statistics	
Variable	x; y
Relationships	r; *SEE*
Norms (mean; standard deviation; percentile)	*M; SD; %ile*
Criterion-reference standard	CRS
Calibration	
Zero (low) point	
Midpoint	
High point	
Tests	
Field	
Field/Lab	
Lab	
Scientific Writing	
Introduction/Purpose	
Method	
Results and Discussion	
Conclusion	

language, the beginner should practice using these terms and units so they become a natural part of the exercise physiology vocabulary.

Selected References

1. American College of Sports Medicine (ACSM). (1986). *Guidelines for graded exercise testing and exercise prescription.* Philadelphia: Lea & Febiger.
2. American College of Sports Medicine (ACSM). (1988). ACSM opinion statement on physical fitness in children and youth. *Medicine and Science in Sports and Exercise, 20,* 422–423.
3. American College of Sports Medicine (ACSM). (1991). *Guidelines for graded exercise testing and exercise prescription.* Philadelphia: Lea & Febiger.
4. American College of Sports Medicine (ACSM). (1991). Information for authors. *Medicine and Science in Sports and Exercise, 23*(7): i–v.
5. American College of Sports Medicine (ACSM). (1995). *ACSM's Guidelines for graded exercise testing and exercise prescription.* Philadelphia: Lea & Febiger.
6. American Psychological Association. (1994). *Publication manual of the American Psychological Association.* Washington, D.C.: Author.
7. Barrow, H. M., & McGee, R. (1971). *A practical approach to measurement in physical education.* Philadelphia: Lea & Febiger.
8. Baumgartner, T. A., & Jackson, A. S. (1987). *Measurement for evaluation in physical education and exercise science.* Dubuque, IA: Wm. C. Brown.
9. Blair, S. N., Falls, H. B., & Pate, R. R. (1983). A new physical fitness test. *The Physician and Sportsmedicine, 11,* 87–91.
10. Blesch, T. E. (1974). *Measurement for evaluation in physical education.* New York: Ronald Press.
11. Bowers, R. W., & Fox, E. L. (1992). *Sports physiology.* Dubuque, IA: Wm. C. Brown.
12. Brooks, G. A., Fahey, T. D., & White, T. P. (1996). *Exercise physiology: Human bioenergetics and its application.* Mountain View, CA: Mayfield Publishing Company.
13. Buskirk, E. R. (1987). Implementation of the use of SI units. *Medicine and Science in Sports and Exercise, 19* (6): 545.
14. Chilakos, A. (1974, December). Cardiovascular endurance training through weight training. *The Physical Educator,* pp. 179–180.
15. Corbin, C. B., & Pangrazi, R. P. (1992). Are American children and youth fit? *Research Quarterly for Exercise and Sport, 63,* 96–106.
16. Cureton, K. J., & Warren, G. L. (1990). Criterion-referenced standards for youth health-related fitness tests: A tutorial. *Research Quarterly for Exercise and Sport, 61*(1): 7–19.
17. Davies, C. T. M. (1968). Limitations to the prediction of maximum oxygen intake from cardiac frequency measurements. *Journal of Applied Physiology, 24,* 700–706.
18. Dintiman, G. B. (1984). *How to run faster.* New York: Leisure Press.
19. Edington, D. W., & Edgerton, V. R. (1976). *The biology of physical activity.* Boston: Houghton-Mifflin.
20. Exercise Science Council of NASPE. (1995, September/October). Basic standards for the programs preparing students for careers in exercise science. *UPDATE,* (NASPE Suppl.), 2.
21. Fitness and Amateur Sport Canada. (1987). *Canadian Standardized Test of Fitness (CSTF) operations manual.* 3d ed. Ottawa, Canada: Author.
22. Fox, E. L., Bowers, R. W., & Foss, M. L. (1993). *The physiological basis for exercise and sport.* Dubuque, IA: Brown & Benchmark.
23. Gardner, J. B., & Purdy, J. G. (1970). *Computerized running training programs.* Los Altos, CA: Tafnews Press.
24. Gutin, B., Manos, T., & Strong, W. (1992). Defining health and fitness: First step toward establishing

children's fitness standards. *Research Quarterly for Exercise and Sport, 63,* 128–132.

25. Jackson, A. S. (1984). Research design and analysis of data procedures for predicting body density. *Medicine and Science in Sports and Exercise, 16,* 616–622.

26. Johnson, B. L., & Nelson, J. K. (1974). *Practical measurements for evaluation in physical education.* Minneapolis: Burgess.

27. Jokl, P., & Jokl, E. (1977). Running and swimming world records. *Journal of Sports Medicine and Physical Fitness, 17*(2): 213–229.

28. Katch, V. L., Sady, S. S., & Freedson, P. (1982). Biological variability in maximum aerobic power. *Medicine and Science in Sports and Exercise, 14*(1): 21–25.

29. Kirk, R. E. (1968). *Experimental design: Procedures for the behavioral sciences.* Belmont, CA: Brooks/Cole Publishing.

30. Knuttgen, H. G. (1978). Force, work, power, and exercise. *Medicine and Science in Sports, 10*(3): 227–228.

31. Knuttgen, H. G. (1984). Information for authors (revised). *Medicine and Science in Sports and Exercise, 16*(6): xviii.

32. Knuttgen, H. G. (1986). Quantifying exercise performance with SI units. *The Physician and Sportsmedicine,* (Dec.): 157–161.

33. Knuttgen, H. G. (1995). Force, work, and power in athletic training. *Sports Science Exchange, 57*(4).

34. Komi, P. V., & Knuttgen, H. G. (1994). Sport science and modern training. In J. D. Halloran, P. V. Komi, H. G. Knuttgen, P. DeKnop, P. Oja, F. Roskam (Eds.), *Sport science studies* (pp. 44–62). Germany: Verlag Karl Hofmann Schondorf.

35. Lang, P. B., Latin, R. W., Berg, K. E., & Mellon, M. B. (1992). The accuracy of the ACSM cycle ergometry equation. *Medicine and Science in Sports and Exercise, 24*(2):272–276.

36. McArdle, W. D., Katch, F. I., & Katch, V. L. (1996). *Exercise physiology: Energy, nutrition, and human performance.* Baltimore: Williams & Wilkins.

37. McGilvery, R. W. (1975). *Biochemical concepts.* Philadelphia: W. B. Saunders.

38. Mechikoff, R., & Estes, S. (1993). *A history and philosophy of sport and physical education.* Dubuque, IA: Brown & Benchmark.

39. Minium, E. W. (1970). *Statistical reasoning in psychology and education.* New York: John Wiley and Sons.

40. Morrow, J. R., & Jackson, A. W. (1993). How "significant" is your reliability? *Research Quarterly for Exercise and Science, 64,* 352–355.

41. Nagle, F. J. (1971). Effects of activity: Metabolic effects. In *Encyclopedia of sport sciences and medicine,* ed. American College of Sports Medicine, 212–215. New York: Macmillan.

42. Newsholme, E. A., Blomstrand, E., & Ekblom, B. (1992). Physical and mental fatigue: Metabolic mechanisms and importance of plasma amino acids. *British Medical Bulletin, 48,* 477–495.

43. Noble, B. J. (1986). *Physiology of exercise and sport.* St. Louis: Times Mirror/Mosby College.

44. Pate, R. (1983). *South Carolina physical fitness test manual.* Columbia: South Carolina Association for Health, Physical Education, Recreation, and Dance.

45. Powers, S. K., & Howley, E. T. (1990). *Exercise physiology.* Dubuque, IA: Wm. C. Brown.

46. Purdy, J. G. (1974). Least squares model for the running curve. *Research Quarterly, 45,* 224–238.

47. Safritt, M. J. (1981). *Evaluation in physical education.* Englewood Cliffs, NJ: Prentice Hall.

48. Safritt, M. J. (1990). *Introduction to measurement in physical education and exercise science.* St. Louis: Times Mirror/Mosby.

49. Serresse, O., Lortie, G., Bouchard, C., & Boulay, M. R. (1988). Estimation of the contribution of the various energy systems during maximal work of short duration. *International Journal of Sports Medicine, 9,* 456–460.

50. Thibault, G., & Peronnet, R. (1988). Physiological analysis of world running records. *Medicine and Science in Sports and Exercise, 20* (2, Suppl.): Abstract #294, p. S49.

51. Thomson, J. M., & Garvie, K. J. (1981). A laboratory method for determination of anaerobic energy expenditure during sprinting. *Canadian Journal of Applied Sport Science, 6,* 21–26.

52. Van Dalen, D. B. (1973). *Understanding educational research.* San Francisco: McGraw-Hill.

53. Vandewalle, H., Peres, G., & Monod, H. (1987). Standard anaerobic exercise tests. *Sports Medicine, 4,* 268–289.

54. Volkov, N. I., & Lapin, V. I. (1979). Analysis of the velocity curve in sprint running. *Medicine and Science in Sports, 11,* 332–337.

55. Wilmore, J. H., & Costill, D. L. (1994). *Physiology of sport and exercise.* Champaign, IL: Human Kinetics.

56. Young, D. S. (1987). Implementation of SI units for clinical laboratory data. *Annals of Internal Medicine, 106*(1): 114–129.

Chapter UN

Units of Measure

Measuring units is the term given to describe the type of measure being made. For instance, in the United States we use pounds to describe our weight, and feet and inches to describe our height. The units most commonly used in exercise physiology are those that measure variables associated with exercise, physiology, and meteorology. Some of these were introduced in Chapter TE Terminology. In accordance with the International System (SI) of nomenclature, numerous variables (characteristics) are described with such measuring units as kilogram, liter, centimeter, milliliter, and millimeter. Many variables combine two or more measuring units to form such units as liters per minute and milliliters per kilogram per minute.

International System (SI)

The quantification of exercise physiology requires that all variables have well-defined units of measure. Americans are already familiar with such units as inches, feet, and pounds, that are used in everyday life. However, the single measuring system that is officially approved worldwide is the International System of Units—often abbreviated SI from its French name, "Système International."[6,23] SI is based upon the decimal and metric systems, thus simplifying the conversion of one unit to another.[18]

With the recent adoption of the metric system by the British, only two other countries in the world, besides the United States, are not using metric units—Burma and a part of an island of Borneo in Indonesia.[12] However, American exercise physiologists have adopted SI's metric units of measure. Although U.S. legislation has discouraged the use of the nonmetric system, it is dying much too slowly according to most American scientists and the general populous in the rest of the world. Most countries have been using metrics for many years. Americans often overlook metric designations on such objects as engine sizes (e.g., cubic centimeters), food containers (e.g., grams), and liquid containers (e.g., liters). Metric markers in America are sometimes found on the outfield fences of baseball fields, on road markers, auto tachometers, and speed-limit signs. In addition, some U.S. buildings display temperature readings in celsius.

Exercise Units

The units used to measure, thus quantify, exercise are force, work, velocity, power, and energy. These terms were introduced in Chapter TE. A detailed description of the units is presented in this chapter, including their interconversion values (Table 1).

Force (F)

The recommended measuring unit for force directed in a linear motion is newton (N), named after a mid-1800's scientist. For angular motion, such as when measuring the strength of leg extensors on an isokinetic machine, the most appropriate term is torque. Its unit of measure is newton meter (N·m). Thus, torque is the product of the force in newtons multiplied by a distance in meters; this distance value is explained in the chapter on leg strength testing.

Although the kilogram (kg) unit should be used only as a weight (mass) unit, it is often used in laboratory situations as a measure of the force necessary to: (a) lift a weight or one's own body weight, (b) crank a bicycle ergometer, and (c) to press against a dynamometer (a strength-measuring device that may be squeezed, pressed, or pulled). Ideally, the kilogram should be replaced by the newton for all force measures in future scientific publications, but the popularity of the kilogram prevents the exclusive use of newtons as force units in this manual.

Work (w)

The unit of measure for work combines the units of measure for the two basic physical quantities—force and distance. Thus, the force unit—(newton) and the distance unit—(meter) combine to produce the work unit—newton meter (N·m). The newton meter is equivalent to another universally approved term, joule (J) or kilojoule (kJ).[4] Although the kilogram meter (kg·m) and newton meter are still common, the preferred expression for work is the joule or kilojoule,[3] because it represents the totality of work rather than its two separate components. In other words, N times m = J; thus, one may as well use the product term, J, rather than its components, N and m.

Velocity (v)

Velocity is commonly measured in miles per hour (mph; $mi \cdot h^{-1}$), but should be reported scientifically as kilometers per hour ($km \cdot h^{-1}$), or meters per minute ($m \cdot min^{-1}$) or per second ($m \cdot s^{-1}$). When the motion is angular, such as actions on an isokinetic machine, the appropriate units of measure are degrees per second ($° \cdot s^{-1}$) and radians per second ($rad \cdot s^{-1}$).

Recommendations for Reporting Measuring Units

Obviously abbreviations are helpful when reporting measuring units. However, abbreviations should only be used when associated with the numeric value. For example, kilogram should not be abbreviated as expressed in this sentence. But the abbreviation should be used if reporting that a person weighs 60 kg. Notice, also, that all abbreviations are not capitalized; the only exceptions are those associated with someone's name, such as N, W, C, and K, for Misters Newton, Watt, Celsius, and Kelvin, respectively, and the unit for liter, L, when it is not combined with its prefixes, such as milliliter. Also, notice that the abbreviations are not pluralized. Thus, 60 kg or 175 cm is not reported as kgs or cms. Abbreviations are followed by a period only for the American abbreviation inches (in.), or at the end of a sentence. A space is also required between the value and the unit, thus 60 kg, not 60kg. The recommended style of expressing per in combined units such as liters per minute, is to use the raised period (bullet) preceding the unit with its negative exponent. Thus, the unit would appear as $L \cdot min^{-1}$, unless this is

impractical for certain computers or typewriters. In that case, one slash (solidus; /) is acceptable (e.g., L/min). However, it is technically incorrect to use more than one solidus per expression, such as "ml/kg/min". The latter could be expressed with one solidus as ml/ (kg·min), but preferably as $ml \cdot kg^{-1} \cdot min^{-1}$. The following provides the mathematical rationale for using the negative exponent in place of the solidus:

$$kg/1 = kg^1 = kg \text{ to a power of 1 (exponent)}$$
$$\text{reciprocal of } kg/1 = 1/kg = kg^{-1} \text{ (negative exponent)}$$
$$ml/kg = ml \times 1/kg = ml \cdot kg^{-1}$$

When expressing the full name, not the abbreviation, of a two-component unit such as newton meter, use a space between the two words, not a hyphen nor linked terms absent of a space. When abbreviating such a two-component unit, use a raised period with no space before or after it, such as in N·m, not the joined Nm.

Power (P)

The following are some common units of measure for power: (a) watts (W), (b) joules per second ($J \cdot s^{-1}$), (c) kilogram meters per minute ($kg \cdot m \cdot min^{-1}$), (d) newton meters per minute ($N \cdot m \cdot min^{-1}$), and horsepower (hp). Many laboratory bike ergometers (e.g., Monark™) use $kg \cdot m \cdot min^{-1}$ or $N \cdot m \cdot min^{-1}$ as the power unit. However, the unit should be converted to watts (W), the accepted unit of measure for power by the scientific community. The watt is equal to the force (N) times the distance (m) that the object moves divided by the time (s) spent moving the object. The symbol for watt is the uppercase W, not to be confused with the lowercase w for work. When the unit watt is spelled out in full it should not begin with a capital letter, despite the fact that the unit was named after Mr. Watt. This rule applies to all units that are proper names (e.g., newton, celsius).

Energy (E)

Although the most popular unit among laypersons is the kilocalorie (kcal), the joule or kilojoule is the universally approved unit of measure for metabolic energy release and its two components—the work (exercise) and the heat equation:[19]

$$\text{Metabolic Energy Release (J) = w (J) + Heat (J)}$$

The exercise physiologist often measures internal energy in terms of the metabolic consumption of oxygen in liters per minute ($L \cdot min^{-1}$)[a] or in relative terms as in mil-

liliters per kilogram body weight ($ml \cdot kg^{-1} \cdot min^{-1}$), or in metabolic equivalents (MET). The term MET denotes a multiple of the resting oxygen consumption. In absolute terms, resting oxygen consumption approximates $0.25 \ L \cdot min^{-1}$, thus, a MET value of 10 represents an oxygen consumption of $2.5 \ L \cdot min^{-1}$. In relative terms, resting oxygen consumption[2] is approximately $3.5 \ ml \cdot kg^{-1} \cdot min^{-1}$ and caloric expenditure is $1 \ kcal \cdot kg^{-1} \cdot h^{-1}$.

There is a close relationship between the exercise units of work and power, and the physiological unit for oxygen consumption. Thus, the steady-state oxygen cost ($\dot{V}O_2$; $ml \cdot min^{-1}$) of cycle ergometry at a person's low or moderate level may be approximated (±6%) from the known power output during cycle ergometry.[2,7,20] This relationship assumes that the exercise intensity is below the person's lactate threshold,[11] thus low and moderate exercise intensities. Equations 1–3 are used for their respective power units of measure: newton meters per minute, kilogram meters per minute,[7] and watts. For a more individualized estimation of oxygen consumption during cycle ergometry, ACSM[5] recommends multiplying the participant's weight (kg) by 1 MET ($3.5 \ ml \cdot kg^{-1} \cdot min^{-1}$), instead of adding the generic resting metabolism value of 300 to the product.

$\dot{V}O_2$ ($ml \cdot min^{-1}$) =

$$[P \text{ (in } N \cdot m \cdot min^{-1}) \times 0.2] + 300 \qquad \text{Eq. 1}$$

$$[P \text{ (in } kgm \cdot min^{-1}) \times 2] + 300 \qquad \text{Eq. 2}$$

$$[P \text{ (in W)} \times 12] + 300 \qquad \text{Eq. 3}$$

For example, if a person is cycling long enough to reach steady state (>3–5 min) at a power level of 100 W,

---

[a]Note: The uppercase "L" is appropriate to denote liters because it can be mistaken for the numeral "1" if printed in lowercase; the lowercase letter "1" is appropriate when following another letter such as in "ml."

Table 1 Common Units and Conversions for Force, Work, Velocity, Power, and Energy

Measuring Unit	Exact Conversion (Research)	Approximate (~) Conversion (Classroom)
Force (F)		
N	1 N = 0.1019 kg	1 N ~ 0.1 kg
kg	1 kg = 9.8066 N	✶ 1 kg ~ 10 N
Work (w)		
kJ	1 kJ = 1000 J	
J; N·m	1 J = 1 N·m = 0.1019 kg·m	1 N·m ~ 0.1 kg·m
kg·m	1 kg·m = 9.8066 N·m	✶ 1 kg·m ~ 10 N·m
Velocity (v)		
m·min^{-1}	1 m·min^{-1} ~ 0.04 mph	
km·h^{-1} (kph)	1 km·h^{-1} = 0.6214 mph	✶ 1 k·h^{-1} ~ 0.6 m·h^{-1}
	= 16.7 m·min^{-1}	
	= 0.28 m·s^{-1}	
mph	1 mph = 26.8 m·min^{-1}	✶ 1 m·h^{-1} ~ 27 m·min^{-1}
	= 0.447 m·s^{-1}	~ 0.45 m·s^{-1}
Power (P)		
W	1 W = 6.118 kg·m·min^{-1}	✶ 1 W ~ 6 kg·m·min^{-1}
	= 0.1019 kg·m·s^{-1}	✶ ~ 0.1 kg·m·s^{-1}
J·s^{-1}; J·min^{-1}	= 1 J·s^{-1} = 60 J·min^{-1}	= 1 J·s^{-1} = 60 J·min^{-1}
N·m·s^{-1}; N·m·min^{-1}	= 1 N·m·s^{-1} = 60 N·m·min^{-1}	= 1 N·m·s^{-1} = 60 N·m·min^{-1}
kg·m·min^{-1}	1 kg·m·min^{-1} = 0.1635 W	1 kg·m·min^{-1} ~ 0.16 W
Energy (E)		
J	1 J = 1 N·m = 0.000239 kcal	
kJ	1 kJ = 1000 J = 0.2389 kcal	1 kJ ~ 0.24 kcal
kcal	1 kcal = 4186 J = 4.186 kJ	✶ 1 kcal ~ 4200 J ~ 4.2 kJ
V̇O$_2$	1 L = 5.05 kcal = 21.14 kJ	✶ 1 L ~ 5 kcal ~ 21 kJ
MET	1 MET = 3.5 ml·kg^{-1}·min^{-1}	
	= 1 kcal·kg^{-1}·h^{-1}	

then the following calculation would estimate that person's total oxygen cost in milliliters per minute:

$$\dot{V}O_2 \ (ml\cdot min^{-1}) = (100 \times 12) + 300$$
$$= 1200 + 300$$
$$= 1500 \ ml\cdot min^{-1} = 1.5 \ L\cdot min^{-1}$$

Once the oxygen cost is known, it is possible to calculate the caloric cost simply by multiplying the liters of oxygen consumed by five (Eq. 4).

$$kcal = 5 \times \dot{V}O_2 \ (L\cdot min^{-1}) \qquad Eq. 4$$

Thus the person in the prior example would burn 7.5 kcal·min^{-1} based on the product of 5 times 1.5 L·min^{-1}.

Table 2 provides the energy values associated with cycling intensities progressing by 25 W intervals. Keep in mind that the table and these equations do not account for the slow component of high intensity exercise that occurs above the lactate threshold.[11] Hence they would underestimate slightly the true oxygen cost for high intensity exercise. What is deemed "high" is determined by the fitness of the exerciser.

Also, the oxygen cost of exercise can be estimated for walking and running, both on a level and sloped terrain.[5] Equation 5 shows that the total oxygen cost (ml·kg^{-1}·min^{-1}) for walking on level ground (or treadmill) is a function of adding resting metabolism to walking metabolism, basically,

the same principle as applied to cycling. Thus, walking is equal to 1 MET (3.5 ml·kg^{-1}·min^{-1}) plus one-tenth of the walking speed (m·min^{-1}).

$$\text{Walking horizontal } \dot{V}O_2 \ (ml\cdot kg^{-1}\cdot min^{-1})$$
$$= 3.5 \ ml\cdot kg^{-1}\cdot min^{-1} + (0.1 \times m\cdot min^{-1}) \qquad Eq. 5$$

Meteorological Units

The primary meteorological concerns of the exercise physiologist are temperature, relative humidity, and barometric pressure. Although the units for these terms are not considered to have metric units, the ones that are presented here are those accepted by the scientific community.

Temperature (T)

The temperature units are apt to be confusing for exercise physiology students because of the three different scales available for temperature—fahrenheit, celsius, and kelvin. In general, fahrenheit/celsius conversions need not be memorized, because most laboratory thermometers have celsius scales. Fahrenheit units are not accepted by the International System; therefore, laboratory students really do not need to convert the celsius value to a fahrenheit value. However, if celsius thermometers are not available, then the fahrenheit value has to be converted to the celsius value. Students are encouraged to make approximate

Table 2 The Energy Cost Measured as Oxygen Consumption ($\dot{V}O_2$) and Joules (J) at Various Power Levels of Cycle Ergometry[a]

Power			Energy[b]		$\dot{V}O_2$
kg·m·min^{-1}	N·m·min^{-1}	W	J	kJ	L·min^{-1}
150	1500	25	1500	1.5	0.6
300	3000	50	3000	3.0	0.9
450	4500	75	4500	4.5	1.2
600	6000	100	6000	6.0	1.5
750	7500	125	7500	7.5	1.8
900	9000	150	9000	9.0	2.1
1050	10 500	175	10 500	10.5	2.4
1200	12 000	200	12 000	12.0	2.8
1350	13 500	225	13 500	13.5	3.1
1500	15 000	250	15 000	15.0	3.5
1650	16 500	275	16 500	16.5	3.8
1800	18 000	300	18 000	18.0	4.2
1950	19 500	325	19 500	19.5	4.6
2100	21 000	350	21 000	21.0	5.0
2250	22 500	375	22 500	22.5	5.3
2400	24 000	400	24 000	24.0	5.7

Notes: [a]Based on approximate conversion values

[b]Spaces, not commas, are sometimes used to separate long numbers into segments of three (e.g., 1 000 000, not 1,000,000; four-digit numbers may use a space or be written without the comma, e.g., 1 000 or 1000. This is especially important in avoiding confusion where some countries use a comma in figures the way other countries use periods.

estimates of celsius values from any given fahrenheit values by using certain mnemonics or by memorizing some of the most important fahrenheit-to-celsius values, such as body temperature, freezing point, and boiling point. Accurate celsius determinations require mathematical conversions. The decimal conversions (0.56 or 1.8), rather than the fractions (5/9 or 9/5), are more compatible with pocket calculators (Eqs. 6 and 7).

$$°F \text{ to } °C: \quad °C = 0.56(°F - 32) \text{ or}$$
$$= (°F - 32)/1.8 \qquad \text{Eq. 6}$$
$$°C \text{ to } °F: \quad °F = (1.8 \times °C) + 32 \qquad \text{Eq. 7}$$

The conversion of celsius to kelvin is made simply by adding the celsius value to 273 °K, or subtracting if the temperature is below 0 °C (Eq. 8).

$$°K = 273 + (°C) \qquad \text{Eq. 8}$$

For example, the following calculation is made to convert the normal body temperature value of 37 °C to kelvin:

$$37 °C = 273 + 37 = 310 °K$$

If an environmental celsius temperature is a minus value, such as −10 °C, then the calculation is

$$−10 °C = 273 + (−10) = 263 °K$$

Relative Humidity (RH)

Many laboratories have a hygrometer to measure relative humidity. These simply state the relative humidity in units of percent. For example, the American College of Sports Medicine[3] recommends that no exercise tests be given in laboratories with above 60% RH. No conversions are necessary because the percent unit is universal. Ideally, laboratories should have instrumentation to record directly or indirectly the WBGT index, a value that considers the interaction between relative humidity and temperature.

Barometric Pressure (P_B)

Usually, laboratory mercury or aneroid barometers measure atmospheric (barometric) pressure in torr units (formerly, mm Hg). At sea level, torr values are 760, the conventional standard value for laboratories throughout the world. Barometric pressures between 700 and 800 torr would not be expected to influence exercise performance. It would be rare to find barometric air pressures exceeding 800 torr within the biosphere. Many barometers in the United States are scaled in inches of mercury. Accordingly, many of the weather reports on U.S. television state the air pressure in inches. Equation 9 converts inches to the universally approved SI torr value.

$$\text{torr} = 25.4 \times \text{in.} \qquad \text{Eq. 9}$$

Some important conversions and mnemonics (memory aids) worth committing to memory for exercise physiology are presented in Table 3.

Metric Conversions

Metric units are much simpler to use than the present United States system. The metric system facilitates the transition (or conversion) from weight and length measures

Table 3 Meteorological Units, Conversions, and Mnemonics for Temperature and Barometric Pressure

Temperature (T)	Barometric Pressure (P_B)
273 °K = 0 °C = 32 °F	1 in. = 25.4 mm = 25.4 torr
−40 °C = −40 °F	760 torr = 29.92 in.[a]
0 °C = 32 °F (freezing)	760 torr = sea level
10 °C = 50 °F	760 torr = 1 atmosphere (atm)
16 °C = 61 °F (60.8 exactly)	
28 °C = 82 °F (82.4 exactly)	
37 °C = 98.6 °F (T_{body})	
22 °C = 72 °F (71.6 exactly)	
100 °C = 212 °F (boiling)	

[a]29.92 reads the same backward.

to volume measures and vice versa. The science community uses metric units exclusively in scientific journals.

The following conversion factors are categorized according to length, weight, and volume measures. Although the conversions from metric to the U.S. system are very helpful in visualizing the size of the object, it is best to think metric. That is, as you learn the metric system, let the metric value itself be meaningful by visualizing it before making a conversion to the U.S. value. For example, when in the presence of a woman who tells you that she weighs 60 kg and is 160 cm (centimeters) tall, let her image linger in your thoughts before making the conversion to the U.S. system . . . whereby she is revealed as being 5 ft, 3 in. tall and weighing 132 lb.

Fortunately, most instruments in an exercise physiology laboratory are labeled in metric units. Thus, there are not many occasions when students need to convert to metrics (see appendix B2). A pocket calculator with basic functions, such as addition, subtraction, multiplication, division, and square root, is adequate for most calculations in this laboratory manual, including those needed for making conversions. Some calculators have automatic functions for metric conversions, but your instructor may not wish you to use these for exam purposes.

Length Measures

Every exercise physiology student is expected to respond quickly and correctly in metric units to the question: "How tall are you and how much do you weigh?" Most Americans cannot express common length measures, such as their height, in metric units. For example, Metropolitan Life tables of 1990 express the average height for adult men and women as about 69 in. (175.3 cm) and 64 in. (162.5 cm), respectively. Americans refer to typical sheets of paper as 8.5 by 11 in. (21.5 by 28 cm). Rarely would Americans refer to a mountain location at an altitude of 9900 ft as being located at 3000 m, nor would they relate a 55-mph (or $m \cdot h^{-1}$) speed limit to about 90 $km \cdot h^{-1}$.

The metric unit of measure for length is the meter. Body height (stature) is often expressed in meters or centimeters. A centimeter is about 40% as long as an inch. To convert the average male's 69 inches to centimeters (cm), the inches may be divided by the metric conversion factor 0.3937, as follows:

$$cm = 69.0 \div 0.3937 = 175.26 = 175.3 \text{ to closest cm}$$

As mentioned previously, the student is encouraged to visualize metric dimensions. For example, Figure 1 shows the size of a 10-cm or 0.1-m line. I encourage you to practice visualizing 10 cm by noting some objects near you that seem about 10 cm in length.

Common metric values and the accepted SI symbols are presented in the following boxes. The metric value of 1 m represents its fractional distance from the equator to the geographic north pole, that is, one-tenth millionth (0.1/1 000 000).

> 1 meter (m) = 100 centimeters (cm) = 1000 millimeters (mm)
> = 39.370 in. = 3.281 ft = 1.0936 yd
> 1 centimeter (cm) = 10 mm = 0.01 m = 0.3937 in.
> 1 millimeter (mm) = 0.001 meter (~1/25 in.)
> 1 kilometer (km) = 1000 m = 0.62137 mile

Weight (Mass) Measures

In responding to the question "How much do you weigh?", exercise physiologists respond using the metric unit called the kilogram. They also describe components of body weight, such as lean weight and fat weight, using the kilogram unit. When measuring underwater weight in order to obtain percent fat, they use the basic mass unit—the gram. The following box relates the gram to its metric counterparts the kilogram and milligram. Additionally, the U.S.-to-metric conversion points out that one kilogram is more than twice as heavy as one pound.

> 1 kilogram (kg) = 1000 grams (g) = 2.2046 lb
> 1 g = 1000 milligrams (mg)

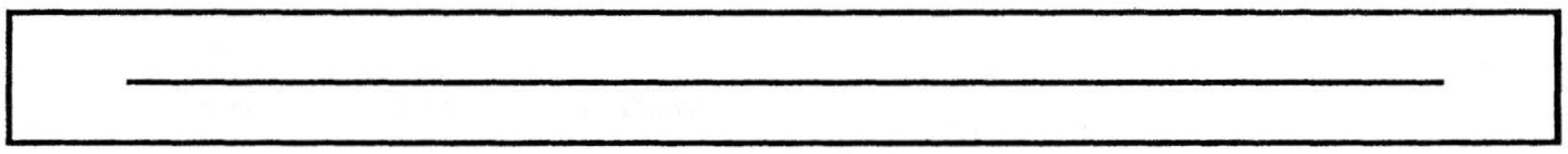

Figure 1 Visualization of a 10-cm line (also 100 mm or 0.1 m).

Typical weights for the average adult American man and woman according to the Metropolitan Life tables of 1990 can be converted to the closest tenth kg by dividing the American value by the approximate conversion factor 2.2.

$$\text{Men: kg} = 172.0 \div 2.2 = 78.0$$

$$\text{Women: kg} = 144.0 \div 2.2 = 65.3$$

Volume (V) Measures

Exercise physiologists use volume measures for such variables as oxygen consumption, lung volumes, sweat loss, fluid replacement, and cardiovascular measures of cardiac output and stroke volume. The basic unit of measure for volume is the liter, which is nearly 6% larger than a quart.

> 1 liter (L) = 1000 milliliters (ml) = 1.0567 quarts (qt)

Interaction of Length, Weight (Mass), and Volume Measures

The metric system facilitates the conversion from weight and length measures to volume measures and vice versa. For example, when a length measure such as a centimeter (cm) is denoted in cubic (cc; cm^3) form, it becomes a volume or capacity measure. Thus, 1000 cm^3 is the same as 1000 ml (or 1 L), a volume measure. Also, the volume measure—1 L—is equivalent to 1 kg, a weight (mass) measure. It is much easier to remember that 1 L is equal to 1 kg than to remember that x amount of quarts or pints equal 1 lb. (I can't remember!)

> 1 cm^3 = 1 cubic centimeter ("cc") = 1 ml
> 1000 cm^3 = 1000 ml (of distilled water at 4 °C) = 1 L = 1 kg

Converting weight to volume has practical significance to an exercise physiologist who is concerned about a performer's water loss via perspiration under hot conditions. Using a sensitive weight scale, the physiologist can calculate the amount (volume) of water lost during exercise by simply subtracting the person's weight after exercise from the weight before exercise. For example, if a person rapidly lost 1 kg of weight while exercising in a sauna, it would require 1 L of fluid to restore normal water balance (assuming that fat loss was insignificant).

Summary of Metric Conversions

Some metric units have sizes that are greater than (>) their respective American sizes. For example, one meter is longer than one yard (1 m>1 yd) by about 10%. Contrarily,

Table 4 Size Comparisons and Conversion Factors for Metric and American Numbers

Physical Variable	Size Comparison	Conversion	Division	
			exact	(~)
Length	1 cm < 1 in.	in. to cm	in. ÷ 0.3937	(0.4)
	1 m > 1 ft	ft to m	ft ÷ 3.281	(3.3)
	1 m > 1 yd	yd to m	yd ÷ 1.0936	(1.1)
	1 km < 1 mile	mile to km	mile ÷ 0.621	(0.6)
Mass	1 g < 1 oz	oz to g	oz ÷ 0.0352	(0.035)
	1 kg > 1 lb	lb to kg	lb ÷ 2.2046	(2.2)
Volume	1 L > 1 qt	qt to L	qt ÷ 1.0567	(1.06)

there are some metric sizes that are less than (<) their respective American (U.S.) sizes, such as the centimeter which is only about 40% the length of an inch.

Table 4 presents other examples of these size comparisons and also provides the necessary values for converting American values to metric ones. In all cases, the listed conversion factor is divided into the American value. For example, if the length of a sprint is 50 yd, then the meter value of 45.7 is found by dividing 50 yd by 1.0936. Rarely is it necessary in exercise physiology to convert metric units to American units, unless the observer has not yet learned to visualize the metric values.

Collection of Basic Data

Nearly all test forms (data collection forms) include basic information about the subjects. This information is sometimes referred to as vital data. It includes such items as (1) name, (2) date and time of test, (3) age, (4) gender, (5) height, and (6) weight. Often, vital data include heart rate and blood pressure; however, they are omitted in this manual whenever they are not significant for the specific test being described. Form UN 1 may be used to record and, in some cases, to calculate conversions for basic data.

Method of Recording and Collecting Basic Data

Names are always written with the last name first, followed by a comma, and then the first name. If confidentiality is a concern, then identification (ID#) numbers should be used instead of names. The test **date** is presented with the month in numerical form at the beginning of the date. For example, September 4, 1995, would be recorded as 9/4/95 (or 09/04/95). Besides recording these on the data collection form (e.g., Form UN 1), they both should be recorded on any type of chart paper such as the electrocardiograph or the isokinetic machine's recording paper. It is important to record test **time** on the data collection form because of the diurnal or circadian variations of certain biological and performance variables.[14,15,16,22] It is best to repeat tests on the same person as close to the original test time as possible.

Age is recorded to the closest year (y), except when it may be important to record to the closest tenth year. For example, if someone turned 72 years of age four months ago, then the age might be recorded as 72.3 y. **Gender** (sex) for an individual is abbreviated as M (male) or F (female). For a group of persons over 17 years of age the recommended group designation is M (men) and W (women).[6]

Height (Stature)

Height, or the more technical term stature, is a variable that is not nearly as significant in most exercise physiology evaluations as weight (mass). However, it is a basic variable that is routinely measured in all labs and, thus, its accurate and standardized measurement should be given serious attention. Our purposes for making height measurements are to: (1) familiarize students with standardized stature measurements; (2) characterize, or describe, the participant; (3) relate the participant's height to U.S. norms; and (4) relate the participant's body weight to height based on U.S. norms.

Stature may be measured on a platform-beam scale (Fig. 2) if the scale's stadiometer (anthropometer) has been checked for accuracy. Most stadiometers now have both centimeter and inch graduations on the sliding vertical bar. The bar has a head lever that the technician can swing upward to a ninety degree angle onto the crown of the participant's head.

An improvised stadiometer can be devised by attaching a metric-graduated tape against a wall that does not have a baseboard. Then any right-angled device can be placed against the crown of a person's head and against the wall. Instead, a mark may be made at the lower edge of the right-angled device, and then the height of that mark can be measured with, ideally, a metal metric tape. It may be convenient to have a short stool, bench, or ladder for the technician to stand on to measure stature. The following procedures may help to standardize and enhance the accuracy of stature measurements:

Preparation

1. If using the platform-beam scale, check its accuracy by confirming the distance from the platform base to the first graduated measure on the stadiometer.
2. The participant is in stocking feet or bare-footed (scantily clothed if weight is to be measured simultaneously).

Procedures

3. The participant steps onto the platform scale and then turns facing away from the balance beam and the stadiometer. The technician, probably standing on a stool, asks the participant to lower his/her head in

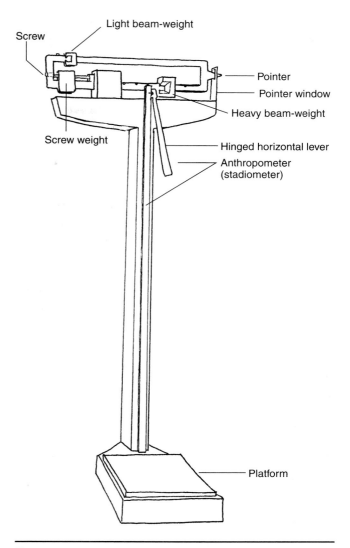

Figure 2 The platform scale for measuring body weight and height; the sliding vertical bar with its head lever for measuring height (stature) is called an anthropometer or stadiometer.

order to clear the swing of the head lever to a horizontal position.

If using a "wall stadiometer," the participant stands facing away from the wall, with heels, scapulae, and buttocks in contact with the wall.[13]

4. The participant stands as tall as possible with heels together and feet angled out to about 60°.[13]
5. As the participant inhales deeply and maintains the designated position, the technician places the right-angled object against the wall and the participant's head (or places the anthropometer's hinged lever on top of the participant's head so that the horizontal lever forms a right angle with the vertical rod).
6. The technician records the height to the nearest 0.1 cm. (If the platform scale's anthropometer is only in inches, the American value is recorded to the nearest one-fourth in. and then converted to the nearest 0.5 cm.)

Accuracy. The test-retest reliability of height measurements is very high. The author has found a correlation of .998 for 28 men tested about one to two weeks apart.

Weight

Weight is probably the most measured variable in exercise physiology laboratories. This basic variable is factored into many of the other variables measured in this laboratory manual, hence its importance cannot be overestimated.

Participants can be weighed in the attire that corresponds to the reference source. For example, if the reference source for comparison allowed 0.3 kg of clothing, such as underwear, shirt, shorts, dress, or trousers, then the person may be weighed accordingly. In the exercise physiology laboratory, often the nude, or nearly nude, weight of the subject is measured for tests that relate the fitness score to body weight. It is always preferred for tests of body composition. If a disposable paper gown is used, it may be deemed as nude weight.[13] Although weighing the nude subject is ideal, it may be more convenient to weigh the clothes prior to weighing the subject wearing those same "weigh-in" clothes. Then the nude weight is found simply by subtracting the weight of the clothes from the weight of the subject wearing those clothes. The exercise-clothed weight should be used for tests that call for the calculation of work or power when the participants are lifting their own weight, such as in stepping, walking uphill, or running uphill. This is because the participants are lifting the weight of the apparel, in addition to their own body weight. The following steps are helpful when measuring a participant's body weight:

Preparation

1. Calibrate the scale (see box insert for calibration of platform scale). In general, the scale should be calibrated monthly.[10]
2. Preferably, the technician weighs as much of the participant's weigh-in clothing as practical.

Procedure

3. The participant, now wearing the weigh-in clothing, stands on and faces the scale; if stature was just measured, then the person simply turns to face the scale while the technician acts as an assistant or spotter (vice versa, if stature is measured after the weight is measured).
4. The technician stands behind the platform scale to read and adjust the beam weights without disturbing the participant. Most platform scales have graduations (readings) on both sides.
5. The technician places the heavy beam-weight (lower lever) to the estimated graduation mark.
6. The technician places the light beam-weight (upper lever) to the graduation mark that causes the pointer to balance in the midair position within the window. If the pointer cannot be balanced with the light beam-weight, then the heavy beam-weight must be readjusted.

7. A technician records the weight on the data collection on Form UN 1.
8. The technician assists the participant off the scale, and thanks that person for being so accommodating.

Accuracy. Weight is a very reliable measure. In two separate studies the author found correlations for weight as high as .99 and .995 in 93 and 28 men, respectively. Others have found similarly high ($r = .99$) values.[8] Weight is often measured on a platform scale that has a balancing beam, two moveable weights, and one tare-screw weight (Fig. 2). These scales are usually only sensitive to the closest quarter pound (0.114 kg), but other types of laboratory scales are sensitive enough to detect weights of 10 g (0.01 kg), about the weight of a U.S. quarter coin. For the platform scale and for basic data purposes, the rounded-off 2.2 conversion for American-to-metric may be used instead of the exact 2.2046 conversion value in order to calculate weight to the closest 0.1 kg.

Results and Discussion

The results section of a scientific report or study simply tells the reader the scores (values) of the measurements. In the Exercise Physiology classroom, the results portion of a report is readily found on the individual data collection form (e.g., Form UN 1) and the group data collection form (e.g., Form UN 2). The latter form may only have the participant's ID number or initials, rather than name. The group results often include the mean *(M),* standard deviation *(SD),* and the range of scores, that is, the lowest to the highest score.

The discussion section of a scientific report provides the reader with an interpretation of these results or measured values. The interpretation of both the individual's score and the average score of the group can be made by referring to the appropriate tables, which give the values from a much larger, but, ideally, a similar, population (e.g., Table 5).

Example of Calibration Procedures for the Platform Scale

Zero Calibration

1. Set both moveable beam weights of the scale to their zero positions on each respective beam's graduated scale.
2. Observe the position of the pointer; it should come to rest in midair between the top and bottom of the pointer window.
3. If necessary, balance the pointer in this midair position by using a dime or screwdriver (or strong thumbnail) to adjust the tare-screw weight of the platform scale. Turning the screw clockwise moves the tare-screw weight toward the screw-head, thus tending to lift the pointer higher in the pointer window.

High-Point Calibration

1. Set the beam weights to the highest position for which you have known calibration weights. Typical platform scales cannot read weights above 159 kg (350 lb). Placing 350 lb of certified weights on the scale would be ideal, but if only 100 kg (220 lb) or more of certified weights are available, set the beam weights accordingly (e.g., set the heavy beam-weight to 200 lb and set the light beam-weight to 20 lb).
2. Place the calibration weights on the scale. (A Cybex™ machine's certified weights can be used as calibration weights).
3. Observe the position of the pointer. Is it in the midair position? . . . the top-of-the-window position? . . . or the bottom position?
4. Adjust the light lever-weight, if necessary, to the pointer's midair position.
5. Record any discrepancy between the original set position and the final balanced position.
6. If needed, derive a correction factor for the high-point readings.

Midpoint Calibration

1. Set the lever weights to a midpoint position for which you have calibrated weights. Balance the pointer to the midair position.
2. Place the calibrated weights on the scale.
3. Adjust the light beam-weight, if necessary, to the pointer's midair position.
4. Record any discrepancy between the original set position and the final midair position.
5. If needed, derive a correction factor for midpoint readings, or readjust the tare-screw weight to the pointer's midair position.

Table 5 Average Stature (cm) and Percentiles (%ile) for American Men Ages 18 to 74 Years

Age (y)	M (cm)	Percentiles (%ile)								
		5th	10th	15th	25th	50th	75th	85th	90th	95th
18–24.9	176.6	165.4	167.8	169.5	171.9	176.6	181.2	183.7	185.5	188.6
25–29.9	176.7	165.1	167.8	169.4	172.0	176.6	181.5	184.0	185.7	188.0
30–34.9	176.2	164.8	167.4	169.0	171.5	176.2	180.9	183.3	184.8	187.2
35–39.9	176.1	164.0	166.8	168.8	171.9	176.1	181.0	183.5	185.0	187.7
40–44.9	175.9	165.0	167.2	168.9	171.4	176.0	180.3	182.7	184.2	186.9
45–49.9	175.2	163.8	166.5	168.0	170.6	174.8	180.2	182.9	184.5	186.6
50–54.9	174.6	164.2	166.4	167.8	170.2	174.6	178.8	181.4	183.2	185.3
55–59.9	173.9	163.2	165.0	166.8	169.3	173.8	178.7	181.0	182.3	184.6
60–64.9	173.0	161.9	165.0	166.4	168.7	173.0	177.4	179.8	181.3	183.7
65–69.9	171.5	159.7	162.9	164.5	166.7	171.6	176.3	178.6	180.1	182.5
70–74.9	170.6	159.5	162.0	163.6	165.8	170.7	175.0	177.4	179.4	182.0

Permission from: Frisancho, A. R. (1990). *Anthropometric Standards for the Assessment of Growth and Nutritional Status.* Ann Arbor, MI: University of Michigan Press.

Stature

An interpretation of body stature may be made by comparing the person's height with that of the same age group and gender. In some cases the stated values for the age categories may differ from one source to another. For example, the Food and Nutrition[9] source gives a higher average height for men between the ages of 18 and 34 than the average from the Frisancho[10] source.

Ages 18–34 y	Average Height (cm)	
	Food and Nutrition	Frisancho
Men	177.8	176.5
Women	162.6	162.9

The average heights for younger men and women are greater than the average heights when all adult ages are included in the norms from the Metropolitan Life tables. Thus it is not unusual for height to decrease starting in middle-age and continuing throughout older adulthood. Average heights (cm) and percentiles (%ile) by age are presented in Tables 5 and 6.[10] For example, if a 24-y-old woman is 171.0 cm tall, Table 6 shows that she is in the 90th %ile, meaning that she is taller than 90% of all women between the ages of 18 and 24.9, and is 8.0 cm taller than the average (50th %ile) for that age group.

Weight

The average weights for U.S. adult men and women are about 78 kg (172 lb) and 65.3 kg (144 lb), respectively, according to the Metropolitan Life tables of 1990. Weights,

Table 6 Average Stature (cm) and Percentiles (%ile) for American Women Ages 18 to 74 Years

Age (y)	M (cm)	Percentiles (%ile)								
		5th	10th	15th	25th	50th	75th	85th	90th	95th
18–24.9	163.0	152.3	154.8	156.4	158.8	163.1	167.1	169.6	171.0	173.6
25–29.9	162.9	152.6	155.2	153.6	156.6	162.8	167.1	169.5	170.9	173.3
30–34.9	162.6	152.9	155.2	156.4	158.4	162.4	166.8	169.2	171.2	173.1
35–39.9	162.8	152.0	155.0	156.4	158.6	162.7	167.0	169.4	171.0	173.5
40–44.9	162.6	151.6	154.3	156.2	158.1	162.7	166.7	168.8	170.5	173.2
45–49.9	162.0	151.7	154.0	155.4	157.9	162.0	166.3	168.4	169.9	172.2
50–54.9	161.2	151.3	153.8	155.3	156.9	161.1	165.1	167.3	169.2	171.0
55–59.9	160.3	149.8	152.7	154.1	156.7	160.3	164.4	166.6	167.8	170.1
60–64.9	159.6	149.2	151.4	153.0	155.6	160.0	163.7	166.1	167.3	169.8
65–69.9	158.6	148.5	150.7	152.4	154.8	158.8	162.6	164.8	166.2	168.1
70–74.9	157.6	147.2	150.0	151.7	153.7	157.4	161.5	163.8	165.5	167.5

Permission from: Frisancho, A. R. (1990). *Anthropometric Standards for the Assessment of Growth and Nutritional Status.* Ann Arbor, MI: University of Michigan Press.

Table 7 Average Weights[a] of American Women Aged 18–74 y by Age and Height

		Age Group (y)												
		18–24		25–34		35–44		45–54		55–64		65–74		
in.	cm	lb	kg	lb	kg	lb	kg	lb	kg	lb	kg	lb	kg
57	144.8	114	51.8	118	53.6	125	56.8	129	58.6	132	60.0	130	59.1
58	147.3	117	53.2	121	55.0	129	58.6	133	60.5	136	61.8	134	60.9
59	149.9	120	54.5	125	56.8	133	60.5	136	61.8	140	63.6	137	62.3
60	152.4	123	55.9	128	58.2	137	62.3	140	63.6	143	65.0	140	63.6
61	154.9	126	57.3	132	60.0	141	64.1	143	65.0	147	66.8	144	65.5
62	157.5	129	58.6	136	61.8	144	65.5	147	66.8	150	68.2	147	66.8
63	160.0	132	60.0	139	63.2	148	67.3	150	68.2	153	69.5	151	68.6
64	162.6	135	61.4	142	64.5	152	69.1	154	70.0	157	71.4	154	70.0
65	165.1	138	62.7	146	66.4	156	70.9	158	71.8	160	72.7	158	71.8
66	167.6	141	64.1	150	68.2	159	72.3	161	73.2	164	74.5	161	73.2
67	170.2	144	65.5	153	69.5	163	74.1	165	75.0	167	75.9	165	75.0
68	172.8	147	66.8	157	71.4	167	75.9	168	76.4	171	77.7	169	76.8

[a]Note: Includes clothing weight between 0.1 to 0.3 kg; pound-to-kg conversion uses 2.2.

Source: Abraham, S., Johnson, C. L., & Najjar, M. F. (1979). *Weight by height and age for adults 18–74 years.* Publication No. (PHS) 79-1656. Hyattsville, MD: U.S. Department of Health, Education, and Welfare. From the NHANES data.

however, are more meaningful if they are categorized according to height and age. The average American weights listed in Tables 7 (women) and 8 (men) are based upon measurements taken by the first National Health and Nutrition Examination Survey (NHANES) in the early 1970s testing 13,645 persons between the ages of 18 and 74 y.[1] The height and weight values are virtually identical to their second survey in the late 1970s on an additional 28,043 persons.[1,10] These weights included clothing weight up to 0.3 kg, but without shoes. The percentage of the population expected for each age-height group is presented in Table 9.

Men appear to weigh about 5 lb (2.3 kg) more for each inch (2.54 cm) of increased height with their greatest weight gain occurring between the ages of 25 and 34 y.

Women weigh about 3 lb (1.4 kg) more for each inch of increased height and their greatest weight gain occurs between the ages of 35 and 44 y. It is important to recognize that the weights listed in these tables are average weights, not recommended weights as are those in Table 10.[17] Based on over 100,000 U.S. women nurses, who were studied over

a 16-y period starting at ages 30 to 55 y, investigators concluded that there is a direct relationship between weight and risk of death.[21] They suggested that optimum weights for women are 85% of the U.S. average for women of the same age and stature as those listed from the NHANES data in Table 7. Using Equation 10, the optimum weight may be calculated from the average weight for women between 18 and 24 y of age and who are 165 cm (65 in.) tall.

$$\text{Optimum Wt for Women}$$
$$= 0.85 \times \text{U.S. ave. for age and ht} \qquad \text{Eq. 10}$$

For example, the average weight of these women is 62.7 (138 lb) based on Table 7. Thus the optimum weight in terms of reduced mortality is:

$$0.85 \times 62.7 = 53.3 \text{ kg } (117.25 \text{ lb})$$

An important factor in mortality that should not be overlooked is a woman's weight gain after the age of 18 y. A gain of 9 kg (20 lb) and 18 kg (40 lb) was associated with a two to three and seven times greater risk of death,

Table 8 Average Weights[a] of American Men Aged 18–74 y by Age and Height

		Age Group (y)											
		18–24		25–34		35–44		45–54		55–64		65–74	
In.	cm	lb	kg	lb	kg	lb	kg	lb	kg	lb	kg	lb	kg
62	157.5	130	59.1	141	64.1	143	65.0	147	66.8	143	65.0	143	65.0
63	160.0	135	61.4	145	65.9	148	67.3	152	69.1	147	66.8	147	66.8
64	162.6	140	63.6	150	68.2	153	69.5	156	70.9	153	69.5	151	68.6
65	165.1	145	65.9	156	70.9	158	71.8	160	72.7	158	71.8	156	70.9
66	167.6	150	68.2	160	72.7	163	74.1	164	74.5	163	74.1	160	72.7
67	170.2	154	70.0	165	75.0	169	76.8	169	76.8	168	76.4	164	74.5
68	172.8	159	72.3	170	77.3	174	79.1	173	78.6	173	78.6	169	76.8
69	175.3	164	74.5	174	79.1	179	81.4	177	80.5	178	80.9	173	78.6
70	177.8	168	76.4	179	81.4	184	83.6	182	82.7	183	83.2	177	80.5
71	180.3	173	78.6	184	83.6	190	86.4	187	85.0	189	85.9	182	82.7
72	182.9	178	80.9	189	85.9	194	88.2	191	86.8	193	87.7	186	84.5
73	185.4	183	83.2	194	88.2	200	90.9	196	89.1	197	89.5	190	86.4
74	188.0	188	85.5	199	90.5	205	93.2	200	90.9	203	92.3	194	88.2

[a]Note: Includes clothing weight between 0.1 to 0.3 kg; pound-to-kg conversion uses 2.2.

Source: Abraham, S., Johnson, C. L., & Najjar, M. F. (1979). *Weight by height and age for adults 18–74 years.* Publication No. (PHS) 79-1656. Hyattsville, MD: U.S. Department of Health, Education, and Welfare. From the NHANES data.

Table 9 Percentiles and Expected Distance from the Mean Weight for All Subjects[a] and for a Sample Group[b]

Percentile	All Subjects ± of the M (kg)	Sample Group (kg)[b]
95th	M + 20.5	83.7
90th	M + 16	79.2 kg
80th	M + 11	74.2
50th	M	63.2
20th	M − 11	52.2
10th	M − 16	47.2
5th	M − 20.5	42.7

[a]Any of the average weights in NHANES tables.
[b]25-y-old women, 160 cm tall, mean weight 63.2 kg from NHANES data.

respectively, from heart disease compared with those women maintaining their weight.[21]

The nomograms in Figures 3 (men) and 4 (women) depict these percentiles based on the combined first and second NHANES reports. However, the nomograms comprise all adult ages from 18 to 74 y, rather than six or ten year categories for this age group as in Tables 7 and 8.

Data Collection Forms

It might be said that data collection is only as good as the forms onto which you record the data. Forms do not only provide a record of the raw data, but can also remind the investigators of the procedural steps to be performed to gather the data. Form UN 1 is a good example of both of these

Table 10 Acceptable Weights for Men and Women 19 Years of Age and Older

Height		Weight			
		Age (y)			
		19–35 y		>35 y	
in.	cm	lb	kg	lb	kg
60.0	152.4	97–128	44.0–58.1	108–138	49.0–62.6
61.0	154.9	101–132	45.8–59.9	111–143	50.3–64.9
62.0	157.5	104–137	47.2–62.3	115–148	52.2–67.1
63.0	160.0	107–141	48.5–64.0	119–152	69.1–68.9
64.0	162.6	111–146	50.3–66.2	122–157	55.3–71.4
65.0	165.1	114–150	51.8–68.0	126–162	57.3–73.5
66.0	167.6	118–155	53.6–70.3	130–167	59.1–75.8
67.0	170.2	121–160	55.0–72.6	134–172	60.8–78.0
68.0	172.8	125–164	56.8–74.4	138–178	62.7–80.7
69.0	175.3	129–169	58.6–76.6	142–183	64.5–83.0
70.0	177.8	132–174	60.0–78.9	146–188	66.4–85.3
71.0	180.3	136–179	61.8–81.2	151–194	68.6–88.0
72.0	182.9	148–195	67.3–88.5	164–210	74.5–95.3

Source: Joint Dietary Guidelines Advisory Committee of U.S. Departments of Agriculture and Health and Human Services. (1990). *Nutrition and your health: Dietary guidelines for Americans.* Home and Garden Bulletin No. 232: U.S. Department of Agriculture.

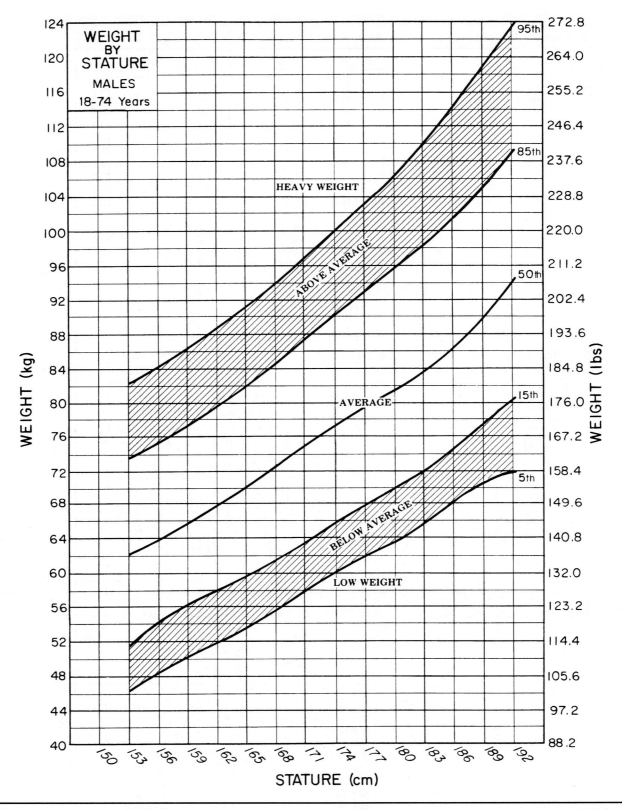

Figure 3 Percentiles of weight (kg/lb) based on the stature (cm) of men between the ages of 18 and 74 y in the NHANE Surveys. From: Frisancho, A. R. (1990). *Anthropometric Standards for the Assessment of Growth and Nutritional Status,* p. 77. Ann Arbor, MI: University of Michigan Press.

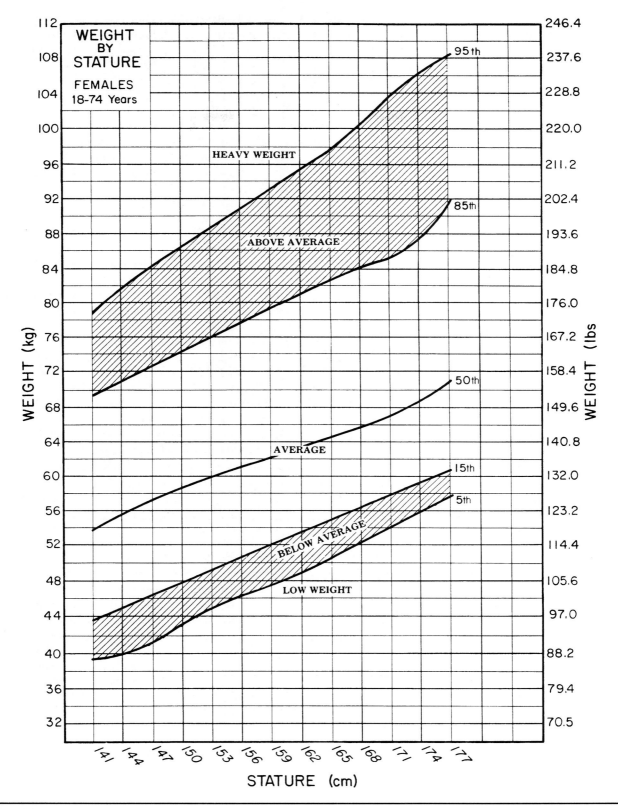

Figure 4 Percentiles of weight (kg/lb) based on the stature (cm) of women between the ages of 18 and 74 y in the NHANE Surveys. From: Frisancho, A. R. (1990). *Anthropometric Standards for the Assessment of Growth and Nutritional Status,* p. 80. Ann Arbor, MI: University of Michigan Press.

characteristics. Form UN 2 provides an example of how a form can facilitate data analysis, such as calculating the mean or the range of scores from a group of participants. Form UN 3 provides an example of a research abstract and allows you to fill in some of the basic data and results. Form UN 4 provides a template that may be used to write your own research abstract. It might be helpful to copy this form before writing on it so that it can be used for future abstracts of test data collected from the later chapters.

References

1. Abraham, S., Johnson, C. L., & Najjar, M. F. (1979). *Weight by height and age for adults 18–74 years.* Publication No. (PHS) 79-1656. Hyattsville, MD: U.S. Department of Health, Education, and Welfare.
2. American College of Sports Medicine (ACSM). (1986). *Guidelines for graded exercise testing and exercise prescription.* Philadelphia: Lea & Febiger.
3. American College of Sports Medicine (ACSM). (1991). *Guidelines for graded exercise testing and exercise prescription.* Philadelphia: Lea & Febiger.
4. American College of Sports Medicine (ACSM). (1991). Information for authors. *Medicine and Science in Sports and Exercise, 23,* i–v.
5. American College of Sports Medicine (ACSM). (1995). *ACSM's Guidelines for graded exercise testing and exercise prescription.* Philadelphia: Lea & Febiger.
6. American Psychological Association. (1994). *Publication manual of the American Psychological Association.* Washington, D.C.: Author, p. 105.
7. Astrand, P. O., & Rodahl, K. (1977). *Textbook of work physiology.* San Francisco: McGraw-Hill.
8. Bemben, M. G., Massey, B. H., Bemben, D. A., Boileau, R. A., & Misner, J. E. (1995). Age-related patterns in body composition for men aged 20–79 years. *Medicine and Science in Sports and Exercise, 27,* 264–269.
9. Food & Nutrition Board, National Academy of Science—National Research Council. (1980). Recommended dietary allowances. 9th ed., revised. In K. L. Jones, L. W. Shainberg, and C. O. Byer (Eds.), *Dimensions* (5th ed.), San Francisco: Harper & Row.
10. Frisancho, A. R. (1990). *Anthropometric standards for the assessment of growth and nutritional status.* Ann Arbor, MI: University of Michigan Press.
11. Gaesser, G. A., & Poole, D. C. (1996). The slow component of oxygen uptake kinetics in humans. In J. O. Holloszy (Ed.), *Exercise and sport sciences reviews* (pp. 35–70). Baltimore: Williams & Wilkins.
12. Garrett, W. E. (1985). Editor's comment. *National Geographic, 167*(6): 693.
13. Gordon, C. C., Chumlea, W. C., & Roche, A. F. (1988). Stature, recumbent length, and weight. In T. G. Lohman, A. F. Roche, & R. Rartorell (Eds.), *Anthropometric standardization reference manual* (pp. 3–8). Champaign, IL: Human Kinetics.
14. Hill, D. W., Borden, D. O., Darnaby, K. M., Hendricks, D. N., & Hill, C. M. (1992). Effect of time of day on aerobic and anaerobic responses to high-intensity exercise. *Canadian Journal of Sport Science, 17,* 316–319.
15. Hill, D. W., Cureton, K. J., & Collins, M. A. (1989). Effect of time of day on perceived exertion at work rates above and below the ventilatory threshold. *Research Quarterly for Exercise and Sport, 60,* 127–133.
16. Hill, D. W., & Smith, J. C. (1991). Circadian rhythm in anaerobic power and capacity. *Canadian Journal of Sport Science, 16,* 30–32.
17. Joint Dietary Guidelines Advisory Committee of U.S. Departments of Agriculture and Health and Human Services. (1990). *Nutrition and your health: Dietary guidelines for Americans.* (Home and Garden Bulletin No. 232). Washington, D.C.: U.S. Department of Agriculture.
18. Knuttgen, H. G. (1986). Quantifying exercise performance with SI units. *Physician and Sportsmedicine,* (Dec.): 157–161.
19. Knuttgen, H. G. (1995). Force, work, and power in athletic training. *Sports Science Exchange, 57*(4).
20. Lang, P. B., Latin, R. W., Berg, K. E., & Mellon, M. B. (1992). The accuracy of the ACSM cycle ergometry equation. *Medicine and Science in Sports and Exercise, 24,* 272–276.
21. Manson, J. E., Willett, W. C., Stampfer, M. J., Colditz, G. A., Hunter, D. J., Hankinson, S. E., Hennekens, C. H., & Speizer, F. E. (1995). Body weight and mortality among women. *New England Journal of Medicine, 333,* 677–685.
22. Wilmore, J. H., & Costill, D. L. (1994). *Physiology of sport and exercise.* Champaign, IL: Human Kinetics.
23. Young, D. S. (1987). Implementation of SI units for clinical laboratory data. *Annals of Internal Medicine, 106,* 114–129.

Form UN 1

Individual Basic Data

Name [   ] Date [   ] Time [   ] a.m. [   ] p.m.
(last)   (first)   (mo/d/y)   (check one)

Age [   ] y   Gender (M or F) [   ]

Ht [   ] in. (closest 0.25 in.) / 0.3937 = [   ] cm (closest 0.5 cm)

Weight Measured on Nonmetric Platform Scale (closest 0.25 lb)

Weight of clothes [   ] lb   Check one: Estimated [   ] Actual [   ]

Body Wt [   ] lb; Body Wt minus Clothes Wt = Nude Wt [   ] lb

Nude Wt / 2.20 = [   ] kg (closest 0.1 kg)

Weight Measured on Sensitive Metric Platform Scale (closest 0.01 kg or 10 g)

Weight of clothes [   ] 0.01 kg (closest 10g)

Body Wt [   ] closest 0.01 kg; Body Wt minus Clothes Wt = Nude Wt [   ] kg

Nude Wt rounded off to the closest 0.1 kg = [   ] kg

Interpretation of Weight: Average [   ]   Above average [   ]   Below average [   ]
(check one of the above using $M = \pm 11$ kg as the average)

Women's Optimum Wt: 0.85 × [   ] kg (U.S. average for age and ht) = [   ] kg [   ] lb

Age 18 wt [   ] kg (Women)

Present wt [   ] kg

kg	lb	Risk>average
≥9	20	2–3
≥18	40	7

Difference [   ] kg

Rest $\dot{V}O_2$ (ml·min^{-1}) = 3.5 ml × [   ] kg = [   ] ml

Form UN 2

Group Data for Age, Height, and Weight

MEN Initials (or ID #)	Age (y)	Height (cm)	Weight (kg)	WOMEN Initials (or ID #)	Age (y)	Height (cm)	Weight (kg)
1.				1.			
2.				2.			
3.				3.			
4.				4.			
5.				5.			
6.				6.			
7.				7.			
8.				8.			
9.				9.			
10.				10.			
11.				11.			
12.				12.			
13.				13.			
M				*M*			
Range				*Range*			

Form UN 3

Fill-In Abstract

Title: Basic Characteristics of Exercise Physiology Lab Students

Name of Investigator: _____
(First & Middle Initial)   (Last name)

Investigator's Affiliation: _____
(University, Institution, etc.)

Introduction & Purpose: The authors of scientific articles describe the persons whom they have studied. Accordingly, the purpose of this investigation was to collect basic data in order to describe the students in the Exercise Physiology Laboratory class.

Method: Name, age, and gender were obtained by a verbal questionnaire. The participants' ($n =$ _____) stature and weight were measured with a platform scale and stadiometer. The men's ($n =$ _____) and the women's ($n =$ _____) heights and weights were measured to the closest _____ cm (_____ in.) and _____ kg (_____ lb), respectively.

Results & Discussion: The average ages of the men and women were _____ y and _____ y, respectively. The men weighed _____ kg and were _____ cm tall compared to the average weight of _____ kg and height of _____ cm for men their age. The women weighed _____ kg and were _____ cm tall compared to the average weight of _____ kg and height of _____ cm for women their age.

Conclusion: The investigator concludes that the men in Exercise Physiology Laboratory weigh (check one) ☐ more than ☐ less than ☐ the same as the average American man based on the age-height-weight tables. The women weigh ☐ more than ☐ less than ☐ the same as the average American woman.

Note: This example of a research abstract includes the headings (e.g., Introduction, Method, etc.), which are not usually included in the published abstract.

Form *UN 4*

Research Abstract[a]

Title	
Investigator	
Introduction	
Purpose	
Method	
Results	
Discussion	
Conclusion	

[a]Form UN 4 may be used as a guide for students in writing abstracts after data have been collected and analyzed for each chapter's variables.

Chapter DS Dynamic Strength

The terms used to describe and quantify exercise are dependent upon the type of muscular action.[20] The two major types of exercise are dynamic and static. Dynamic exercise consists of muscle actions that are concentric or eccentric, depending on whether the muscles are shortened (concentric) or lengthened (eccentric). During most dynamic exercises, the speed of movement is variable throughout the movement, such as when lifting a barbell. Thus the load being lifted changes speed, due to biomechanical, physiological, and anatomical factors of the lifter, but the absolute load itself (the mass of the load) does not change. The other type of exercise—static—utilizes a muscular action that is isometric. The muscles do not change their length, except that caused by the elasticity of the muscle and connective tissues. Another type of muscle action called isokinetic may be proposed on the basis of the isokinetic apparatus. These machines alter the resistance of the load, causing the load to move at a constant speed,[13] although the muscle movement itself may not always be constant.[20]

Strength may be defined as the maximal force generated at a given velocity of exercise.[21] The velocity of exercise may include muscle actions that cause muscle fibers to lengthen (eccentric), remain the same length (isometric), or shorten (concentric). At zero velocity the exercise is static, whereas all other velocities of exercise include muscle actions that are dynamic. Therefore, the ideal profile of a person's strength would include measurements of that person's forces under all possible velocities. The practical approach, however, would be to measure strength during a movement at variable speed, during muscle action at zero speed, and during movements at designated constant speeds. Chapter DS focuses on dynamic strength (free-weights), that is, strength during a movement in which the body part is changing its speed of movement.

Three popular free-weight exercises that are described as dynamic strength tests in this chapter are (1) the bench press, (2) the standing overhead (military) press, and (3) the two-arm curl. Depending on the controlled or standardized conditions, the free-weight field tests described here could be classified also as field/lab or, possibly, laboratory tests.[35] This chapter includes a description of both direct and indirect (predicted; estimated) measures of dynamic strength for the muscle groups used in performing the three free-weight exercises.

Rationale

One of the most operational (easily applied) definitions for dynamic strength states that it is manifested as a person's *one repetition maximal,* or *1-RM,* for a specific movement.

Direct 1-RM

A direct measure of strength is the maximal weight that a person can lift in the prescribed manner only one time. A brief preview of the traditional 1-RM test would show that it requires a person to exert maximally on a selected weight, chosen as close as possible to the person's expected 1-RM weight. If the person cannot lift it with correct form, then a lower weight is tried after a rest interval; if the person properly lifts the weight twice, then the performer stops. After a rest interval, a small additional weight is added, and the person tries again. This process is repeated until only one repetition is possible.[26] Obtaining the 1-RM value for the first time in a person may be inaccurate and time consuming because of the number of attempts at achieving one, and only one, repetition at a given weight[23] and a lack of standardizing the lifting position or procedures. Direct 1-RM measurements also may be injurious for some persons, especially the elderly[33] and children.[16] The American Academy of Pediatrics[1] and the National Strength and Conditioning Association[31] endorse this sentiment in not recommending 1-RM performances by children.

Indirect 1-RM

Fortunately, the 1-RM value may be approximated by knowing any number of maximal repetitions from two to twenty for any given weight lifted. Thus, the 1-RM may be calculated from equations based upon either a linear or a slightly curvilinear (exponential) relationship between the percent of 1-RM (% 1-RM) and less than 20 repetitions maximal (RM). Although a performer may become fatigued during this procedure, a single maximal repetition is avoided.

When the indirect 1-RM method is based on a **linear relationship** between % 1-RM and the number of RM, the 1-RM can be estimated from measuring the number of RM at intensities between 80% and 100% 1-RM,[15,17,22,24] and possibly extended from intensities as low as 60% RM.[15,28] In general, the percent of a 1-RM load decreases by about 2 to 2.5% for each increase in the number of maximal

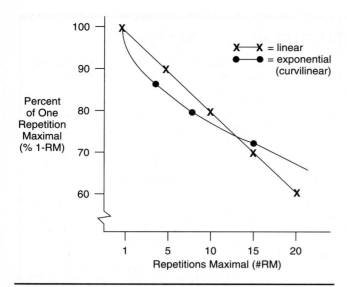

X—X = linear
●—● = exponential (curvilinear)

Percent of One Repetition Maximal (% 1-RM)

Repetitions Maximal (#RM)

Figure 1 The curvilinear[26] and linear relationships between the percent of one repetition maximal (% 1-RM) and the number of repetitions maximal (#RM). The curved line is drawn for conceptual purposes only, i.e., not drawn at the reference's precise data points.

repetitions (Fig. 1). Thus, the 1-RM load represents 100% 1-RM that can be lifted only once, whereas a 90% 1-RM load could be lifted about five times. The equation and its calculation are presented at the end of the Method section of this chapter.

The reverse is also true; if the 1-RM is known, it is possible to predict the approximate load that can be lifted a given number of times. For example, if a person's 1-RM is 100 kg, it is likely that about 75%–80% of 100 kg (then 75–80 kg) could be lifted no more than nine to twelve times (9-RM to 12-RM), or about ten times.[22]

The **curvilinear-based equation**[26] to predict the 1-RM is more complicated, but is particularly applicable for the bench press. It really consists of two equations, the first predicting the % 1-RM by an exponential regression, and the second predicting the 1-RM. The methods require that the maximal number of bench-press repetitions be timed for one minute (1-min RM). Its calculation also requires more advanced math, but if the calculator has the proper functions, it can be performed easily. An advantage of this equation is that it is reasonably accurate when the load for the bench press dips as low as 55% 1-RM. The equations and their calculation are presented at the end of the Method section of this chapter.

Bioenergetic Rationale

The biochemical pathway for maximal muscle actions, that is, strength, is the phosphagenic pathway. Even the longest of 1-RM movements is completed in less than 10 s; this includes the time spent holding the weight prior to the move-

ment, raising the weight, holding it in the lifted position, and lowering the weight.[30] Thus, the actual time spent raising the weight is usually less than three seconds. As illustrated in the fitness continuum (Figs. 2 and 3 in Chapter TE), maximal exercise efforts of this duration are placed within the strength fitness category.

Anatomical Rationale

Anatomically, the major muscles that are used to execute the three strength tests described here are presented in Table 1. All three of these popular strength training exercises emphasize the upper body musculature, particularly the arms, shoulders, and chest.[8,11,40]

Purpose of the Free-Weight Strength Tests

Strength testing serves purposes related to both health and performance. Inconclusive research suggests that persons, especially women, who habitually exert forcefully against resistances may protect themselves from losing some bone density.[2,4] It seems plausible that stronger persons are more likely to provide the necessary forces to prevent the advent of porous bones, associated with osteoporosis. Before embarking on strength-training programs it is meaningful to evaluate participants in order to prescribe their programs and monitor their progress. For example, a trainee's exercise prescription may include performing two or three sets of maximal repetitions at 80% of the 1-RM load.

Additionally, the purpose of the Free-Weight Tests as performed in *Exercise Physiology Laboratory Manual* goes beyond the mere measurement of strength. Because of the distinct terminology and measurements in exercise physiology, another purpose of these tests is to familiarize the student with common exercise terms and measurements associated with work and power. Thus, in addition to learning how to administer the strength tests, students will learn how to measure positive (concentric) work, negative (eccentric) work, total work, and power.

Table 1 Primary Muscles for Three Free-Weight Strength Tests

Standing Overhead Press	Two-Arm Curl	Bench Press
Shoulders	Arms	Shoulders
anterior deltoid	biceps brachii	anterior deltoid
coracobrachialis	brachioradialis	coracobrachialis
serratus anterior	brachialis	Chest
trapezius		sternocostal/
levator scapulae		clavicular
		pectoralis
Chest		Arms
upper pectoralis major		triceps brachii
Arms		
triceps brachii		

Accuracy of 1-RM Testing

Regardless of the accuracy of the equipment and the diligence of the examiner and participant, strength scores in participants will vary due to daily biological variability; this may cause strength scores in an individual to change by 2–12%.[37] When the 1-RM strength was determined for a two-arm curl performed two days apart on a custom-made weight machine, the test-retest correlation was .98. This correlation may not be as high, however, for two-arm curls performed with free-weights because of less standardization of body position and movement.[36] The test-retest variation of 1-RM and predicted 1-RM ranges from ±5–15%.[3] Thus, if on one day a person lifts 50 kg, or is predicted to lift 50 kg, then on a subsequent day that person's 1-RM, or predicted 1-RM, may be any value between 47.5 to 52.5 kg if at the least variability, and 42.5 to 57.5 kg at the most variability. Test-retest reliability is likely to be higher if the average of a few trials is used rather than the highest score of a few trials.[27]

The traditional direct method of measuring dynamic strength is not without its inconsistencies, especially for inexperienced lifters. Because 1-RM strength trials may increase significantly from trial one to trial two, especially in older adults,[34] the second trial of another day should be used as the baseline for strength-training intervention studies. It would be inappropriate to attribute all strength gains to the resistance training program on the basis of strength scores from trial one.

Although the National Football League's (NFL) test of strength for prospective players is not exactly like the predictive ones described here, it is similar enough to provide some input as to the accuracy of such predictive 1-RM tests. The NFL prescribes an absolute weight of 225 lb (~100 kg) to be bench pressed as many times as possible (repetitions maximal; RM). Their valid test ($r = .96$) predicted 1-RM strength in college football players, who required about seven repetitions to fatigue. The prediction appeared to be most accurate for those players who performed 10 RM or less.[6]

When predicting 1-RM from repetitions maximal, some inaccuracy may occur in assuming that there is a 2 to 2.5% decrease in any given person's 1-RM mass for each single increase of repetitions maximal. For example, this would assume that 10 RM is approximately equal to 80% of 1-RM mass. However, one reviewer reported a range from 60% to 90% for persons performing 10 repetitions maximal.[29] The initial strength and resistance training experience of the performer can affect the prediction of 1-RM.[5] This negative linear relationship also appears to vary with different muscle groups.[7]

The measurement of power for the bench press, using a 90% 1-RM method, revealed a test-retest correlation of .97.[3]

Method

The method section of a research paper should enable the readers to duplicate the researcher's study. This means that the equipment (instruments and materials), procedures, and calculations (analysis) should be described accordingly.

Equipment

The equipment for the dynamic strength test includes the following: (1) weighing scale (e.g., platform scale or electronic scale); (2) barbell; (3) assorted free-weights ranging from 1 kg (~2.5 lb) to 10 kg (~25 lb) each; (4) barbell collars (unless weights are welded onto the barbell); (5) stopwatch capable of measuring to a tenth of a second.

Weighing scales, used to measure the mass and force components, were discussed in Chapter UN. The barbell and weights, needed to measure the force component of work and power, are found in most weight rooms. A total weight of about 90 kg (~200 lb) should accommodate most performers. One bench is needed for one of the three strength exercises described here. Most exercise physiology laboratories have measurement tapes (preferably metric) and stopwatches to measure the distance and time components of work and power. Although the calculations of work and power may be performed without a calculator, the proper use of a pocket calculator minimizes time and assures accuracy. Students are encouraged to bring their own pocket calculators to every laboratory session.

Executing the Three Free-Weight Strength Movements

The accuracy of free-weight strength testing is enhanced if the execution of the lifts is standardized. The prescribed positions of the standing overhead press, two-arm curl, and bench press are illustrated in Figures 2, 3, and 4, respectively. Ideally, each subject should perform the three exercises according to the sequence presented here in order to assure recovery from fatigue of specific muscle groups.

Standing Overhead Press

1. The participant stands with the feet parallel and shoulder width apart.
2. Two technicians, or spotters, place the barbell in the hands of the participant at shoulder level and in front of the chest.
3. The participant grasps the barbell with a pronated grip (thumbs medial) and with the hands separated about shoulder width.
4. The elbows are pointed downward with the hands in a semi-hyperextended position as the bar rests along the clavicles during this preparatory position.
5. The participant then raises the bar over the head without bending the legs or back.
6. After straightening the arms the participant returns the bar to the preparatory position.

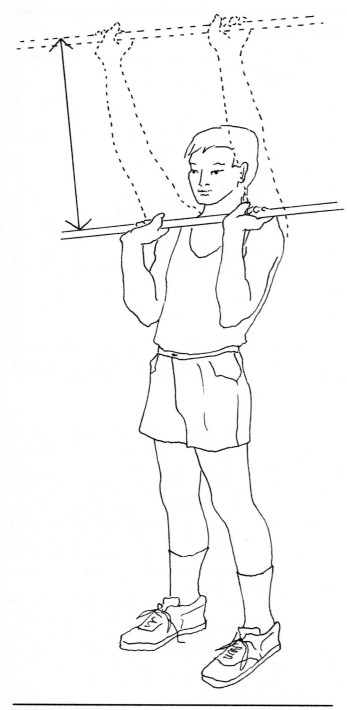

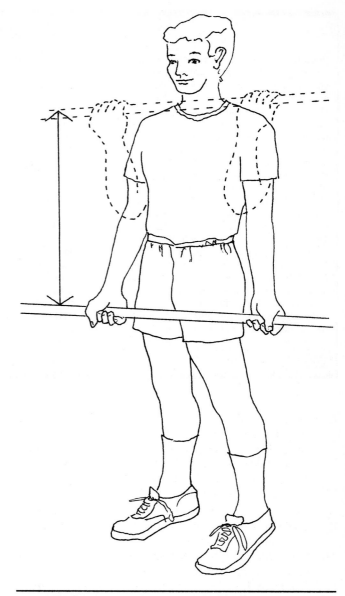

Figure 3 The beginning and end positions for the two-arm curl. The arrow denotes the distance measurement needed for calculating work.

Figure 2 The beginning and end positions for the standing overhead press; the arrow denotes the distance measurement needed for calculating work.

Two-Arm Curl

1. The participant stands with the feet parallel and shoulder width apart.
2. With arms hanging down at the sides and with the hands taking a supinated grip (palms facing out, thumbs lateral), the bar is held with straightened arms and against the thighs.
3. The participant then raises the bar to the chest by flexing at the elbow joint and without bending the legs and back. (By standing with the back near the wall, it might ensure that the participant does not lean backwards.)
4. After reaching the fully flexed position, the participant returns the bar to the preparatory position.

Bench Press

1. The participant lies supine on a wide bench with the knees bent and the soles of the feet on the bench. However, if the subject is in jeopardy of toppling

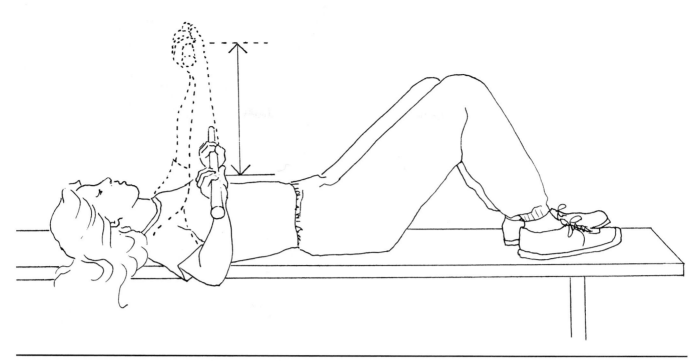

Figure 4 The beginning and end positions for the bench press. An alternate bench position places the participant's feet on the floor. The arrow denotes the distance measurement needed for calculating work.

from the bench, the feet may be on the floor and straddling the bench as in power-lifting competitions. Some might argue that by placing the feet on the floor, it causes the back to arch, thus placing it in jeopardy of injury.[9,25]

2. Two technicians, or spotters, place the barbell in the participant's pronated hands (thumbs medial) spaced about shoulder width apart and at chest level.

3. The participant raises the weight to a straightened-arms position directly above the chest.

4. The participant returns the barbell to the preparatory position.

Preparation

As with all of the tests performed in this manual, the first step is to record the **basic data.** Thus, the name, date, time, age, gender, height, and weight are recorded on Form DS 1. An additional factor, specific for free-weight testing, might be the recording of the performer's experience in lifting free-weights. The body weight should be as close to the nude weight as possible, and measured according to the procedures described in Chapter UN. Usually, it is not necessary to record meteorological data for the strength tests, because it is unlikely that environmental conditions will affect the strength measures.

The second step is to **calibrate** the test equipment. The calibration of the platform scale was described in the cali-

bration box of Chapter UN. Usually, the stopwatch can be assumed to be accurate, but to be sure, it might be compared to another from a reputable dealer.

It is not unusual for the poundage of commercial weights to be labeled inaccurately. For example, in one instance a weight that was marked as 8.8 lb, really weighed 10.4 lb. Hence, the weights, barbells, and collars that are to be used for testing should be verified on an accurate scale prior to testing. The actual pounds or kilograms should be labeled with an appropriate marking device (e.g., chalk) on the barbells or weights.

In some instances **mass** is considered equal to the force lifting the mass, such as when lifting a barbell against gravitational forces. The mass (free-weights), which in this case is the **force,** should be weighed on a metric scale to the closest tenth kilogram, or be converted to metrics after being weighed on a nonmetric scale. All values are recorded on Form DS 1.

Before the subject performs the maximal repetitions for a given weight, **distance (D)** measurements must be made for each of the three exercises in order to calculate the work ($w = F \times D$) accomplished. The distances are measured to the closest centimeter with a metric tape and are recorded on Form DS 1. They can be made with the performer using an imaginary or unloaded bar at two points: the preparatory and endpoints of each movement. The criteria for measuring these distances are illustrated in Figures 2, 3, and 4 and outlined in Table 2.

Table 2 Landmarks for Measuring Distances for the Three Free-Weight Exercises

Test	Bar Preparatory Point	Bar Endpoint
Standing Overhead Press	Near upper chest	Straightened-arms position over head
Two-Arm Curl	Against thighs	Fully flexed arm-curl position near chest
Bench Press	On chest	Straightened-arms position over head

Table 3 Suggested Weights for the Indirect 1-RM Test

Free-Weight Test	Suggested Weight
Standing Overhead Press	1/3 body wt + 5 kg or 10–11 lb
Two-Arm Curl	1/3 body wt
Bench Press	1/2 body wt

After the distance measures are made, the performer should be given 5–10 min of **prior exercise,** consisting of loosening-up and warming-up exercises. Obviously, these exercises should incorporate the muscles to be used in the three strength tests. Thus, the loosening-up exercises should stretch the upper body muscles and tendons. One warmup set of about eight repetitions should mimic the executions of each lift, but with weights that are about 40% or less of an estimated one repetition maximal. This can be followed by another set of three repetitions between 50% and 70% of estimated 1-RM.[38] However, it should be recognized that these preliminary estimates are rather exploratory for first-time performers.

Summary of Preparatory Steps

Technician (Tester/Examiner/Investigator/Researcher)

1. Calibrate the platform scale or electronic scale. (Refer to the calibration box in Chapter UN).
2. Weigh and mark the barbells and assorted weights. Labeling them in newton (N) units can simplify work and power calculations.
3. Record basic data on Form DS 1. Ask performer about experience with free-weights. Weigh the performer and record "nude" body weight to the closest 0.1 kg and height to closest 0.5 cm. (Refer to Chapters TE and UN. See following steps 1 and 2 for performer.)
4. Explain and demonstrate the proper execution of the three free-weight lifts using only the barbell (see step 3 of performer).
5. Measure and record (Form DS 1) the vertical distance for one concentric action of each barbell lift of the performer (refer to illustrations and Table 2).
6. Load the barbell with an appropriate weight for the performer (see Table 3). The suggested weight for the standing overhead press by inexperienced lifters = 1/3 body wt + 5 kg; record this weight on Form DS 1.
7. As the final preparatory step, the technician prescribes a prior-exercise regimen similar to that previously described and found in the "prior exercise" box.

Performer (Participant/Subject)

1. Provide technician with basic data factors such as name, age, and experience with free-weights.
2. Provide technician with clothes to be worn during weigh-in, or be scantily-clothed so that weight is near nude-weight value.
3. Practice the three lifts until performance is satisfactory.
4. Hold the preparatory and endpoint positions for each lift so that the technician can record the distance measurements.
5. As the final preparatory step, the performer loosens up and warms up by following the prior exercise regimen described previously and summarized in the box.

Prior Exercise Regimen

Loosen-up routine:
2–3 min spent stretching (ballistic and static) the muscle groups to be used in the three lifts. (Refer to Table 1 for appropriate muscle groups.)

Warm-up routine:
Set 1: 8 reps at ~40% of estimated 1-RM
Rest 2–3 min
Set 2: 3 reps at 50–70% of estimated 1-RM
Rest 2–3 min

Test Procedures for 1-RM, Work and Power

Procedures for both the direct and indirect methods of determining 1-RM strength are described here. The direct method is the traditional trial-and-retrial method in which the results may be compared with the results of the indirect method. Hence, the comparison can serve as a validation of the indirect method. The direct method will not include those procedures associated with familiarization of exercise terms, such as work and power, and their respective measuring units.

Direct 1-RM. The procedures outlined here[32,38] should be preceded by similar preparatory considerations as described earlier, except that the distance measures need not be made and the prior-exercise regimen may be altered slightly. The procedural steps for the traditional direct measurement of 1-RM are as follows:

1. The performer warms up with three to four repetitions at an estimated load that is about 40–60% of the perceived 1-RM.

2. Then the performer rests for 2–3 min.
3. The performer continues the warmup by repeating three to four repetitions, but this time at 60–80% of perceived 1-RM.
4. Again, the performer rests for 2–3 min.
5. The performer attempts a single lift at a load that is 95% of perceived 1-RM.
6. Most performers would need a recovery period of 2–7 min. Although as little as 1-min rest may be enough for some persons, recovery as long as 5–10 min may be necessary for others.[38]
7. If the performer feels the previous load was close to the actual 1-RM load, then 5-lb (~2.5 kg) increments are added to the prior load; if the performer feels that the prior estimate of 95% was considerably off from the actual 1-RM, then >5-lb increments are added.
8. If the performer can properly execute a single lift, but no more than one repetition, on the second, third, or fourth retrial, then this load should be recorded as the 1-RM on Form DS 1.
9. If more than four attempts at the 1-RM value are needed, then the performer should be retested on another day with the advantage of having the knowledge gained from this session's trials.[38]

Indirect 1-RM. As mentioned previously, the prediction of 1-RM may be made based on either a linear relationship or a curvilinear relationship between % 1-RM and RM. The focus of the following is based on the more popular, but not necessarily more accurate, linear relationship. The ultimate step in predicting 1-RM is to determine the performer's maximal number of repetitions for a given weight (force). Repetitions maximal is defined as the number of repetitions, without a rest interval, performed until no other properly executed repetition can be completed. In order to comply with the linearity rationale, it is best if the number of maximal repetitions does not exceed twenty. If it is apparent that the subject is about to exceed twenty repetitions, then the subject should stop and wait for 5–10 min before repeating the exercise at a heavier weight. The suggested weights presented in Table 3, which are similar to those suggested by others,[23] may be helpful for persons with little idea of their 1-RM weights.

Power Measurement. Timing the durations of each of the three free-weight lifts is necessary when calculating power because power is the rate of doing work. The timer should start the stopwatch at the first visible movement of the performer during the test. For the indirect measurement of 1-RM for all three free-weight lifts that are based on the linear equation, the timer stops the watch when the subject returns the weight after the last complete or partial repetition. The timer records the time to the closest whole second(s). The performer should execute the repetitions at a comfortable

pace because the purpose of the power measurement is not to rate and compare the quality of the performer's peak power. If the latter were the goal, the performer would need to execute the maximal repetitions as fast as possible; however, the author is not aware of any norms for such a test. The primary purpose of the power "test" is to become familiar with the concept of power and its calculation.[19] Power is calculated according to Equation 5 ($P = w/t$) in Chapter TE. The conversions for the various force, work, and power units may need to be reviewed on Table 1 of Chapter UN.

Calculations

Calculating Indirect 1-RM Based on Linear Relationship

The equation for calculating 1-RM based on the linear relationship between % 1-RM and RM is presented in Equation 1.

$$\text{1-RM (lb or kg)} = \frac{\text{lb or kg at RM between 2–20}}{[100\% - (\text{RM} \times 2)]} \qquad \text{Eq. 1}$$

For example, if a person could lift 100 kg (220 lb) only once, then the 100 kg would represent one repetition maximal or 1-RM, or 100% 1-RM. However, if this person lifted 80 kg ten times, then the 1-RM value of 100 kg is derived without directly measuring it by using Equation 1 as follows:

$$\begin{aligned} \text{1-RM (kg)} &= 80 \text{ kg} / [100\% - (10 \times 2)] \\ &= 80 \text{ kg} / (100\% - 20) \\ &= 80 \text{ kg} / 80\% \text{ or } 0.80 \\ &= 100 \text{ kg} \end{aligned}$$

Calculating 1-RM Based on Curvilinear Relationship

Two equations are used for calculating 1-RM based on the curvilinear (exponential) relationship between % 1-RM and 1-min RM for the bench press.[26] The performer bench presses a weight that is estimated to be about 55% to 95% of 1-RM. Rest breaks are allowed as the performer attempts a maximal number of lifts in one minute. By including the multiplication of the 1-min RM for the bench press by a constant negative exponent in the first equation (Eq. 2), the percentage of 1-RM can be predicted for the bench press. The predicted % 1-RM can be used in the second equation (Eq. 3) to predict the 1-RM for the bench press. The test-retest reliability correlation is .97.

$$\% \text{ 1-RM} = 52.2 + (41.9 \text{ e}^{-0.055 \text{ 1-minRM}}) \qquad \text{Eq. 2}^a$$

where:

52.2 and 41.9 are constants
e = the rounded-off natural logarithm value of 2.72
–0.055 = the constant negative exponent
1-minRM = the number of repetitions in 1 min

$$\text{1-RM (kg)} = \text{repetition wt in kg} \div (\% \text{ 1-RM}/100) \qquad \text{Eq. 3}$$

---

^{a}Calculator requires the y^x or x^y function

For example, if a person bench presses 50 kg thirty times by the end of 1 min, then the following calculations can predict, first, the % 1-RM, and, secondly, the 1-RM:

$$\% \text{ 1-RM} = 52.2 + (41.9 \text{ e}^{-0.055 \text{ 1-minRM}})$$
$$= 52.2 + (41.9 \times 2.72^{-0.055 \times 30})$$
$$= 52.2 + (41.9 \times 2.72^{-1.65})$$
$$= 52.2 + (41.9 \times 0.192)$$
$$= 52.2 + 8.0$$
$$= 60.2\% = 60\% \text{ rounded-off value}$$

$$\text{1-RM (kg)} = \text{repetition wt in kg} \div (\% \text{ 1-RM}/100)$$
$$= 50 \text{ kg} \div (60/100)$$
$$= 80/0.60$$
$$= 83 \text{ kg}$$

Calculating Work

Equation 4 is used to calculate the **positive work** from the mass lifted (force, F), the distance of a single repetition (D for 1 rep), and the number of maximal repetitions (#RM). The latter will, presumably, consist of more than one repetition, and will also include a somewhat subjective estimate of the fraction for the attempt of the final incomplete repetition. For example, if the performer properly executed nine complete repetitions, but attempted a tenth lift that only went half the proper distance, then record this as 9.5 RM.

$$^{+}w = F \times (D \text{ for 1 rep} \times \#RM) \qquad \text{Eq. 4}$$

Thus, if a person bench pressed a weight (F) of 50 kg (110 lb) no more than six times (6 RM), to a height of 0.5 m, then the positive work could be calculated from these values as follows:

$$^{+}w = 50 \text{ kg} \times (0.5 \text{ m} \times 6 \text{ RM})$$
$$= 50 \text{ kg} \times 3 \text{ m}$$
$$= 150 \text{ kg·m}$$

Because force and work are expressed scientifically as newtons (N) and newton meters (N · m) or joules (J), respectively, the conversion of kilograms and kilogram meters (see Table 1 in Chapter UN) is made as follows:

$$\text{F (in N)} = 50 \text{ kg} \times 10 = 500 \text{ N}$$
$$^{+}w \text{ (in N·m or J)} = 150 \text{ kg·m} \times 10 = 1500 \text{ N·m};$$
$$\text{or } 500 \text{ N} \times 3 \text{ m} = 1500 \text{ N·m}$$
$$= 1500 \text{ J (1.5 kJ)}$$

Positive work, however, accounts only for the concentric muscle action lifting the weight vertically against gravity. To measure the total work of these dynamic exercises, the eccentric muscle action, or **negative work,** must be considered. Although the estimate of negative work is quite variable, it might be assumed to be approximately one-third of positive work for the purposes of appreciating the concept of total work. Thus, using the hypothetical example of 1500 J for positive work, the calculation of **total work** is made by using Equation 3 from Chapter TE ($w = 1.33 \times {}^{+}w$):

$$w = 1.33 \times 1500 \text{ J} = 2000 \text{ J (2 kJ)}$$

Calculating Power

If the performer accomplishes 200 kg·m (2000 N·m; 2000 J) of total work in 15 s (or 0.25 min), then **power** can be calculated from the examples listed here in units of kilogram meters per second (#1; $kg·m·s^{-1}$) or per minute (#2; $kg·m·min^{-1}$), or in units of newton meters per second (#3; $N·m·s^{-1}$) or per minute (#4; $N·m·min^{-1}$).

#1 $P (kg·m·s^{-1}) = 200 \text{ kg·m} / 15 \text{ s} = 13.3$

#2 $P (kg·m·min^{-1}) = 200 \text{ kg·m} / 0.25 \text{ min} = 800$

#3 $P (N·m·s^{-1}) = 2000 \text{ N·m} / 15 \text{ s} = 133$

#4 $P (N·m·min^{-1}) = 2000 \text{ N·m} / 0.25 = 8000$

Because power is most appropriately expressed scientifically as watts (W), the approximate conversions of kilogram meters per second or minute, and of newton meters per second or minute are made as follows:

$$P \text{ (W)} = 13.3 \text{ kg·m·s}^{-1} / 0.1 = 133 \text{ W}$$
$$P \text{ (W)} = 800 \text{ kg·m·min}^{-1} / 6 = 133 \text{ W}$$
$$P \text{ (W)} = 133 \text{ N·m·s}^{-1} / 1 = 133 \text{ W}$$
$$P \text{ (W)} = 8000 \text{ N·m·min}^{-1} / 60 = 133 \text{ W}$$

These work and power calculations may appear complicated at first, but they can be simplified quite easily by labeling the lifted weight in newtons (simply adding a zero to the end of the kilogram value). This converts kilograms to newtons, thus the work units N·m and J (remember, 1 N·m = 1 J) are easily derived. Power units ($N·m·s^{-1}$ or W), can then be easily calculated from Equation 3 by dividing the number of seconds (e.g., 15) into the N·m (e.g., 2000). In this example, the watt and $N·m·s^{-1}$ value is 133 W or $N·m·s^{-1}$ (1 W = 1 $N·m·s^{-1}$).

Summary of Testing Procedures for Determining the Indirect 1-RM and Its Associated Work and Power

Except for the preparatory steps that have been mentioned previously, the following summary includes procedural steps by the technician and performer during the indirect 1-RM test. It also indicates that calculations need to be made by the technician after the collection of the data.

Procedures

1. Ask the performer to lift the weight as prescribed for the movement and as many times as possible at a comfortable pace, but without a rest interval. Start the stopwatch at the subject's first movement and stop it after the last attempt of a repetition; record the time to the closest second on Form DS 1.

2. Count and record the number of repetitions maximal including the fraction of a possible partial repetition on the last attempt.

3. Provide a retrial, after a 5–10 min recovery period, if the performer exceeds or would appear to exceed twenty RM.
4. Calculate and record (Form DS 1) ^+w, w, and P.

Results and Discussion

Strength categories are often selected on the basis of absolute 1-RM and relative 1-RM values. Indeed, a person with a very high absolute 1-RM is strong, but a person of lower body weight and lower 1-RM may also be relatively strong when the 1-RM is related to body weight. Guidelines for the interpretation of strength scores (1-RM) based upon percent body weight for men and women are found in Table 4.[39] These percentages are not based on the necessary data to derive standards; nevertheless, they are intended to indicate optimal values. These guidelines suggest that women should achieve a percentage that is 70% of the men's percentage for the three movements. For example, if a 60 kg woman's 1-RM for the bench press is 42 kg (~92 lb), then she has met a suggested criterion by benching 70% of her body weight.

Women's norms for the standing overhead press and the bench press are presented in Table 5.[18] These are based on a large number of college-aged women who underwent

10 weeks of strength training. In general, the 1-RM values increase as body weight increases, with a couple of minor exceptions. The means of the bench press in Table 5 closely agree with the proposed optimal guidelines presented in Table 4, but the means of the standing press are greater than those in Table 4. Thus, because these values represent strength-trained women and reflect the guidelines in Table 4, they may be used as suggested goals, but not as typical values for untrained college women.

Norms for bench-press strength in adult men and women in three age categories (<30 y; 30–50 y; >50 y) are presented in Table 6.[14]

Persons who know their bench press 1-RM on a **variable resistance machine,** such as the Universal, could compare their scores with those from a large sample of men and women tested at the Cooper Clinic.[21] The women, average age of 39.5 ($SD = 9.6$), could bench press about 33 kg ($SD = 7.7$), and the men, average age of 41.6 ($SD = 9.2$) could bench press about 73 kg ($SD = 17.4$). The women's 1-RM represented about 55% of their body weight, whereas the men's represented about 87% of their body weight.

Standard values for a wide age range in free-weight bench-press strength relative to body weight are presented in Table 7.[2,10] For example, if a 25-year-old man, weighing 100 kg (220 lb), benches 120 kg (264 lb), then the strength (S):weight (W) ratio is calculated according to Equation 5:

$$S:W = 1\text{-RM}/W \qquad \text{Eq. 5}$$
$$= 120/100 = 1.20$$

Thus this man would be classified in the high end of the "good" strength fitness category. The ratios are the same

Table 4 Optimal Free-Weight Strength in Men and Women Based on % Body Weight

	Standing Press	Two-Arm Curl	Bench Press
Men	67%	50%	100%
Women	47%	35%	70%

Source: Percentages derived from Wilmore and Costill, p. 377, 1988.

Table 5 Free-Weight Strength (1-RM in lb) of Bench Press (BP) and Standing Press (SP) in College Women of Various Body Weights (kg)

						Body Weight								
kg	43–47		48–51		52–56		57–61		62–65		66–70		70	
~lb	95–104		105–114		115–124		125–134		135–144		145–154		>154	
						1-RM (lb)								
%ile	BP	SP	BP	SP	BP	SP	BP	SP	BP	SP	BP	SP	BP	SP
99	98	80	112	100	116	95	123	98	117	101	143	115	166	137
90	85	69	96	84	99	80	104	83	100	85	118	97	140	117
80	80	64	89	77	91	74	96	78	93	79	108	90	130	108
70	76	60	84	72	86	70	90	73	88	74	101	84	122	102
60	72	57	79	68	81	66	85	69	83	70	94	80	115	97
50	69	55	76	64	77	63	80	66	79	66	88	76	109	92
40	66	52	72	60	73	59	76	62	75	62	83	72	103	87
30	63	49	67	56	68	56	71	59	71	58	76	67	96	82
20	58	45	62	51	63	51	65	54	65	53	69	62	88	76
10	53	40	56	44	56	45	57	48	58	47	59	55	78	67

Source: Kindig, L. E., Soares, P. L., Wisenbaker, J. M., & Mrvos, S. R. (1984). Standard scores for women's weight training. *The Physician and Sportsmedicine, 12*(10): 67–74. Permission of McGraw-Hill © 1984.

Table 6 Free-Weight 1-RM Bench Press Strength (lb and kg) in Adult Men and Women Under 30 y to Over 50 y of Age

	Age (y)											
	<30				30–50				50+			
%ile	Men		Women		Men		Women		Men		Women	
	1-RM											
	lb	~kg	lb	~kg	lb	~kg	lb	~kg	lb	~kg	lb	~kg
95	203	92	105	48	183	83	95	43	161	73	84	38
90	191	87	100	45	172	78	91	41	151	69	81	37
80	175	80	95	43	158	72	86	39	139	63	76	35
70	164	75	91	41	148	67	83	38	130	59	73	33
60	155	70	88	40	139	63	80	36	122	55	71	32
50	146	66	85	39	131	60	77	35	115	52	68	31
40	137	62	82	37	123	56	74	34	108	49	66	30
30	128	58	79	36	114	52	71	32	100	45	63	29
20	117	53	75	34	104	47	68	31	91	41	60	27
10	101	46	70	32	90	41	63	29	79	36	55	25
5	89	40	65	30	79	36	59	27	69	31	52	24
Mean	146	66	85	39	131	60	77	35	115	52	68	31
SD	35	16	12	5	32	15	11	5	28	13	10	5

Note: The kilogram values may be converted to newton values by simply attaching a zero at the end of each kilogram value.

Source: R. V. Hockey, Physical Fitness: The Pathway to Healthful Living, 1989. Copyright C. W. Mosby Year Book, Inc., St. Louis, MO 63146.

Table 7 Standard Categories for the Ratio (lb:lb; kg:kg) of 1-RM Bench-Press Strength to Body Weight

	Men				
Category	Age (y)				
	20–29	30–39	40–49	50–59	60+
Excellent	>1.26	>1.08	>0.97	>0.86	>0.78
Good	1.17–1.25	1.01–1.07	0.91–0.96	0.81–0.85	0.74–0.77
Average	0.97–1.16	0.86–1.00	0.78–0.90	0.70–0. 80	0.64–0.73
Fair	0.88–0.96	0.79–0.85	0.72–0.77	0.65–0.69	0.60–0.63
Poor	<0.87	<0.78	<0.71	<0.64	<0.60

	Women				
Category	Age (y)				
	20–29	30–39	40–49	50–59	60+
Excellent	0.78	0.66	0.61	0.54	>0.55
Good	0.72–0.77	0.62–0.65	0.57–0.60	0.51–0.53	0.51–0.54
Average	0.59–0.71	0.53–0.61	0.48–0.56	0.43–0. 50	0.41–0.50
Fair	0.53–0.58	0.49–0.52	0.44–0.47	0.40–0.42	0.37–0.40
Poor	<0.52	<0.48	<0.43	<0.39	<0.36

From unpublished data from Institute for Aerobics Research (1985) by Gettman. Prescription Resource Manual, p. 161. Reprinted by permission of The Cooper Institute for Aerobics Research, Dallas, TX.

when both 1-RM and body weight are either presented in nonmetric (lb:lb) or metric (kg:kg) units. The percentiles associated with each qualitative category are:

>75th %ile = Excellent
65–74 = Good
35–64 = Average
10–34 = Fair
<10th = Poor

Comparative scores for ratios between the two-arm curl 1-RM and body weight have been derived from data on 250 college-age men and women.[12] Table 8 categorizes the data into strength categories.

Norms for the power measurement as described here are not available. If, however, a large number of performers were instructed to execute the repetitions as fast as possible, the data could generate meaningful power comparisons.

Table 8 1-RM Two-Arm Curl Strength to Body Weight Ratios for College-Aged Men and Women

Two-Arm Curl 1-RM Ratios (lb:lb; or kg:kg)		
Category	Men	Women
High	0.70	0.50
	0.65	0.45
Above Average	0.60	0.42
	0.55	0.38
Average	0.50	0.35
	0.45	0.32
	0.40	0.28
Below Average	0.35	0.25
	0.30	0.21
	0.25	0.18

Source: Data from Heywood, *Advanced Fitness Assessment and Exercise Prescription*, 1991, Human Kinetics.

References

1. American Academy of Pediatrics. (1983). Weight training and weight lifting: Information for the pediatrician. *The Physician and Sportsmedicine, 11*(3): 157–161.

2. American College of Sports Medicine (ACSM). (1995). *ACSM's Guidelines for graded exercise testing and exercise prescription.* Philadelphia: Lea & Febiger.

3. Berger, R. A., & Smith, K. J. (1991). Effects of the tonic neck reflex in the bench press. *Journal of Applied Sport Science Research, 5,* 188–191.

4. Block, J. E., Smith, R., Friedlander, G., & Genant, H. K. (1989). Preventing osteoporosis with exercise: A review with emphasis on methodology. *Medical Hypotheses, 30*(1): 9–19.

5. Braith, R. W., Graves, J. E., Leggett, S. H., & Pollock, M. L. (1993). Effect of training on the relationship between maximal and submaximal strength. *Medicine and Science in Sports and Exercise, 25*(1): 132–138.

6. Chapman, P. P., Whitehead, J. R., & Brinkhert, R. H. (1996). Prediction of 1-RM bench press from the 225 lbs reps-to-fatigue test in college football players. *Medicine and Science in Sports and Exercise, 28,* Abstract #393, S66.

7. Claiborne, J. M., & Donolli, J. D. (1993). Number of repetitions at selected percentages of one repetition maximum in untrained college women. *Research Quarterly for Exercise and Sport, 64*(Suppl): (Abstract).

8. Clarke, D. H. (1975). *Exercise physiology.* Englewood Cliffs, NJ: Prentice-Hall.

9. Corbin, C. B., & Lindsey, R. (1996). *Physical fitness concepts.* Dubuque, IA: Brown & Benchmark.

10. Gettman, L. R. (1988). Fitness testing. In S. Blair, P. Painter, R. Pate, L. Smith, & C. Taylor (Eds.), *Resource manual for guidelines for exercise testing and prescription.* Philadelphia: Lea & Febiger.

11. Hay, J. G., & Reid, J. G. (1982). *The anatomical and mechanical bases of human motion.* Englewood Cliffs, NJ: Prentice-Hall.

12. Heywood, V. H. (1991). *Advanced fitness assessment and exercise prescription.* Champaign, IL: Human Kinetics.

13. Hislop, H. J., & Perrine, J. J. (1967). The isokinetic concept of exercise. *Physical Therapy, 47,* 114–117.

14. Hockey, R. V. (1989). *Physical fitness: The pathway to healthful living.* St. Louis: Times Mirror/Mosby College Publishers.

15. Hoeger, W. K., Barette, S. L., Hale, D. F., & Hopkins, D. R. (1987). Relationship between repetitions and selected percentage of one repetition maximum. *Journal of Applied Sports Science Research, 1,* 11–13.

16. Invergo, J. J., Ball, T. E., & Looney, M. (1991). Relationship of push-ups and absolute muscular endurance to bench press strength. *Journal of Applied Sport Science Research, 5,* 121–125.

17. Johnson, P. B., Updyke, W. F., Schaefer, M., & Stollberg, D. C. (1975). *Sport, exercise, and you.* San Francisco: Holt, Rinehart, and Winston.

18. Kindig, L. E., Soares, P. L., Wisenbaker, J. M., & Mrvos, S. R. (1984). Standard scores for women's weight training. *The Physician and Sportsmedicine, 12*(10): 67–74.

19. Knuttgen, H. G. (1995). Force, work, and power in athletic training. *Sports Science Exchange, 8*(4): 1–5.

20. Knuttgen, H. G., & Kraemer, W. J. (1987). Terminology and measurement in exercise performance. *Journal of Applied Sport Science Research, 1,* 54–68.

21. Kohl, H. W., Gordon, N. F., Scott, C. B., Vaandrager, H., & Blair, S. N. (1992). Musculoskeletal strength and serum lipid levels in men and women. *Medicine and Science in Sports and Exercise, 24,* 1080–1087.

22. Kraemer, R. R., Kilgore, J. L., Kraemer, G. R., & Castracane, V. D. (1992). Growth hormone, IGF-1, and testosterone responses to resistive exercise. *Medicine and Science in Sports and Exercise, 24,* 1346–1352.

23. Kuramoto, A. K., & Payne, V. G. (1995). Predicting muscular strength in women: A preliminary study. *Research Quarterly for Exercise and Sport, 66,* 168–172.

24. Landers, J. (1985). Maximum based on repetitions. *National Strength and Conditioning Association Journal, 6,* 60–61.

25. Liemohn, W. S. et al. (1988). Unresolved controversies in back management. *Journal of Orthopaedic and Sports Physical Therapy, 9,* 239–244.

26. Mayhew, J. L., Ball, T. E., Arnold, M. D., & Bowen, J. C. (1992). Relative muscular endurance performance as a predictor of bench press strength in college men and women. *Journal of Applied Sport Science Research, 6,* 200–206.
27. McArdle, W. D., Katch, F. I., & Katch, V. L. (1996). *Exercise physiology: Energy, nutrition, and human performance.* Baltimore: Williams & Wilkins.
28. McCarthy, J. J. (1991). *Effects of a wrestling periodization strength program on muscular strength, absolute endurance, and relative endurance.* Master's thesis, California State University, Fullerton.
29. McComas, A. J. (1994). Human neuromuscular adaptations that accompany changes in activity. *Medicine and Science in Sports and Exercise, 26,* 1498–1509.
30. Murray, J. A., & Karpovich, P. V. (1956). *Weight training in athletics.* Englewood Cliffs, NJ: Prentice-Hall.
31. National Strength and Conditioning Association. (1985). Position paper on prepubescent strength training. *NSCA Journal, 7*(4): 27–31.
32. *Penn State Sports Medicine Newsletter.* (1992). The RM prescription. *1*(2): 7.
33. Pollock, M. L., Graves, J. E., Leggett, S. H., Braith, R. W., & Hagberg, J. M. (1991). Injuries and adherence to aerobic and strength training exercise programs for the elderly. *Medicine and Science in Sports and Exercise, 23,* 1194–1200.
34. Rikli, R. E., Jones, C. J., Beam, W. C., Duncan, S. J., & Lamar, B. (1996). Testing versus training effects on 1-RM strength assessment in older adults. *Medicine and Science in Sports and Exercise, 28*(5, Suppl.), Abstract #909, S153.
35. Rutherford, W. J., & Corbin, C. B. (1994). Validation of criterion-referenced standards for tests of arm and shoulder girdle strength and endurance. *Research Quarterly for Exercise and Sport, 65,* 110–119.
36. Sale, D. G. (1991). Testing strength and power. In J. D. MacDougal, H. A. Wenger, & H. J. Green (Eds.), *Physiological testing of the high-performance athlete.* (pp. 21–106). Champaign, IL: Human Kinetics.
37. Wakim, K. G., Gersten, J. W., Elkins, E. C., & Martin, G. M. (1950). Objective recording of muscle strength. *Archives of Physical Medicine, 31,* 90–100.
38. Weir, J. P., Wagner, L. L., & Housh, T. J. (1994). The effect of rest interval length on repeated maximal bench press. *Journal of Strength and Conditioning Research, 8,* 58–60.
39. Wilmore, J. H., & Costill, D. L. (1988). *Training for sport and activity.* Dubuque, IA: Wm. C. Brown.
40. Yessis, M. (1992). *Kinesiology of exercise: A safe and effective way to improve performance.* Indianapolis, IN: Masters Press.

Form DS 1

Individual Free-Weight Strength Test Form

Basic Data

Name _____ (last) _____ (first) Date _____ (mo/ d / y) Time _____ a.m. _____ p.m. _____

Age _____ y   Gender (M or F) _____   Free-wt experience _____ Y _____ N

Ht _____ in.   _____ cm   Body Wt _____ lb _____ kg

Free-Weight Test Data

Test	Vertical Distance (D)				Force (F)			Work (w)		
	+ D (1 Rep)		Reps	+D				^{+}w		Total w^b
	cm	m	RM	m	lb	kg	N	kg·m	N·m; J	J
Standing Press										
Two-arm Curl										
Bench Press										

	Total Time (t) RM		Power (P)			Interpretation of 1-RM		
	s	min	$N·m·s^{-1}$	$N·m·min^{-1}$	W^a	%Body Wt^c	%ile	ratio
Standing Press		0.						
Two-arm Curl		0.						
Bench Press		0.						

^{a}W = 6.12 kgm·min^{-1} = 1 N·m·s^{-1} = 60 N·m·min^{-1}
^{b}1.33 × $^{+}$w
^{c}(1-RM ÷ body wt) × 100 = %

1-RM (lb or kg) = lb or kg at RM between 2–20/[100% – (RM × 2)]

= _____ lb or kg/[100% – (_____ RM × 2)]

= _____ lb or kg/(100% – _____ %)

= _____ lb or kg/ 0. _____ = _____ lb or kg

Form DS 2

Group Form for MEN'S Free-Weight Strength (kg), Work (w; kJ), and Power (P; W) for Standing Press (SP), Bench Press (BP), and Arm Curl (AC)

Initials or ID #	Direct 1-RM			Indirect 1-RM			Ratio		w	P
	SP	2-AC	BP	SP	2-AC	BP	2-AC	BP	(kJ)	W
1.										
2.										
3.										
4.										
5.										
6.										
7.										
8.										
9.										
10.										
11.										
12.										
13.										
M										

Form DS 3

Group Form for WOMEN'S Free-Weight Strength (kg), Work (w; kJ), and Power (P; W) for Standing Press (SP), Bench Press (BP), and Arm Curl (AC)

Initials or ID #	Direct 1-RM			Indirect 1-RM			Ratio		w	P
	SP	2-AC	BP	SP	2-AC	BP	2-AC	BP	(kJ)	W
1.										
2.										
3.										
4.										
5.										
6.										
7.										
8.										
9.										
10.										
11.										
12.										
13.										
M										

Chapter SS Static Strength

The importance of handgrip strength is not just to have an impressive handshake. Good handgrip strength may prevent people from dropping various objects such as jars, bottles, and cans, in addition to allowing them to open the lid of a jar. Especially for older persons, good handgrip strength may prevent a fall down stairs or in bathtubs by enabling them to grasp a rail; it may also permit them to squeeze the gas pump at the service station. In summary, handgrip strength is important for successful performance in activities of daily living.

The monitoring of handgrip strength is meaningful in the diagnosis and prognosis of neck injuries. Thus, the measurement of handgrip strength has implications concerning people's safety, convenience, and neuromuscular assessment.

Rationale

The rationale for the measurement of strength may be categorized into three areas—anatomical, physiological, and biochemical. All of these are interrelated.

Anatomical Rationale

Grip strength is related ($r = .60$) to muscle mass.[13] Handgrip strength is mainly a function of the muscles in the forearm, in addition to those in the hand. Eight muscles serve as the prime movers and stabilizers for handgrip strength; eleven other muscles within the hand itself assist in the contraction.[4]

Physiological Rationale

Strength is found at the very beginning of the fitness continuum that was described and illustrated in Chapter TE (Figs. 1 and 2). Some performers can reach their peak force of a static handgrip test of strength in 0.3 s,[20] whereas others may take 2.7 s.[2] Some people may be able to hold the peak force for only 1 s,[12] whereas others might hold it for a few seconds[20] (Fig. 1).

Biochemical Rationale

Based upon this rapid onset and decay of peak force, it should be obvious that the energy pathway predominantly involved in maximal muscle actions (strength) is the phosphagen system. Thus, the primary biochemical reaction for strength, or any muscle action, is

$$\text{Adenosine triphosphate (ATP)} \xrightarrow{\text{ATPase}} \text{ADP} + \text{P} + \text{Energy}$$

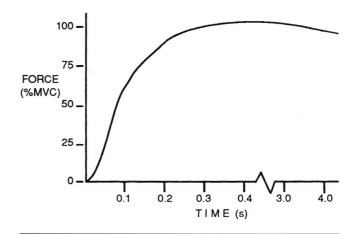

Figure 1 A typical force (%MVC) curve during a maximal isometric contraction (strength).

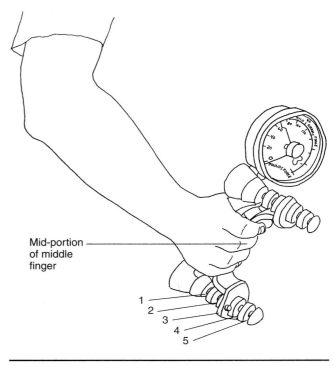

Figure 2 The proper positioning of the body, upper arm, forearm, and hand during handgrip strength testing.

Accuracy of Handgrip Strength Testing

Muscular strength is highly affected by the nervous system. Thus, emotional or mental factors play an important role in strength testing. If the motivation of the subject is consistent, strength variability should be minimized. Individual daily variations in strength range from 2 to 12% in women and 5 to 9% in men.[24] Reliability coefficients for strength testing are usually .90 or higher.

For the average person, handgrip strength correlates quite highly ($r = .69$) with the total strength of twenty-two other muscles of the body.[5] Static tests of strength are more valid for static muscle actions than they are for dynamic actions.

Because the need for large amounts of ATP is so urgent, the ATP and its quick rejuvenator, creatine phosphate (CP), must be immediately available for the interacting muscle filaments—actin and myosin. However, the stores of ATP and PC are very limited. Because they cannot be resupplied adequately by the slower glycolytic and oxidative systems, the actin and myosin filaments cannot interact in order to continue contracting forcefully. Consequently, a rapid decay occurs in the peak force despite the effort to sustain it.

Method

As mentioned previously, the method of field/lab testing of strength is quite simple. The procedures of handgrip dynamometry can be learned quickly by watching a brief demonstration and then practicing for a few minutes.

Equipment for Handgrip Strength Testing

Various instruments may be used to measure muscle strength. Some of these are (a) free weights (e.g., barbells), (b) dynamometers, (c) cable tensiometers, (d) load cells (electromechanical devices), and (e) isokinetic devices. In clinical settings, physicians and therapists often evaluate strength by using a manual testing method by which they subjectively determine the resistance they feel when the patient exerts against them. Also, they have used hand-held dynamometers which they place against the limb of the patient's muscle group, and, again, the test requires both patient and examiner to resist each other.[25]

The word *dynamometer* comes from the Greek word meaning *power measure*. Because time is not measured in the strength tests described here, the more apt description of the handgrip dynamometer would be as a force-measuring device, rather than as a power-measuring one. Dynamometers were used as early as 1798.[21]

A common laboratory dynamometer, the Jamar™, uses a sealed hydraulic system to activate its force indicator during an isometric contraction. For example, the movement of the grip for the Jamar instrument (Fig. 2) cannot be perceived; however, spring dynamometers, such as the Stoelt-ing™, the Lafayette™, and the Smedley™ grip, may move up to 1.5 cm during a maximal handgrip contraction.[11]

Strength is usually measured in units of force or torque. The force units for static dynamometry should be expressed, preferably, in newtons (N); although kilograms (kg) and pounds (lb) are commonly printed on the dials of most handgrip dynamometers, the scientific community encourages the use of newtons.[14] Most handgrip dynamometers provide scales that read up to 200 to 220 lb, or 90 to 100 kg. Most grip dynamometers have double pointers, one pointer holding the maximal reading until it is reset; some (e.g., Lafayette™) have a floating pointer that holds its position until reset.

Calibration of Grip Dynamometers

The accuracy of the dynamometer or load cell may be calibrated periodically by hanging a known weight from the instrument. This tends to work better with the Jamar™ dynamometers than the spring-loaded dynamometers. Although this method can tell you if the dynamometer is accurate, the manufacturers suggest you return it to them for readjustment if there is an inaccuracy.

Procedures for Handgrip Dynamometry

The procedures for handgrip strength testing are summarized as follows:

1. The performer should be in the standing position.
2. The performer's head should be in the midposition (facing straight ahead).
3. The grip size should be adjusted so that the middle finger's midportion (second phalanx) is approximately at a right angle.
   a. Grip adjustments on some dynamometers (e.g., Jamar) are made by slipping off the moveable handle and repositioning it into the five manufactured slots:
      #1 = the slot at the innermost position for the smallest grip size (see Fig. 2).
      #5 = the slot at the outside position for the largest grip size.
   b. Grip adjustments for some dynamometers (e.g., Lafayette and Smedley) are made by lifting the hinge, if present, on the side of the fixed outer handle of the dynamometer and then twirling the inner stirrup to the desired setting.
4. The technician should record the grip setting (1–5 for Jamar; 10–40 mm on inner scale for Smedley) on Form SS 1.
5. The performer's forearm may be placed at any angle between 90° and 180° (right angle to straight) of the upper arm; the upper arm is in a vertical position. (See Fig. 2.)
6. The performer's wrist and forearm should be at the midprone position.
7. The performer should exert maximally and quickly.

8. The performer should make two[18,22] or three[23] trials alternately with each hand, with at least 30 s between trials for the same hand.[16]
9. The technician should record the force in kg, then convert the circled best score to newtons simply by multiplying the kg value by 10.
10. The technician resets the indicator hand of the dynamometer to approximately zero after each trial.
11. The technician thanks the performer for his/her cooperation and effort.

Comments on the Procedures

The midposition of the head is recommended in order to avoid the bias of the tonic neck reflex.[3,10] Although this natural reflex may be diminished in adults, it causes the flexors of the opposite side (contralateral) of the body to be the most strong when the head is turned laterally away from the forearm being tested.[8,9]

Grip sizes do not make much difference except in performers with large hands who are tested at small grip settings, or subjects with small hands who are tested at large settings.[17]

The midpronated arm position was used by investigators whose norms are presented in this manual. However, norms are available for grip testing in the palm-up position while the forearm rests on a table.[1]

Although performers should make powerful exertions at the start of each trial, they should be careful to avoid jerking the dynamometer. No movement from the initial body position can take place during the trial, nor can the hand touch any other part of the body.

The performer should not gradually approach maximal; in fact, it is counterproductive to take more than five seconds to reach maximal contraction, especially in older persons.[15]

Based on the recovery rate of the phosphagens,[7] 30 s to 1 min should be sufficient as a rest interval between trials for the same hand, especially if each contraction is less than 3 s. When in doubt of sufficient rest, a rest interval of one minute is recommended.[22]

The chosen score has varied among investigators. Most investigators have used the best of two[18,22] or three[23] untimed trials, or the average of the last 2 s of two 3-s trials.[1]

Results and Discussion

The norms for grip strength are usually categorized according to age because grip strength is just as strongly correlated with age (−.64) as with muscle mass.[13] The decline in men's strength after the forties follows a curvilinear regression (Eq. 1).[13]

$$\text{Grip Sum (kg)} = 90.6 + (0.84 \times \text{Age}) - (0.014 \times \text{Age}^2) \quad \text{Eq. 1}$$

where:

Grip Sum is the sum of the best right and left grip forces

The norms in Tables 1–4 are derived from grip forces measured by a Stoelting/Smedley dynamometer, a spring-type

Table 1 Percentiles (%ile) for Sum (R + L) of Grip Strength (kg) in Men and Women Ages 18–59 y

Ages (y)	18	19	20–24	25–29	30–34	35–39	40–44	45–49	50–59
%ile				Men's Grip Strength (kg)					
90	111	110	122	123	124	121	121	110	110
80	106	113	115	115	115	115	115	108	102
70	101	109	110	110	110	109	108	104	96
60	98	104	105	107	106	106	103	99	93
50	96	101	102	103	102	102	100	95	89
40	93	98	99	100	98	98	97	91	85
30	90	94	94	95	95	93	93	82	81
20	86	90	89	90	90	88	87	81	75
10	81	84	80	81	82	79	81	75	66
M	97.1	102.0	102.9	103.6	103.4	101.9	101.4	95.6	89.4
SD	15.5	13.7	16.8	15.6	16.8	17.3	16.1	16.1	16.1
Ages (y)	18	19	20–24	25–29	30–34	35–39	40–44	45–49	50–59
%ile				Women's Grip Strength (kg)					
90	59	63	61	67	65	66	64	64	57
80	55	59	57	62	60	59	58	57	52
70	52	54	53	57	57	55	54	53	48
60	49	50	50	53	53	53	51	52	45
50	46	48	48	49	49	51	49	49	43
40	43	46	45	48	47	49	47	47	40
30	39	42	42	46	44	46	43	44	38
20	36	39	38	43	41	43	40	40	34
10	31	36	34	37	36	36	36	34	30
M	47.1	49.9	48.7	52.2	51.5	51.9	50.0	50.0	44.0
SD	9.7	10.3	9.8	10.7	11.4	11.6	11.1	10.7	9.8

From H. J. Montoye and D. E. Lamphiear, "Grip and Arm Strength in Males and Females Age 10 to 69," *Research Quarterly, 48*(1), Table 3, p. 113, 1977. Copyright © American Alliance for Health, Physical Education, Recreation and Dance, 1900 Association Dr., Reston, VA 22091.

Table 2 Norms for the Ratio of the Sum of Right and Left Grip Strengths to Body Weight ($kg \cdot kg^{-1}$ wt) in Men and Women Ages 18–59 y

Ages (y)	18	19	20–24	25–29	30–34	35–39	40–49	50–59
%ile				Men's Ratios ($kg \cdot kg^{-1}$ body wt)				
90	1.62	1.75	1.73	1.72	1.64	1.62	1.54	1.39
80	1.50	1.54	1.59	1.54	1.52	1.51	1.41	1.30
70	1.47	1.44	1.53	1.47	1.45	1.42	1.34	1.22
60	1.44	1.36	1.45	1.40	1.39	1.35	1.28	1.10
50	1.37	1.33	1.39	1.35	1.33	1.28	1.24	1.14
40	1.33	1.29	1.32	1.28	1.29	1.23	1.19	1.10
30	1.31	1.24	1.26	1.20	1.24	1.17	1.14	1.03
20	1.22	1.17	1.18	1.12	1.18	1.11	1.07	0.98
10	1.16	1.12	1.08	1.01	1.10	1.02	0.99	0.89
M	1.37	1.37	1.39	1.34	1.35	1.30	1.25	1.14
Ages (y)	**18**	**19**	**20–24**	**25–29**	**30–34**	**35–39**	**40–49**	**50–59**
%ile				Women's Ratios ($kg \cdot kg^{-1}$ body wt)				
90	1.02	1.10	1.04	1.12	1.05	1.07	1.02	0.90
80	0.95	1.04	0.97	1.02	1.00	1.00	0.93	0.83
70	0.90	0.94	0.91	0.97	0.94	0.93	0.87	0.78
60	0.82	0.85	0.86	0.91	0.89	0.87	0.81	0.71
50	0.78	0.80	0.81	0.86	0.83	0.84	0.77	0.68
40	0.72	0.77	0.77	0.82	0.78	0.80	0.73	0.63
30	0.69	0.74	0.72	0.75	0.72	0.75	0.69	0.69
20	0.65	0.69	0.68	0.68	0.68	0.69	0.68	0.52
10	0.58	0.64	0.61	0.61	0.60	0.60	0.54	0.48
M	0.79	0.85	0.82	0.86	0.83	0.84	0.78	0.68

From H. J. Montoye and D. E. Lamphiear, "Grip and Arm Strength in Males and Females Age 10 to 69," *Research Quarterly, 48*(1), Table 6, p. 116, 1977. Copyright © American Alliance for Health, Physical Education, Recreation and Dance, 1900 Association Dr., Reston, VA 22091.

Table 3 Summed Grip Strength in Males 30–89 y of Age ($n = 355$)

Age (y)	Right + Left Grip Strength (kg)	~SD
30–39	104	1.6
40–49	101	1.3
50–59	95	1.0
60–69	88	1.0
70–79	75	1.0
80–89	66	1.6

Adapted from Kallman, D. A., Plato, C. C., & Tobin, J. D. (1990). The role of muscle loss in the age-related decline of grip strength: Cross-sectional and longitudinal perspectives. *Journal of Gerontology: Medical Sciences, 45*, M82–88. Permission from The Gerontological Society of America, Copyright ©.

dynamometer (e.g., Lafayette™). The first two tables are based on the 1970s epidemiological study of over 6,000 persons in Tecumseh, Michigan,[18] and are similar to the 1990 report on a smaller, but extended to an older, population.[13] Table 2 provides the strength/body weight ratios, whereby the sum of the right and left grip strength scores is divided by the person's body weight (kg ÷ kg body wt).

This ratio becomes important when evaluating a person's ability to lift his/her own body weight or to assume and support certain body positions (e.g., hanging from a chin-up bar, or grasping a rail). The scores in Table 3 include an older population of 60 to 89 y-olds.[13] The Canadian norms presented in Table 4 are based on data from the 1981 Canada Fitness Survey, and show higher values than the Michigan norms.

Some conclusions that may be made from these and other norms are as follows: (1) Boys and girls have similar grip strengths until puberty; (2) Men's grip sums are between 1.75 and 2.0 times greater than women's for the ages represented in these norms; (3) Grip strength increases rapidly with age for males between the onset of puberty and the twenties; and (4) Grip strength declines slowly with age between the thirties to the late fifties for both sexes. Also, it appears that the sum of the right and left grip strengths averages about 1.3 times higher than the body weight for the men, and about 80% of the body weight for the women in most of the age groups presented in Table 2.[18] An intriguing sidenote that needs confirmation is the finding that 8–17-y-old right-handers are stronger in their right hand grip, but professed left-handers often show no superiority in their left handgrip.[19]

Table 4 Percentiles for the Sum of Right and Left Grip Strengths in Canadian Men (M) and Women (W) Ages 20–69

Age (y)	20–29		30–39		40–49		50–59		60–69	
Gender	M	W	M	W	M	W	M	W	M	W
%iles										
95	136	78	135	80	128	80	119	72	111	67
90	127	74	127	76	123	76	114	69	106	62
85	124	71	123	73	119	73	110	65	102	60
80	120	70	120	71	117	71	108	63	99	58
75	118	68	117	69	115	69	105	62	96	56
70	115	67	115	68	112	67	103	60	94	55
65	113	65	113	66	110	65	102	59	93	54
60	111	64	111	65	108	64	100	58	91	53
55	109	63	109	63	106	62	99	57	89	52
50	107	62	107	62	104	61	97	56	88	52
45	106	61	105	61	102	59	96	55	86	51
40	104	59	104	60	100	58	94	54	84	50
35	102	58	101	59	98	57	92	53	82	49
30	100	56	99	58	96	56	90	53	81	49
25	97	55	97	56	94	55	87	51	79	48
20	95	53	94	55	91	53	85	50	76	47
15	91	52	91	53	89	51	83	48	73	45
10	87	50	87	51	84	49	80	46	69	43
5	81	47	81	48	76	46	74	42	62	39

Source: Data from Fitness and Amateur Sport, Canada, 1987.

References

1. Baumgartner, T. A., & Jackson, A. S. (1987). *Measurement for evaluation in physical education and exercise science.* Dubuque, IA: Wm. C. Brown.
2. Bemben, M. G., Clasey, J. L., & Massey, B. H. (1990). The effect of the rate of muscle contraction on the force-time curve parameters of male and female subjects. *Research Quarterly for Exercise and Sport, 61*(1): 96–99.
3. Berntson, G. G., & Torello, M. W. (1977). Expression of Magnus tonic neck reflexes in distal muscles of prehension in normal adults. *Physiology and Behavior, 19,* 585–587.
4. Buck, J. A., Amundsen, L. R., & Nielsen, D. H. (1980). Systolic blood pressure responses during isometric contractions of large and small muscle groups. *Medicine and Science in Sports and Exercise, 12*(3): 145–147.
5. deVries, H. A. (1980). *Physiology of exercise in physical education and athletics.* Dubuque, IA: Wm. C. Brown.
6. Fitness and Amateur Sport, Canada. (1987). *Canadian standardized test of fitness: Operations manual.* 3d ed. Ottawa, Ontario, Canada: Fitness and Amateur Sports Directorate.
7. Fox, E. L., Bowers, R. W., & Foss, M. L. (1988). *The physiological basis of physical education and athletics.* Philadelphia: Saunders College Publishing.
8. George, C. O. (1970). Effects of the asymmetrical tonic neck posture upon grip strength of normal children. *Research Quarterly, 41,* 361–364.
9. George, C. O. (1972). Facilitative and inhibitory effects of the tonic neck reflex upon grip strength of right- and left-handed children. *Research Quarterly, 43,* 157–166.
10. Gesell, A., & Ames, L. B. (1947). The development of handedness. *Journal of Genetic Psychology, 70,* 155–175.
11. Heyward, V., McKeown, B., & Geeseman, R. (1975). Comparison of the Stoelting handgrip dynamometer and linear voltage differential transformer for measuring maximal grip strength. *Research Quarterly, 46*(2): 262–266.
12. Hislop, H. J. (1963). Quantitative changes in human muscular strength during isometric exercise. *Journal of the American Physical Therapy Association, 43,* 21–38.
13. Kallman, D. A., Plato, C. C., & Tobin, J. D. (1990). The role of muscle loss in the age-related decline of grip strength: Cross-sectional and longitudinal perspectives. *Journal of Gerontology: Medical Sciences, 45,* M82–88.
14. Knuttgen, H. G. (1986). Quantifying exercise performance with SI units. *The Physician and Sportsmedicine* (Dec): 157–161.

15. Kroll, W., Clarkson, P. M., & Melchionda, A. M. (1981). Age, isometric strength, rate of tension development and fiber type composition. *Medicine and Science in Sports and Exercise 13,* Abstract, 87.

16. Lind, A. R., & McNicol, G. W. (1967). Circulatory response to sustained handgrip contractions performed during other exercise, both rhythmic and static. *The American Journal of Cardiology, 38,* 46–51.

17. Montoye, H. J., & Faulkner, J. A. (1975). Determination of the optimum setting of an adjustable grip dynamometer. *The Research Quarterly, 35,* 30–36.

18. Montoye, H. J., & Lamphiear, D. E. (1977). Grip and arm strength in males and females, age 10 to 69. *Research Quarterly, 48,* 109–120.

19. Montpetit, R. R., Montoye, H. J., & Laeding, L. (1967). Grip strength of school children, Saginaw, Michigan: 1899–1964. *Research Quarterly, 38,* 231–240.

20. Morris, A. F., Clarke, D. H., & Dainis, A. (1983). Time to maximal voluntary isometric contraction (MVC) for five different muscle groups in college adults. *Research Quarterly for Exercise and Sport, 54,* 163–168.

21. Regnier, C. (1798). Description and use of the dynamometer, or instrument for ascertaining the relative strength of men and animals. *Philosophical Magazine, 1*(1): 399–404.

22. Sale, D. G. (1991). Testing strength and power. In J. D. MacDougal, H. A. Wenger, & H. J. Green (Eds.), *Physiological testing of the high-performance athlete.* (pp. 21–106). Champaign, IL: Human Kinetics.

23. Stoelting, C. H. (1970). Smedley Instruction Manual. Chicago: Author.

24. Wakim, K. G., Gersten, J. W., Elkins, E. C., & Martin, G. M. (1950). Objective recording of muscle strength. *Archives of Physical Medicine, 31,* 90–100.

25. Wikholm, J. B., & Bohannon, R. W. (1991). Hand-held dynamometer measurements: Tester strength makes a difference. *The Journal of Orthopaedic and Sports Physical Therapy, 13,* 191–193.

Form **SS 1**

Individual Data for Handgrip Strength

Name [   ] Date [   ] Time [   ] a.m. [   ] p.m. [   ]

Age [   ] y Gender (M or F) [   ] Ht [   ] cm Wt [   ] kg

Dominant Hand (check): Right (R) [   ] Left (L) [   ]

Instrument

[Hydraulic (e.g., Jamar)]

Grip Setting (circle):

1st; 2nd; 3rd; 4th; 5th

[Spring (e.g., Lafayette)]

(mm setting on handle): [   ] mm

[Other type _____]

Force (kg) (circle best trial of each hand)

Trial #1		Trial #2		Trial #3	
R	L	R	L	R	L
___	___	___	___	___	___
R	L	R	L	R	L
___	___	___	___	___	___
R	L	R	L	R	L
___	___	___	___	___	___

Best Trials	Right Hand		Left Hand		Sum of R and L	
Hydraulic	[ ]	+	[ ]	=	[ ] kg; × 10 =	[ ] N
Spring	[ ]	+	[ ]	=	[ ] kg; × 10 =	[ ] N
Other	[ ]	+	[ ]	=	[ ] kg; × 10 =	[ ] N

Ratio of Grip Sum to Body Wt ($kg \cdot kg^{-1}$ wt):

Grip Sum [   ] kg/ [   ] kg body wt = [   ] ratio

Age-Predicted Grip Sum (kg) = $90.6 + (0.84 \times$ [   ] y$) - (0.014 \times$ [   ] $y^2)$

$= 90.6 +$ [   ] $- (0.014 \times$ [   ] $)$

$= 90.6 +$ [   ] $-$ [   ]

$=$ [   ] kg $=$ [   ] N

Form **SS 2**

Group Data for Handgrip Strength

Handgrip Strength[a]

MEN Initials (or ID #)	R kg	L kg	Sum kg	Sum:Wt kg·kg⁻¹
1.				
2.				
3.				
4.				
5.				
6.				
7.				
8.				
9.				
10.				
11.				
12.				
13.				
14.				
15.				
16.				
17.				
18.				
19.				
20.				
21.				
22.				
Mean				

WOMEN Initials (or ID #)	R kg	L kg	Sum kg	Sum: Wt kg·kg⁻¹
1.				
2.				
3.				
4.				
5.				
6.				
7.				
8.				
9.				
10.				
11.				
12.				
13.				
14.				
15.				
16.				
17.				
18.				
19.				
20.				
21.				
22.				
Mean				

[a]Best trial

Chapter IS

Isokinetic Strength

The laboratory test selected for the measurement of leg strength requires the performer to perform an isokinetic movement on a specially designed machine. The isokinetic measurement of leg strength is classified as a laboratory test because the apparatus does not lend itself to simultaneous testing of individuals and due to the cost, size, and complexity of the apparatus. Despite the high cost of the isokinetic instrument, the description has been included in this manual because of the prevalence of such machines in many athletic training facilities on college campuses and in sophisticated fitness and rehabilitation clinics.

Leg strength diminishes faster than upper body strength as one ages past young adulthood.[22] Thus, leg strength training and periodic monitoring are important for middle and older age persons if they intend to keep functioning optimally in activities of daily living.

In addition to determining the state of training of the legs, testing the legs may provide insight into the risk of injuring them. Muscle strength asymmetry (difference in strength between right and left legs) may be a predisposing factor in muscle strains,[44] especially in the weaker leg.[16] This asymmetrical leg strength may also lead to knee injuries.[6] A **bilateral imbalance** whereby the non-dominant leg is only 90–95% as strong as the dominant leg could lead to strains.[25,47] The 90% (or 0.90 ratio) strength–balance criterion is also recommended as a guide for lower limb stress fracture.[29]

Similarly, an **ipsilateral imbalance** between the strength of the antagonist (hamstrings) and agonist (quadriceps) of the same leg could lead to a higher risk of leg injury.[29,44] Hamstring (H) strength should be at least 50%[34] or 75%[17,32] of quadriceps (Q) strength, producing an H:Q ratio greater than 0.50 and 0.75, respectively.

However, not all investigators support this relationship between imbalanced strength and injury susceptibility.[3,21] Another group reported no difference in knee injury rate when bilateral imbalances were <90% for right versus left.[55]

Rationale

The rationale for isokinetic testing of leg strength may be categorized into mechanical and anatomical rationales.

Mechanical Rationale for Isokinetic Testing

The term *isokinetic* refers to the constant speed of such movements; thus, no momentum is gathered throughout a truly isokinetic movement.[26] Once the performer reaches the set speed, an increase in force by the performer causes the isokinetic device to counteract this force with an accommodating increase in resistance. Conversely, a decrease in the application of force results in a corresponding decrease in the resistance.[41] Thus, the movement does not change speed significantly. The testing apparatus controls the angular velocity of the exercise, thus allowing the musculature to elicit maximal tension for each angle within the movement range.

The laboratory measurement of isokinetic strength provides torque measurements throughout the active range of motion during this maximal effort. The unit of measure for isokinetic strength is a torque value, commonly referred to as foot-pounds or newton meters (N·m) (see Chapter TE). **Torque** indicates the force rotating about an axis, that is, the turning or twisting force,[23] such as the force produced by a wrench when tightening the nut on a bolt. Because isokinetic devices have lever arms connected to strain gauges, torque is produced and recorded from the angular motion. *Peak torque* is the term that indicates muscular strength. Torque (τ), or moment, as presented in Equation 1, is the product of force (F) and the distance (D) of the lever arm.[13]

$$\tau \text{ (ft-lb or N·m)} = F \text{ (lb or N)} \times D^{lever} \text{ (ft or m)} \qquad \text{Eq. 1}$$

The distance of the lever arm is measured from the center of rotation to the point where the external force is applied. This distance is often referred to as the **moment arm.** For example, if a force of 50 lb (22.7 kg or 223 N based on 1 kg = 9.8 N) is applied at the end of a moment arm measuring 2 feet (0.61 m) in length (Fig. 1), then the torque is calculated as

$$\tau \text{ (ft-lb)} = 50 \text{ lb} \times 2 \text{ ft} = 100 \text{ ft-lb}$$

$$\tau \text{ (N·m)} = 223 \text{ N} \times 0.61 \text{ m} = 136 \text{ N·m}$$

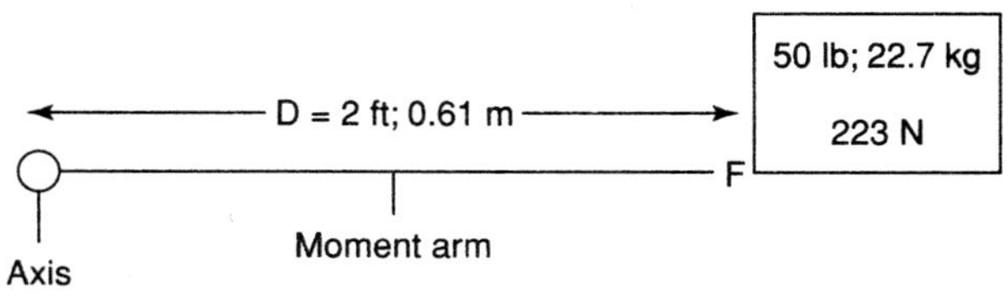

Figure 1 Torque production (136 N·m) as a function of the external force (F; 223 N) applied at the end-length of the moment arm (D; 0.61m).

The U.S. system's product (ft-lb) could have been converted to the metric unit (N·m) by using the conversion factor (Eq. 2):

$$1 \text{ ft-lb} = 1.3560 \text{ N·m} \qquad \text{Eq. 2}$$

Thus: 1.3560×100 ft-lb $= 135.6$ N·m (or 136 N·m to the closest whole N·m)

Anatomical Rationale

Although isokinetic dynamometers are capable of measuring the torque of various muscle groups, only those muscles that flex and extend the lower leg are discussed here. Knee extension is represented by the strength of the quadriceps muscle group, which is made up of four muscles—the rectus femoris and the three vasti muscles—vastus medialis, lateralis, and intermedius. Knee flexion is represented by the strength of the hamstring muscle group, which consists of three muscles—the biceps femoris, the semitendinosus, and the semimembranosus.

Fiber type plays an important role in determining the peak torque and duration of isokinetic contractions. For example, persons with higher percentages of fast-twitch fibers produce more torque ($r = .69$) at moderate ($180° \cdot s^{-1}$) speeds, but have greater fatigability ($r = .86$), than persons with lower percentages.

Calibration of Isokinetic Machine

The manufacturers' manuals that accompany isokinetic instruments provide detailed calibration procedures. The instrument's torque values, both statically and dynamically, can be checked by attaching known weights to the dynamometer's lever arm at a known distance.[36,38,48] The accuracy of the velocity settings on the Cybex™ can be checked by counting the number of complete turns of the input shaft in one minute.[36,38] Ideally, to correct for the effect of gravity on the Cybex II, the performer should place the tested leg in an extended position and then relax the leg while it passively (no contraction) flexes. The technician will later add this value (N · m) to the extension score and subtract it from the flexion score.[12]

Method

The methods of testing isokinetic leg strength are much more elaborate than those for testing handgrip strength. Compared to handgrip dynamometers, the equipment for isokinetic testing is very expensive and complex.

Equipment

There are various instruments to test isokinetic leg strength, such as Ariel™, Biodex™, Hydra-Fitness™, LIDO™, Kin-Com™, Merac™, and Cybex II™ (Fig. 2). The Kin-Com™ and Biodex™ machines can test both concentric and eccentric strength.

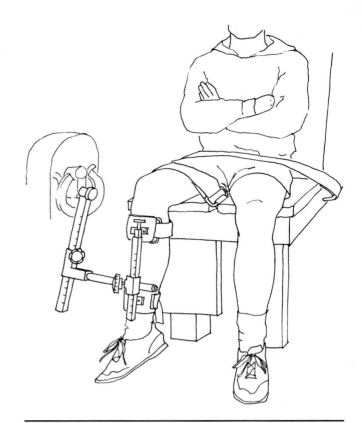

Figure 2 The position of the performer for isokinetic testing of leg strength with the Cybex II.

Following are four common torque scales:[50]

ft-lb	N·m
30	40.7
90	122
180	244
360	488

Popular isokinetic speeds are 60, 180, and 300 degrees per second ($°·s^{-1}$); these are often referred to as slow, medium, and fast speeds. However, the fast speed may be construed as slow compared to the speeds required in many sport's movements, such as sprinting, throwing, striking, kicking, and jumping. Some models (e.g., Cybex II⁺) provide speed increments of $15°·s^{-1}$ from zero to 300 and may be controlled with an electronic remote device. When the speed is set to 0, static (isometric) strength is measured. Researchers often express speed as rads per second ($rad·s^{-1}$) by dividing degrees per second by 57.3 (Eq. 3).[18,20]

$$rad·s^{-1} = °·s^{-1} \div 57.3 \qquad \text{Eq. 3}$$

where $rad·s^{-1}$ = radial velocity

rad = radian = 0.5π = radius of circle = $57.3°$

$1° = 0.01745$ radian

$\pi = 3.1416 =$ ratio of the circumference of a circle to its diameter

The conversion of $°\cdot s^{-1}$ to $rad\cdot s^{-1}$ is much simpler than it appears. For example, the calculation for finding the $rad\cdot s^{-1}$ for a velocity of $300°\cdot s^{-1}$ is

$$300°\cdot s^{-1} = 300 \div 57.3$$
$$= 5.23 \ rad\cdot s^{-1}$$

Accuracy of Isokinetic Testing

The reliability and validity of various isokinetic devices are acceptable.[5,11,42,48]

Reliability

The test-retest reliabilities of isokinetic testing on the Cybex™ ranges from good to high, with reported r values for leg extension of .84 and .85 for peak torques of the left and right leg[49] to .97.[8] The repeatability of torque measurement ranges from 1 to 2 ft-lb at the four torque scales of 30 (40.7 N·m), 90 (122 N·m), 180 (244 N·m), and 360 (488 N·m) ft-lb of a Cybex II™ isokinetic machine.[10] Greater variability occurs at the higher velocities of contraction than at the lower speeds.[52] Peak torques measured on the Kinetic Communicator™ (Kin-Com) machines have reliabilities in the high .80s or low .90s.[37]

Validity

Most velocity settings on isokinetic machines are much lower than an unrestricted (unloaded) knee extension velocity. For example, the lower leg moves at about $700°\cdot s^{-1}$ (12 rad·s⁻¹) when kicking a football,[56] more than twice as fast as the highest velocity for the Cybex II™ machine. Although isokinetic movements are not sustained very long in most physical activities, isokinetic strength scores have been able to discriminate between strength and endurance athletes. The validity of isokinetic testing appears to be supported by a high correlation between lean body weight (muscle mass) and strength of hip/knee extension as measured by peak isokinetic torque.[2] The strength of leg extension is highly correlated ($r = .89$) with general body strength when measured isotonically.[59] Although equivocal, some researchers have found a close relationship between isotonic, isometric, and isokinetic voluntary strength, especially if the joint angles are similar.[1,33]

Procedures

The procedures for testing the isokinetic strength of the legs include a description of the preparations in addition to the actual testing of the performer. They also include proper reading of the instrument and the graphic recording of torque. Most of the procedures relate to the Cybex II⁺ but are often applicable to the Kin-Com, Biodex, and LIDO-Active. Some differences are noted with respect to the number of trials, rest interval, and activation force. As with most laboratory procedures, adequate preparations include those concerned with the equipment and the performer.

Instrument Preparations

1. Procedures for periodic calibration are found in the calibration box or in the manufacturer's manual.
2. The recording apparatus should be readied for testing by setting the Damp to the No. 2 position; this smooths the printed curve that is generated by the performer's forces.
3. The technician selects an appropriate torque scale on the recorder—30, 180, or 360 ft-lb—based upon the estimated output of the performer; usually 180 ft-lb (244 N·m) is chosen. The Kin-Com machine may be set to a certain preload or activation force (e.g., 20–100 N) which means that this preset force must be applied by the performer before the lever arm will move.[30,37]
4. The technician sets the Input Direction to CW (clockwise) for left limb or CCW (counter-clockwise) for right limb.
5. The position scale should be placed at the 150° mark, representing the approximate range of motion for testing of knee extension/flexion.

Performer Preparations

1. The performer sits in an upright position with the hips flexed to 90° (see Fig. 2).
2. The technician uses pelvic and thigh straps to stabilize the hips and thighs, respectively.
3. The technician identifies the axis of rotation of the knee joint and visually aligns the input shaft of the dynamometer with this axis of rotation at the lateral epicondyle.
4. The technician adjusts the length of the lever arm so that the inferior rim of the shin pad contacts the tibia just above the malleoli of the ankle; the technician secures the shin/ankle strap. It may be advisable to standardize the length of the lever arm at a fixed length to avoid possible alteration of torque output.[52]
5. With the performer's knee at full flexion as limited by the chair, the performer's range of motion is about 105–135°.
6. The performer grasps the chair's handles if available, or folds arms across the chest, and maintains this position throughout the warmup and the test.
7. The technician explains and demonstrates the leg movements for the strength test. Aside from assuring that the performer understands that maximal efforts are made, no further encouragement during the test is advised so that uniformity in tester-performer interaction is maintained.[40]
8. The performer warms up by making 5 to 10 submaximal repetitions (about 50% MVC), both during flexion and extension at each speed setting (60, 180, and $300°\cdot s^{-1}$).
9. The performer then rests for 2–5 min before the initial test, while the technician sets the velocity to $60°\cdot s^{-1}$ and sets the paper recording speed to 5 or 25 mm·s⁻¹.

The Test

1. With the recorder on, the performer makes three maximal repetitions at $60°\cdot s^{-1}$.[3,10,28,29]

2. After a 30^{39}–60^{51} s rest, the performer makes three maximal repetitions at $180°\cdot s^{-1}$. Instead of three consecutive contractions without a pause, technicians may allow rest intervals of 1–3 min for one-to-two slow velocity ($<180°\cdot s^{-1}$) actions, and as little as 20–30 s between three trials at higher velocities.[52] However, be consistent if comparing performers. Performers on the Kin-Com machine may use four alternating test contractions—two concentric and two eccentric—with a 5 s rest between muscle actions.[30]

3. Again after a 30–60 s rest, the performer makes three maximal repetitions at $300°\cdot s^{-1}$.

4. The highest torque of each group of three trials is recorded on Form IS 1. See the examples in Figures 3 and 4.

5. The technician rearranges the apparatus for testing the other leg, and repeats the steps.

6. The performer should statically stretch the quadriceps and hamstrings after the testing session.

7. The technician calculates the relative torque ($N\cdot m\cdot kg^{-1}$), and the ratios for ipsilateral (H:Q), and bilateral (L:R; or nondominant:dominant) strength.

For estimation of **fast-twitch fiber type:**

8. The technician sets the machine to $180°\cdot s^{-1}$.

9. The performer makes 50–55 maximal knee extension repetitions; the rest interval between each repetition is about 0.7 s,[57] or about the time required for the submaximal flexion movement.

10. The technician counts each repetition and then averages the peak torque for the first to third and 48th to 50th repetitions.

11. The technician obtains the percent fast-twitch (%FT) fibers from Equation 4[57] by finding the decline ($\%\downarrow$) in average peak torque (P-τ) values of the first to third repetitions and 48th to 50th repetitions of maximal knee extensions at $180°\cdot s^{-1}$.

$$FT\% = (0.90 \times \%\downarrow) + 5.2 \qquad \text{Eq. 4}$$

where:

$$\%\downarrow = \left[\frac{(P\text{-}\tau \text{ at } 1\text{–}3) - (P\text{-}\tau \text{ at } 48\text{–}50)}{P\text{-}\tau \text{ at } 1\text{–}3}\right] \times 100$$

For example, if a person's average peak torques for the first three repetitions and the 48th–50th repetitions are 200 and 110 N·m, respectively, then the fast-twitch fiber percentage is calculated as follows:

$$\%\downarrow = [(200\ N\cdot m - 110\ N\cdot m) \div (200\ N\cdot m)] \times 100$$

$$= (90\ N\cdot m \div 200\ N\cdot m) \times 100$$

$$= 0.45 \times 100$$

$$= 45\%$$

Thus,

$$\%FT = (0.90 \times 45) + 5.2$$

$$= 40.5 + 5.2$$

$$= 45.7\% \text{ (or 46\% to nearest whole \%)}$$

12. For estimation of **slow-twitch fiber type (%ST)** use Equation 5:

$$\%ST = 100 - FT\% \qquad \text{Eq. 5}$$

$$= 100 - 45.7$$

$$= 54.3\% \text{ (or 54\% to the nearest whole \%)}$$

Comments on Isokinetic Procedures

Static (isometric) strength is measured by performing one repetition at $0°\cdot s^{-1}$ and then resting for about 30 s. The sequence of the testing for leg extension and flexion at different speeds is usually from slowest to fastest (e.g., 60, 180, and 240 or $300°\cdot s^{-1}$). Athletes involved in power sports could be tested at the higher speeds. If a detailed analysis of the relationship between torque and angle is desired, then the tracing is usually recorded at a speed of $25\ mm\cdot s^{-1}$; however, for routine testing the recording speed is usually $5\ mm\cdot s^{-1}$. The dual tracings provide a recorded replay of the movement, one tracing showing the torque values and another showing the position (angle in degrees) of the lower leg. It is not within the scope of this manual to analyze the strength at the various positions, thus the angle recording is deleted here.

The recording paper for the torque tracing is divided from top to bottom into 30 divisions with a bold line at every third line and two fainter lines between the bold lines. If the 180 ft-lb (244 N·m) torque scale is selected (Fig. 3), then the top line represents 180 ft-lb (244 N·m); when 180 is divided by the 30 divisions then each intervening horizontal line is equivalent to 6 ft-lb (8.14 N·m), and the interval between each of the ten bold lines equivalent to 18 ft-lb (24.4 N·m). In Figure 3, the highest "x" on the graph paper represents the peak torque of a hypothetical performer. The peak torque is read as 174 ft-lb (about 236 N·m) because the highest "x" is at the next-to-highest line. Because each line is worth 6 ft-lb and the top line is equivalent to 180 ft-lb, it is apparent that the next-to-highest line represents 174 ft-lb. Figure 4 is an actual tracing of the quadriceps during extension (higher curve) and hamstrings during flexion (lower curve).

Results and Discussion

One of the strongest angles for the measurement of *static* leg extension (quadriceps) is $50°^{43}$ ($0°$ = full extension), whereas the strongest angle for static knee flexion (hamstrings) is $30°$.[60] The greatest torque for *dynamic isokinetic* actions is generated at speeds of $30°\cdot s^{-1}$ for both knee

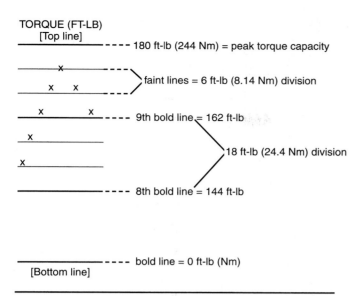

Figure 3 Schematic representation of the horizontal lines on the graph paper of an isokinetic recorder (e.g., Cybex II) with a drawn peak torque (x) value of 174 ft-lb (236 N·m).

Table 1 Strength of the Knee Extensors and Flexors at an Isokinetic Speed of $60° \cdot s^{-1}$ in Healthy Men and Women Ages 45–78 y

Age (y)	Extension		Flexion	
	Men			
	(N·m)	(SD)	(N·m)	(SD)
45–54	180	35	100	21
55–64	163	30	94	20
65–78	144	30	78	19
	Women			
	(N·m)	(SD)	(N·m)	(SD)
45–54	108	22	58	14
55–64	98	20	52	10
65–78	89	15	49	10

Adapted from Frontera, W. R., Hughes, V. A., Lutz, K. J., & Evans, W. J. (1991). A cross-sectional study of muscle strength and mass in 45- to 78-yr-old men and women. *Journal of Applied Physiology, 71,* 644–650.

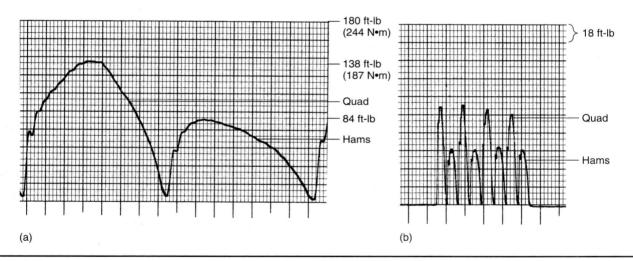

Figure 4 An actual isokinetic tracing scaled at 180 ft-lb (244 N·m) and recorded at (a) 25 mm·s⁻¹, and (b) another person at 5 mm·s⁻¹. Peak torque in (a) for the quadriceps is 138 ft-lb or 187 N·m, and for the hamstrings is 84 ft-lb or 114 N·m. In (b), peak torque for the quadriceps is 96 ft-lb.

extension and flexion. By its very nature, torque is indirectly related to the speed of the movement; that is, the slower the movement, the greater the torque. The hamstring/quadriceps (H/Q), or flexion/extension (Fl/Ex) ratios are lowest at the highest torques, and the highest torques are at the lowest speeds.[44,53]

Absolute and Relative Isokinetic Strength

Prior to 1983 no acceptable norms existed for isokinetic testing.[10] However, in 1991 investigators reported the isokinetic strength of the knee flexors and extensors on 200 healthy men and women between the ages of 45 and 78 years (Table 1).[14]

Comparative values are presented in absolute (N·m) and relative (N·m·kg⁻¹ body wt) terms in Table 2. The women collegiate athletes' absolute strength was about 60% as strong as the men's, whereas their relative strength was 80% of the men's.

The strength of athletes playing different sports or positions is expected to differ due to the specificity of training. This was demonstrated in differentiating between power performers and endurance performers in elite adolescent female track/field athletes.[29] Also, college football players had greater relative leg extension strength (2.13 N·m·kg⁻¹) than sedentary persons (1.9), orienteers (1.7), and racewalkers (2.0).[28] However, the

Table 2 Comparative Isokinetic Values for Knee Extension (Ex;Q) and Flexion (Flex;H) at $180°·s^{-1}$

Reference/Group	Torque				Ratio	
	N·m		$N·m·kg^{-1}$		H/Q	L/R
	Flex	Ex	Flex	Ex		
A. Reference #4						
Athletic College Men			1.36	1.95	0.70	
Athletic College Women			1.11	1.58	0.70	
B. Reference #15						
High School Footballers	105	133	1.42	1.80	0.79	
C. Reference #24						
Elite Alpine Skiers				2.2		
D. Reference #28						
Elite Adolescent Female						
Track/Field Athletes	80	107	1.29	1.79	0.80	
E. Reference #29						
College Footballers	157	200	1.66	2.13	0.78	0.97
F. Reference #58						
Sedentary Subjects				1.9		
Orienteers				1.7		
Racewalkers				2.0		
Downhill Skiers				2.3		
Sprinters/Jumpers				2.7		
G. Reference #61						
Nonathletic Men			1.34	1.71	0.78	
Nonathletic Women			1.07	1.36	0.79	

Adapted from data of Beam et al., 1985; Gilliam et al., 1979; Haymes & Dickinson, 1980; Housh et al., 1984; Housh et al., 1988; Thorstensson et al., 1977; Wyatt and Edwards, 1981.

footballers had smaller ratios than elite alpine skiers (2.2),[24] sprinters/jumpers (2.7) and downhill skiers (2.3).[58] The college footballers also were stronger in both absolute and relative terms than high school football players.[15] In both football studies the linemen were stronger than the backs.

Bilateral Leg Strength

Each football players' left and right (L/R) legs differed in strength by an average of 3%, well within either the 5% or 10% criterion of acceptability.[47] However some authorities advise athletes to seek a zero percent difference between their right and left leg strength.[27]

Ipsilateral Leg Strength

The ipsilateral (hams vs. quads; H/Q) ratios of the university football players were 0.77 and 0.89 at $180°·s^{-1}$ and $300°·s^{-1}$, respectively.[28] These values are similar to those reported for collegiate distance runners[44] and high school football players,[15] but higher than the 0.64 ratio of male ballet dancers.[45]

Fiber Type

Table 3 summarizes various studies[7,9,19,35,58] on fiber type distribution in men and women who are sedentary or

Table 3 Fiber Type Distribution in Sedentary and Athletic Men and Women

Men		Women	
Activity	%Fast Twitch	Activity	%Fast Twitch
Sedentary	52	Sedentary	50
Marathoners	19	800-m Runners	39
Distance Runners	30	X-Country Skiers	40
X-Country Skiers	36	Shot-Putters	50
Race Walkers	40	Cyclists	50
Cyclists	40	Long/High Jumpers	52
800-m Runners	51	Sprinters	73
Downhill Skiers	51	Weightlifters	53
Shot-Putters	62	Sprinters/Jumpers	63

Source: Based on data from Burke et al., 1977; Costill et al., 1976; Gollnick et al., 1972; Komi et al., 1977; and Thorstensson et al., 1977.

participants in various sports. The large variations in percentages within each group testify to the influence of other factors besides fiber type in predicting success for each sport. The prediction of fiber type is enhanced by adding other influencing factors, such as fat-free thigh mass, to the equation.[54]

References

1. Abernethy, P. J., & Jurimae, J. (1996). Cross-sectional and longitudinal uses of isoinertial, isometric, and isokinetic dynamometry. *Medicine and Science in Sports and Exercise, 28,* 1180–1187.
2. Abler, P., Foster, C., Thompson, N. N., Crowe, M., Alt, K., Brophy, A., & Palin, W. D. (1986). Determinants of anaerobic muscular performance. *Medicine and Science in Sports and Exercise, 18,* (supplement): Abstract #3, S1.
3. Beam, W. C. (1982). *The influence of body composition, aerobic capacity and muscular strength on the incidence of injury in athletics.* Unpublished doctoral diss., Ohio State University, Columbus.
4. Beam, W. C., Bartels, R. L., Ward, R. W., Clark, N., & Zuelzer, W. A. (1985). Multiple comparisons of isokinetic leg strength in male and female collegiate athletic teams. *Medicine and Science in Sports and Exercise, 17*(2): Abstract #20, 269.
5. Bemben, M. G., Grump, K. J., & Massey, B. H. (1988). Assessment of technical accuracy of the Cybex II isokinetic dynamometer and analog recording system. *Journal of Orthopaedic and Sports Physical Therapy, 19,* 12–17.
6. Bender, J. A. (1964). Factors affecting the occurrence of knee injuries. *Journal of Association of Physical and Mental Rehabilitation, 18,* 130–134.
7. Burke, E., Cerny, F., Costill, D., & Fink, W. (1977). Characteristics of skeletal muscle in competitive cyclists. *Medicine and Science in Sports and Exercise, 9,* 109–112.
8. Clarkson, P. M., Johnson, J., Dextradeur, D., Leszcyznski, W., Wai, J., & Melchionda, A. (1982). The relationships among isokinetic endurance, initial strength level, and fiber type. *Research Quarterly, 53,* 15–19.
9. Costill, D., Fink, W., & Pollock, M. (1976). Muscle fiber composition and enzyme activities of elite distance runners. *Medicine and Science in Sports and Exercise, 8,* 96–100.
10. Cybex. 1983. *Isolated joint testing and exercise.* Ronkonona, NY: Cybex.
11. Farrell, M., & Richards, J. G. (1986). Analysis of the reliability and validity of the kinetic communicator exercise device. *Medicine and Science in Sports and Exercise, 18,* 44–49.
12. Ford, W. J., Bailey, S. D., Babich, K., & Worrell, T. W. (1994). Effect of hip position on gravity effect torque. *Medicine and Science in Sports and Exercise, 26,* 230–234.
13. Fox, E. L. (1984). *Sports physiology.* Philadelphia: W. B. Saunders.
14. Frontera, W. R., Hughes, V. A., Lutz, K. J., & Evans, W. J. (1991). A cross-sectional study of muscle strength and mass in 45- to 78-yr-old men and women. *Journal of Applied Physiology, 71,* 644–650.
15. Gilliam, T. B., Sady, S. P., Freedson, P. S., & Villanacci, J. (1979). Isokinetic torque levels for high school football players. *Journal of Sports Medicine, 60,* 110–114.
16. Gleim, G. W., Nicholas, J. W., & Webb, J. N. (1978). Isokinetic evaluation following leg injuries. *The Physician and Sportsmedicine,* (Aug.): 74–82.
17. Glick, J. M. (1980). Muscle strains: Prevention and treatment. *The Physician and Sportsmedicine,* (Nov.): 74–82.
18. Golden, C. L., & Dudley, G. A. (1992). Strength after bouts of eccentric or concentric actions. *Medicine and Science in Sports and Exercise, 24,* 926–933.
19. Gollnick, P. D., Armstrong, R. B., Saubert, C. W., et al. (1972). Enzyme activity and fiber composition in skeletal muscle of untrained and trained men. *Journal of Applied Physiology, 33,* 312.
20. Grabiner, M. D., & Hawthorne, D. L. (1990). Conditions of isokinetic knee flexion that enhance isokinetic knee extension. *Medicine and Science in Sports and Exercise, 2,* 235–240.
21. Grace, T. G., Sweetser, E. R., Nelson, M. A., et al. (1984). Isokinetic imbalance and knee-joint injuries. *Journal of Bone and Joint Surgery, 66-A,* 734–740.
22. Grimby, G., & Saltin, B. (1983). The ageing muscle. *Clinical Physiology, 3,* 209–218.
23. Hay, J. G. (1978). *The biomechanics of sports technique.* Englewood Cliffs, NJ: Prentice-Hall.
24. Haymes, E. M., & Dickinson, A. L. (1980). Characteristics of elite male and female skiracers. *Medicine and Science in Sports and Exercise, 12,* 153–158.
25. Hinson, M. M. (1977). *Kinesiology.* Dubuque, IA: Wm. C. Brown.
26. Hislop, H. J., & Perrine, J. J. (1967). The isokinetic concept of exercise. *Physical Therapy, 47,* 114–117.
27. Hough, D. O., & Ray, R. (1994). Stress fractures. *Sports Science Exchange, 7*(1), Gatorade Sports Science Institute.
28. Housh, T. J., Johnson, G. O., Marty, L., Eischen, G., Eischen, C., & Housh, D. J. (1988). Isokinetic leg flexion and extension strength of university football players. *Journal of Orthopaedic and Sports Physical Therapy, 9,* 365–369.
29. Housh, T. J., Thorland, W. G., Tharp, G. D., Johnson, G. O., & Cisar, C. J. (1984). Isokinetic leg flexion and extension strength of elite adolescent female track and field athletes. *Research Quarterly for Exercise and Sport, 55,* 347–350.
30. Jensen, R. C., Warren, B., Laursen, C., & Morrissey, M. C. (1991). Static pre-load effect on knee extensor isokinetic concentric and eccentric performance. *Medicine and Science in Sports and Exercise, 23,* 10–14.
31. Klein, K. K. (1974). Muscular strength and the knee. *The Physician and Sportsmedicine,* (Dec.): 29–31.
32. Knapik, J. J., Bauman, C., Jones, B. H., & Vaughan, L. (1989). Preseason screening of female collegiate athletes: Strength measures associated with athletic injuries. *Medicine and Science in Sports and Exercise, 21* (Suppl. 2), Abstract #388, 565.

33. Knapik, J. J., Wright, J. E., Mawdsley, R. H., & Braun, J. M. (1983). Isokinetic, isometric and isotonic strength relationships. *Archives of Physical Medicine and Rehabilitation, 64,* 77–80.

34. Knight, L. K., & Cage, J. B. (1980, March). Strength imbalance and injury. *The Physician and Sportsmedicine,* p. 140.

35. Komi, P. V., & Karlsson, J. (1977). Physical performance, skeletal muscle enzyme activities, and fiber types in monozygous and dizygous twins of both sexes. *Acta Physiologica Scandinavica, 105,* Suppl. 462.

36. Koutedakis, Y., Frischknecht, R., Vrbova, G., Sharp, N. C. C., & Budgett, R. (1995). Maximal voluntary quadricep strength patterns in Olympic overtrained athletes. *Medicine and Science in Sports and Exercise, 27,* 566–572.

37. Kramer, J. F., Vaz, M. D., & Hakansson, D. (1991). Effect of activation force on knee extensor torques. *Medicine and Science in Sports and Exercise, 23,* 231–237.

38. Lesmes, G. R., Costill, D. L., Coyle, E. F., & Fink, W. J. (1978). Muscle strength and power changes during maximal isokinetic training. *Medicine and Science in Sports, 10,* 266–269.

39. Marcinik, E. J., Potts, J., Schlabach, G., Will, S., Dawson, P., & Hurley, B. F. (1991). Effects of strength training on lactate threshold and endurance performance. *Medicine and Science in Sports and Exercise, 23,* 739–743.

40. Messier, S. P., Edwards, D. G., Martin, D. F., Lowery, R. B., Canon, D. W., James, M. K., Curl, W. W., Read, H. M., & Hunter, D. M. (1995). Etiology of iliotibial band syndrome in distance runners. *Medicine and Science in Sports and Exercise, 27,* 951–960.

41. Moffroid, M., Whipple, R., Hofkosh, J., Lowman, E., & Thistle, H. (1969). A study of isokinetic exercise. *Physical Therapy, 49,* 735–746.

42. Molczyk, L, Thigpen, L. K., Eickhoff, J., Goldgar, D., & Gallagher, J. C. (1991). Reliability of testing the knee extensors and flexors in healthy adult women using a Cybex II isokinetic dynamometer. *Journal of Orthopaedic and Sports Physical Therapy, 14,* 37–41.

43. Morris, A. F. (1974). Myotatic reflex effects of bilateral leg strength. *American Corrective Therapy Journal* (Jan.–Feb.): 24–29.

44. Morris, A. F., Lussier, L., Bell, G., & Dooley, J. (1983). Hamstring/quadriceps strength ratios in collegiate middle-distance and distance runners. *The Physician and Sportsmedicine* (Oct.): 71, 72, 75–77.

45. Mostardi, R. A., Porterfield, J. A., Greenberg, B., Goldberg, D., & Lea, M. (1983). Musculoskeletal and cardiopulmonary characteristics of the professional ballet dancer. *The Physician and Sportsmedicine, 11,* 53–61.

46. Murray, D. A., & Harrison, E. (1986). Constant velocity dynamometer: An appraisal using mechanical loading. *Medicine and Science in Sports and Exercise, 18,* 612–624.

47. Nicholas, J. A., Strizak, A. M., & Veras, G. (1976). A study of thigh muscle weakness in different pathological states of the lower extremity. *The American Journal of Sports Medicine, 4,* 241–248.

48. Patterson, L. A., & Spivey, W. E. (1992). Validity and reliability of the LIDO active isokinetic system. *Journal of Orthopaedic and Sports Physical Therapy, 15,* 32–36.

49. Perrin, D. H. (1986). Reliability of isokinetic measures. *Athletic Training, 21,* 319–321.

50. Perrin, D. H. (1993). *Isokinetic exercise and assessment.* Champaign, IL: Human Kinetics.

51. Petersen, S. R., Bagnall, K. M., Wenger, H. A., Reid, D. C., Castor, W. R., & Quinney, H. A. (1989). The influence of velocity-specific resistance training on the in vivo torque-velocity relationship and the cross-sectional area of quadriceps femoris. *The Journal of Orthopaedic and Sports Physical Therapy, 10,* 456–462.

52. Sale, D. G. (1991). Testing strength and power. In J. D. MacDougal, H. A. Wenger, & H. J. Green (Eds.), pp. 21–106. *Physiological testing of the high-performance athlete.* Champaign, IL: Human Kinetics.

53. Stafford, M. G., & Grana, W. A. (1984). Hamstring/quadriceps ratios in college football players. A high velocity relationship. *American Journal of Sports Medicine, 12,* 290–311.

54. Suter, E., Herzog, W., Sokolosky, J., Wiley, J. P., Macintosh, B. R. (1993). Muscle fiber type distribution as estimated by Cybex testing and by muscle biopsy. *Medicine and Science in Sports and Exercise, 25,* 363–370.

55. Sweetser, E. R., Grace, T. G., Nelson, M. A., Ydens, L. R., & Skipper, B. J. (1983). Pre-season isokinetic muscle testing in high school athletes and relationship to knee injuries. *Medicine and Science in Sports and Exercise, 15,* Abstract, 154.

56. Thorstensson, A. (1976). Muscle strength, fibre type and enzyme activities in man. *Acta Physiologica Scandinavica, 98* (Suppl. 443), 1–45.

57. Thorstensson, A., & Karlsson, J. (1976). Fatigability and fiber composition of human skeletal muscle. *Acta Physiologica Scandinavica, 98,* 318–322.

58. Thorstensson, A., Larsson, L., Tesch, P., & Karlsson, J. (1977). Muscle strength and fiber composition in athletes and sedentary men. *Medicine and Science in Sports and Exercise, 9,* 26–30.

59. Tornvall, G. (1963). Assessment of physical capabilities. *Acta Physiologica Scandinavica, 53* (Suppl. 210), 1–102.

60. Williams, M., & Stutzman, L. (1959). Strength variation through the range of motion. *The Journal of Orthopaedic and Sports Physical Therapy, 10,* 456–462.

61. Wyatt, M. P., & Edwards, A. M. (1981). Comparison of quadriceps and hamstring torque values during isokinetic exercise. *Journal of Orthopaedic and Sports Physical Therapy, 3,* 48–56.

Form IS 1

Individual Data for Isokinetic Leg Strength

Name [JAY] Date [9-13-99] Time [1:55 PM] a.m. [ ] p.m. [X]

Age [ ] y   Gender (M or F) [M]   Ht [ ] cm   Wt [68] kg

Dominant Leg (check): Right (R) [X] Left (L) [ ]

Speed: (°·s⁻¹)   60   180   300

Peak Torque:		N·m		N·m·kg⁻¹		N·m		N·m·kg⁻¹		N·m		N·m·kg⁻¹	
	L	R	L	R	L	R	L	R	L	R	L	R
Knee Flexion (H)		146.8		~~2.2~~ 2.2		101.0		1.5		84.6		1.2

	L	R	L	R	L	R	L	R	L	R	L	R
Knee Extension (Q)		196.9		2.9		188.9		1.7		103.7		1.5

Ratios: 60   180   300

Ipsilateral (Dominant) [.75]   [.85]   [.82]
(Flex:Ex; H/Q)

Bilateral [ ]   [ ]   [ ]
(L:R)

Fiber Type: Repetition   Average

Peak Torque (N·m)   1st [122.9]   2nd [136.5]   3rd [145.6]   [135]

Peak Torque   48th [12.2]   49th [12.2]   50th [59.3]   [27.9]

% Decline = [$\dfrac{135 \text{ N·m Ave. of 1 to 3} - 27.9 \text{ N·m Ave. 48 to 50}}{135 \text{ N·m Ave. of 1 to 3}}$] × 100

= 79.3 % Decline

%FT = (0.90 × 79.3 % Decline) + 5.2 = ~~76.6~~ %; %ST = 100 − %FT ~~76.6~~ = ~~23.4~~ %

Form IS 2

Group Data for Isokinetic Leg Strength

Isokinetic Speed ($°·s^{-1}$)

	60				180				300			
MEN **Initials** **(or ID #)**	Nm	Nm/kg	H/Q	L/R	Nm	Nm/kg	H/Q	L/R	Nm	Nm/kg	H/Q	L/R
1.												
2.												
3.												
4.												
5.												
6.												
7.												
8.												
9.												
10.												
11.												
Mean												
WOMEN **Initials** **(or ID #)**												
1.												
2.												
3.												
4.												
5.												
6.												
7.												
8.												
9.												
10.												
11.												
Mean												

Chapter SP

Speed—40-, 50-, and 60-Yard Sprints

Exhibitions of strength are dependent upon the anaerobic pathway. As noted previously, however, strength performance was completed in less than 3 s. Predominantly anaerobic tasks can be sustained longer than 3 s, but less than 1.5 to 3 min. Contrary to aerobic exercise, anaerobic tasks do not rely predominantly upon the transport and extraction of oxygen by the cardiovascular and respiratory systems. Anaerobic fitness and its corresponding anaerobic activities are primarily dependent upon the energy sources already existing within the muscular system. Although a popular term for anaerobic fitness is *muscle endurance,* its use is discouraged because muscle endurance may be applied justifiably to the aerobic fitness component.

Anaerobic fitness may be categorized into three components: (a) short, (b) long, and (c) mixed. These are based upon the time limits for maximal performance and the predominant energy source(s) for each (see the anaerobic fitness continuum in Fig. 1).

Short-anaerobic fitness refers to exercise performed at a maximal pace for about 10 s in most persons and up to about 30 s in a few elite athletes. Short anaerobic fitness is a dominant fitness component of the principal activity displayed in such popular sports as football, baseball, basketball, and soccer. Performers of such tasks often attempt to accelerate toward 100% of maximal velocity (see Fig. 4 in Chapter TE). Primarily, short anaerobic fitness is biochemically dependent upon two factors: (1) the muscles' storage capacity (mol) of adenosine triphosphate (ATP) and creatine phosphate (CP), and (2) the muscles' rate $(mol \cdot min^{-1})$ of resynthesizing and splitting ATP and CP.[14] The most rapid resynthesis of ATP occurs by energy released from the desynthesis of CP. Secondarily, short anaerobic fitness is partially dependent upon glycogen energy sources from the glycolytic system.

Long-anaerobic fitness is a term used to indicate the ability to achieve and sustain maximal efforts that are slightly longer than those within the short-anaerobic category; however, long-anaerobic activities are of lesser intensity and velocity than the short-anaerobic activities. Thus, maximal efforts ranging from a minimum of 10 to 30 s to a maximum of about 60 to 90 s are long-anaerobic activities that rely predominantly upon the anaerobic pathway.[17,18,19,20] For example, some persons running at optimal paces for distances between 250 and 600 m would likely finish between 30 and 90 s, respectively. Biochemically, these long-anaerobic activities are primarily dependent upon

the anaerobic glycolytic system, and, secondarily, upon the anaerobic phosphagenic system. The aerobic pathway makes a smaller, but significant, contribution to ATP production during long-anaerobic exercise. In addition to enhancing one trial of long-anaerobic performance, long-anaerobic fitness enhances performance in a series of short- and long-anaerobic trials.

Mixed fitness indicates a person's performance for optimally paced exercise efforts that can be sustained slightly longer than long-anaerobic activities but are shorter than aerobic activities. Thus, maximal efforts ranging from a minimum of about 60 to 90 s to a maximum of about 2 to 3 min are categorized as mixed fitness on the fitness continuum. Mixed fitness is dependent rather equally upon the glycolytic pathway and the aerobic pathway for ATP production—with those events closest to 90 s favoring the glycolytic pathway and those closest to 3 min favoring the aerobic pathway.

One of the physiological objectives of anaerobic tests is to hint at the levels of anaerobic substrates, such as ATP and PC, available for successful high intensity performance. Although noninvasive muscle biopsy measures of substrate concentrations are now possible through nuclear magnetic resonance (NMR) spectroscopy,[4] NMR is much more expensive than other anaerobic field, field/lab, or lab tests, such as the Sprint Tests, Wingate Cycle Test, and Treadmill Tests, respectively.

Some of the numerous popular anaerobic field tests are (a) sprints or runs of less than 800 m; (b) shuttle runs; (c) standing broad jump; (d) situps; and (e) upper body tests, such as pullups, pushups, and dips. The 40-, 50-, and 60-yd sprints are popular tests among college recruiters and professional scouts, who often administer them in order to evaluate or screen baseball and football players. The 60-yd sprint is used by baseball scouts because it is the approximate distance a base runner covers when trying to score from second base on a batter's single. The 40-yd sprint is used by football coaches because it represents the typical punt-coverage distance. Because these two sports are so "American," it is unlikely that in the near future these American units will be changed to their respective metric units rounded off to 37 m and 55 m.

Biomechanical Rationale

Technically speaking, anaerobic power is not measured in these sprints. This is because of the lack of a true vertical

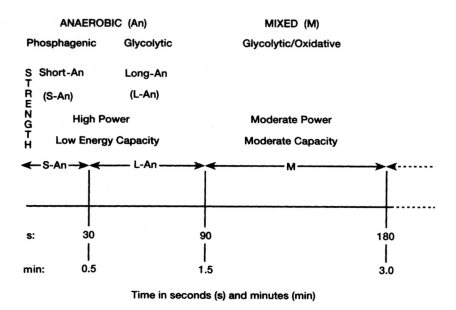

Figure 1 The anaerobic fitness continuum of short and long anaerobic fitness, in addition to the fitness component (mixed) that is a mixture of aerobic and anaerobic fitness.

distance component; only the horizontal distance is known, but it cannot be used to calculate work (or power) as defined by a physicist ($w = F \times D$). However, an estimate of relative horizontal power may be made by multiplying the sprint velocity (v) by the weight (F) of the performer (Eq. 1).

$$\text{"Horizontal P"} = \text{"F"} \times v \qquad\qquad \text{Eq. 1}$$

where:
P = power in $kg \cdot m \cdot s^{-1}$ or $N \cdot m \cdot s^{-1}$
"F" = body weight in kg or N
v = velocity = $D \div t = D/t = m \cdot s^{-1}$

Tests for running speed are not exact estimates of anaerobic power because speed and power are not identical. The contribution of mass (weight) to power may be visualized as a dropped ping-pong ball versus a golf ball contacting a pane of glass. Obviously, the golf ball is more powerful.

The contribution of velocity may be visualized by comparing the power of two thrown baseballs—one going 50 mph and the other going 100 mph; although they both have the same mass, the faster one is more powerful. The concept of horizontal power is applicable to the collisions often encountered between competitors in such sports as football and hockey.

Physiological Rationale

The duration of these sprints ranges from a minimum of about 4.3 s in the 40-yd sprint for a world-class runner to about 11 s in the 60-yd sprint for a slow college student. Thus, they are considered short-anaerobic tests because they are performed usually within the time frame of short-anaerobic fitness.

Accuracy of Sprint Tests

Validity

The validity of sprint tests is supported by moderate correlations reported[6,16] between 40-yd sprint times and other leg-power tests such as the Vertical Jump (r = .625, .48) and the vertical velocity component of the Margaria Stair-Run Test (r = .711, .88). There is a high relationship (r = .91) between the 40-m (43.7-yd) sprint and peak anaerobic power of the Wingate Cycle Test.[13] As with many performance tests (e.g., sprint tests) that purport to measure physiological performance such as phosphagenic ability, the performer's coordination for such activity is a contributing factor.

Reliability

It is possible to test running speed by administering sprints even shorter than 40 yards. However, greater reliability is likely in sprints longer than 20 yards.[3] The reliability of the 40-yd sprint is reported to be as high as .970.[7] Timing errors may range up to 1–2% when using a stopwatch.[8]

Biochemically, the tests are highly dependent upon the capacity and rate of splitting the phosphagens—adenosine triphosphate and creatine phosphate. A submaximal force, but high velocity, activity such as sprinting is probably more dependent upon the *rate* of myosin-actin interactions than upon the *number* of myosin-actin interactions.[11]

Method

All three of the sprint tests may be administered simultaneously (see Fig. 2). The facility can be any level terrain—

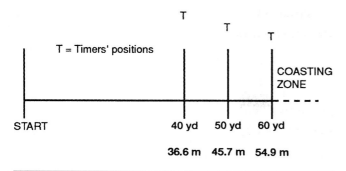

Figure 2 The sprint "layout" for measuring the times for the 40-yd (36.6-m), 50-yd (45.7-m), and 60-yd (54.9-m) sprints.

marked-off football field, track, baseball diamond, gymnasium—that has an accurately measured sprint distance. For example, if you are using a baseball diamond, simply add 10, 20, and 30 yd to the distance between the bases in order to create 40, 50, and 60 yd, respectively. There should be a minimum of 25 yd beyond the 60-yd marker in order to provide the sprinter with ample space to slow down; this is called the **coasting** or **deceleration zone.**

Administrative Procedures

The procedures for administering the sprint tests should include time for prior exercise and postexercise to prevent injuries and muscle soreness. The performers need to know the proper starting technique, while the technicians should become familiar with the timing of the event.

Prior Exercise (PE)

Prior exercise is recommended before all anaerobic tests because they are more apt to cause injury than aerobic tasks. The term *prior exercise* is preferred over the term *warmup* because of the technical distinction between warmup and loosening up. When people loosen up, usually by stretching, there is very little change in body temperature; thus, the term warmup is misleading. Table 1 provides a prescription (Rx) for prior exercise.

Sprinter's Starting Technique

In order to reduce the effect of skill or past experience, participants should not use the specialized sprint-start technique of a track athlete. However, the starting position should assume a lower center of gravity and a forward lean. Ideally, the performer should have shoes that will not slip upon starting. Starting blocks of any sort, such as holes or another person's feet, are not prescribed.

Timing of the Sprint

The three timers should use a stopwatch capable of measuring in tenths of a second. If strap-stopwatches are used, the strap should be securely wrapped around the technician's wrist or hung around the neck. After becoming familiar with the stopwatches, the timers should position themselves

Table 1 Prior Exercise Prescription (PE-Rx) for the Sprint Tests

Time (min)	Activity
0:00–3:00	Warmup—Low Intensity (1st phase)
	(1) Jogging in place; (2) Slow, relaxed jog
3:00–5:00	Loosen up (Stretching)
	Static stretch: hip-groin area, "gastrocs," "quads," and "hams"
	Ballistic stretch: Same muscle groups as above
5:00–10:00	Warmup—Moderate Intensity (2nd phase)
	(1) Short hops/jumps; (2) 10-, 40-, 50-yd runs of moderate speed
10:00–12:00	Recovery Interval between PE-Rx and First Trial of Sprint Test
	(1) Walking or walking in place; (2) Loosening up (ballistic and static)

at the 40-, 50-, and 60-yd markers to allow an optimal view of the runner when starting and when breaking the plane of the finish line (see Fig. 2). The timers should acknowledge a "Ready" signal of the runner. As soon as the runner makes the first movement to sprint, all timers start their watches. Thus, a "GO" signal is **not** given because reaction time is not a consideration in this power test. As soon as the runner's trunk breaks the plane of the respective finish lines, technicians stop their watches. They record the times to the closest tenth of a second on Form SP 1. The best time of the two or three trials is used as the individual's score for group statistical purposes.

Number of Trials

Unless the performer has not been sprint-training, no more than three trials should be performed in one day. Three trials are recommended only if the difference in times between trials is greater than 0.20 s. Regardless of the non-sprint-trained performer's feelings about the muscles or motivational status, strict adherence to the three-trial rule should prevail. Otherwise, delayed onset muscle soreness (DOMS) is likely. To avoid DOMS or injury and to allow restoration of the phosphagens, there should be a rest period between trials of at least 1–2 min if only sprinting 40 m,[2] and 3–8 min if performing 60-m sprints. Active recovery, such as fast walking or slow jogging, is superior to passive recovery, such as sitting or standing, during the relief interval for short-anaerobic activity.[21]

Prevention of Muscle Soreness

Unaccustomed anaerobic activity is conducive to delayed onset muscle soreness, whereby DOMS occurs as early as 6, but usually 8 to 24 hours postexercise.[22] In addition to adhering to the prior exercise prescription and the three-trial maximum, the following two recommendations are made in order to eliminate or minimize stiffness:

1. Immediately following the sprint trials, the sprinter should repeat the first 5 min (warmup and loosening up) of the prior exercise regimen.

2. The sprinter should repeat the static stretching exercises periodically throughout the next three days.[5]

Calculation of Horizontal Power

By using Equation 1, horizontal power may be calculated from velocity and body weight as follows:

1. Convert the American distances of the sprints into their respective meter units by dividing the yards by 1.0936, or simply by consulting Figure 2 or Form SP 1.
2. Calculate the velocity (v) by dividing the time (s) into the metric distance ($v = m \div s$).
3. Multiply the kilogram body weight by ten to obtain newtons.
4. Multiply newtons by velocity to obtain horizontal power expressed as $N \cdot m \cdot s^{-1}$.

Results and Discussion

In general, the norms for the 40- and 60-yd sprint tests are ill defined for the average person. The 50-yd norms are applicable to boys and girls younger than college age (Table 2; AAHPERD, 1976). The average times in the 50-yd sprint for college-aged men and women, including reaction time, have been reported as 6.8 s and 8.2 s, respectively.[12]

A large group of college football players averaged 5.35 s ($SD = 0.30$) in the 40-yd sprint.[6] Additionally, there are various criteria that have been used often by scouts or coaches of football and baseball organizations that might be helpful in interpreting sprint times. Testimonies of running speed have been presented in such popular media as newspapers, magazines, TV, and radio (Table 3). Cautious interpretation of sprint times for specific sports or positions is warranted considering the fact that, although football players are often timed in the 40-yd sprint, linemen rarely run 40 yd on any given play. Despite this reservation, however, it appears that the correlation between 5- or 15-yd times and 40-yd times is very high.[7]

Table 2 AAHPERD Norms for 17+-Year-Old High School Boys and Girls in the 50-Yd Sprint

| | 50-Yd Time (s) | | |
Category	Percentile	Boys	Girls
	95	5.9	6.8
Excellent		6.1	7.0
	75	6.3	7.4
Good		6.4	7.4
Average	50	6.6	7.9
Fair		7.0	8.3
	25	7.0	8.4
Low		7.5	8.9
	5	7.9	9.5

Reprinted by permission of the American Alliance for Health, Physical Education, Recreation and Dance, 1900 Association Dr., Reston, VA 22091.

Table 3 Comparative Times (s) for the 40-, 50-, and 60-Yd Sprints

40-Yd	Time	50-Yd	Time	60-Yd	Time
Football[a]		Track		Baseball	
College Players	5.35	Men's WR[b]	5.15	Top criteria:	
Fast Running Back[10]	4.35	Women's WR	5.74	High school	7.2
				College	7.0
Fast NFL Lineman	4.56	50 m (55 yd)		Professional	6.8 or 6.9
		Men's WR	5.55		
Fast High Schoolers		Women's WR	6.06		
Guards	4.75				
Tackles	4.9				
Pro Flanker Time[9]	4.4–4.6			Fastest in NFL	6.18
Female College Athletes[15]	5.96			55 m (60 yd)	
Gladiator Criterion	≤4.8			Men's WR	5.99

[a]NFL scouts sometimes allow "rolling" starts
[b]WR = former world record; Data from Dintiman, 1984, p. 166; Fox & Mathews, 1974, p. 202, Mayhew et al., 1994.

References

1. AAHPERD. (1976). *AAHPERD youth fitness test manual.* Washington, D.C.: AAHPERD Publications.

2. Balsom, P. D., Seger, J. Y., Sjodin, B., & Ekblom, B. (1992). Maximal-intensity intermittent exercise: Effect of recovery duration. *International Journal of Sports Medicine, 13,* 528–533.

3. Baumgartner, T. A., & Jackson, A. S. (1987). *Measurement for evaluation in physical education and exercise science.* Dubuque, IA: Wm. C. Brown.

4. Brooks, G. A., Fahey, T. D., & White, T. P. (1996). *Exercise physiology: Human bioenergetics and its applications.* Mountain View, CA: Mayfield.

5. Chen, T. C., & Hsieh, S. S. (1996). The effects of stretching and cryotherapy on delayed onset muscle soreness. *Medicine and Science in Sports and Exercise, 28* (Suppl., 5), Abstract #1077, p. S181.

6. Costill, D. L., Miller, S. J., Myers, W. C., Kehoe, F. M., & Hoffman, W. M. (1968). Relationship among selected tests of explosive leg strength and power. *The Research Quarterly, 39*(3): 785–787.

7. Crews, T. R., & Meadors, W. J. (1978). Analysis of reaction time, speed, and body composition of college football players. *Journal of Sports Medicine and Physical Fitness, 18,* 169–172.

8. deVries, H. A., & Housh, T. J. (1994). *Physiology of exercise for physical education, athletics, and exercise science.* Dubuque, IA: Brown & Benchmark.

9. Dintiman, G. B. (1984). *How to run faster.* Champaign, IL: Leisure Press.

10. Fox, E. L., & Mathews, D. K. (1974). *Interval training: Conditioning for sports and general fitness.* Philadelphia: W. B. Saunders.

11. Green, H. J. (1991). What do tests measure? In J. D. MacDougall, H. A. Wenger, & H. J. Green (Eds.), *Physiological testing of the high performance athlete* (pp. 7–19). Champaign, IL: Human Kinetics.

12. Johnson, P. B., Updyke, W. F., Schaefer, M., & Stolberg, D. C. (1975). *Sport, exercise, and you.* New York: Holt, Rinehart, and Winston.

13. Kaczkowski, W., Montgomery, D. L., Taylor, A. W., & Klissourous, V. (1982). The relationship between muscle fiber composition and maximal anaerobic power and capacity. *Journal of Sports Medicine and Physical Fitness, 22,* 407–413.

14. Mathews, D. K., & Fox, E. L. (1976). *The physiological basis of physical education and athletics.* Philadelphia: W. B. Saunders.

15. Mayhew, J. L., Bemben, M. G., Rohrs, D. M., & Bemben, D. A. (1994). Specificity among anaerobic power tests in college female athletes. *Journal of Strength and Conditioning Research, 8,* 43–47.

16. McArdle, W. D., Katch, F. I., & Katch, V. L. (1991). *Exercise physiology.* Philadelphia: Lea & Febiger.

17. Medbo, J. I., & Burgers, S. (1990). Effect of training on the anaerobic capacity. *Medicine and Science in Sports and Exercise, 22,* 501–507.

18. Medbo, J. I., Mohn, A. C., Tabata, I., Bahr, R., Vaage, O., & Sejersted, O. M. (1988). Anaerobic capacity determined by maximal accumulated O_2 deficit. *Journal of Applied Physiology, 64,* 50–60.

19. Medbo, J. I., & Sejersted, O. M. (1985). Acid-base and electrolyte balance after exhausting exercise in endurance-trained and sprint-trained subjects. *Acta Physiologica Scandinavica, 125,* 97–109.

20. Medbo, J. I., & Tabata, I. (1989). Relative importance of aerobic and anaerobic energy release during shortlasting, exhausting bicycle exercise. *Journal of Applied Physiology, 67,* 1881–1886.

21. Signorile, J. F., Ingalls, C., & Tremblay, L. M. (1993). The effects of active and passive recovery on short-term high intensity power output. *Canadian Journal of Applied Physiology, 18,* 31–42.

22. Smith, L. L., Brunetz, M. H., Chenier, T. C., McCammon, M. R., Houmard, J. A., Franklin, M. E., & Israel, R. G. (1993). The effects of static and ballistic stretching on delayed onset muscle soreness and creatine kinase. *Research Quarterly for Exercise and Sport, 64,* 103–107.

Form *SP 1*

Individual Data for Sprint Tests

Name _____ Date _____ Time _____ a.m. ☐ p.m. ☐

Gender (M or F) ☐   Ht ☐ cm   Wt ☐ kg $\times 10 =$ ☐ N

Location: Field ☐   Track ☐   Diamond ☐   Gym ☐   Other ☐

Footwear: Jog ☐   Track ☐   Baseball ☐   Tennis ☐

Bare ☐   Other ☐   Air v ☐ Calm ☐ Breezy

Sprint Times (to closest 0.1 s)

40-YD (36.6 m)	50-YD (45.7 m)	60-YD (54.9 m)
Trial #1 _____ s	#1 _____ s	#1 _____ s
Trial #2 _____ s	#2 _____ s	#2 _____ s
Trial #3 _____ s	#3 _____ s	#3 _____ s
(If #1−#2>0.2 s)		

[Circle best trial of each sprint distance; use best trial to calculate v]

Velocity ($v = D/t$) _____ m·s^{-1} _____ m·s^{-1} _____ m·s^{-1}

Horizontal Power (P) for 50-Yd (45.7 m) Sprint

Body Wt (F) _____ N $\times$ Velocity (v) _____ m·s^{-1} $=$ "Power" (P) _____ N·m·s^{-1}

Form SP 2

Group Data for Sprints

Initials	Sprint Times (closest 0.1 s)			Horizontal Power
Men	40 yd	50 yd	60 yd	50-yd N·m·s^{-1}
1.				
2.				
3.				
4.				
5.				
6.				
7.				
8.				
9.				
M				
Women	40 yd	50 yd	60 yd	50-yd N·m·s^{-1}
1.				
2.				
3.				
4.				
5.				
6.				
7.				
8.				
9.				
M				

Chapter VP Vertical Power

To a biomechanist the vertical jump test is a more true power test than a sprint test on a level terrain. The current test is a modification of one developed by Dr. Dudley Sargent in the early 1900s—the Sargent Jump Test.[43] His test simply required a measurement of the difference between the standing-reach height and the jump-height. Because no true expression of anaerobic power, only jumping distance, was made in the original test, it would not qualify as a laboratory test. However, because the modified version does include a power measurement, and because of the simple equipment and procedures, the present vertical jump test would qualify as a field/lab test.

Several anaerobic tests may be performed in the lab or in the field. Equation 6 ($P = w/t$) in Chapter TE is used to calculate power in such field/lab tests as Vertical Jump, Wingate Cycle, and Anaerobic Power Step. The force component can be taken from the weight (kg; N) of the jumper; the time component can be measured electronically as the time in air from an electronic contact mat attached to a special timer.[25,45] Also, time may be estimated from the law of falling bodies or acceleration of gravity,[4,16,45] based upon the difference in the original height of the center of gravity (g) and its height at the peak of the jump (Eq. 1).

$$\text{acceleration of } g = 9.81 \text{ m·s}^2 \qquad \text{Eq. 1}$$

The height of a jump is dependent on the vertical speed of the body's center of gravity at the moment of leaving the terrain.

Physiological Rationale

Although the vertical jump has been called an explosive strength test,[33] partly because the single jumping movement itself is accomplished in less than a second, it is not a true strength measure because a maximal force is not elicited. Conceivably, repeated jumps within a 10-s period would have little decrement. Thus, the ability to perform well on this test may be more related to short-anaerobic fitness rather than strength.

Correlations between strength and vertical jump have been quite variable. The ballistic act of vertical jumping correlated moderately high ($r = .74$; .81) with peak *relative* isokinetic torque[8] (N·m·kg^{-1}) and static force[22] of the leg extensors, respectively. However, others have found insignificant[9,11,27] or low[12,14] ($r < .2$) or moderate[19,41] ($r = .4–.6$) correlations between strength and jumping. Two

reviewers[32] provide a rationale for this low strength vs. jump relationship, especially when the comparative strength measure is a static or slow muscle action. For example, a 1-RM is much slower than the vertical jump in which the feet are in contact with the terrain for only about 350 ms (0.35 s). The reviewers conclude that the ability to generate the highest dynamic rate of force development is a very significant factor in such an explosive movement as the vertical jump. Thus, it appears that short-anaerobic fitness is a fitness component that is too complex to be predicted by strength alone.

Disregarding the skill factor, jumping ability is dependent biochemically upon the individual's phosphagen capacity and the ability to use these phosphagen stores at a rapid rate.

Biomechanically, the jump test combines hip and knee extension with ankle plantar flexion.[20,44] The percentage of fast twitch fibers in the vastus lateralis—one of the four quadricep muscles—is significantly related ($r = .48$) to jump height as measured from a force platform.[6]

Method

The methods of conducting the vertical jump test consider (a) equipment, (b) prior exercise, (c) body positions and measurements, and (d) calculations.

Equipment

An accurate platform scale may be used to measure the weight of the jumper in their "jumping" clothes and shoes. An anthropometer or stadiometer may be used to measure height, but the height of the jumper is of no significance in the calculation of anaerobic power nor in the interpretation of the norms. However, adding the jump height to the individual's height will produce the distance from the floor to the jumping point; this would be significant, for example, for basketball and volleyball players. A calculator with square-root capability is convenient for making the power calculations.

The vertical jump test may be conducted with or without special electronic equipment. If the nonelectronic method is used, then a flat measuring scale about 1 ft wide and 3–4 ft long, with horizontal lines at 1-in. intervals, can be attached to a wall or post (e.g., a basketball backboard). It is possible to use a simple yard/meter stick as the

Accuracy of the Vertical Jump

Validity

A validity coefficient of .78 has been reported based upon the sum of four track and field event scores.[28] Sprint times appear to be low to moderately correlated with the vertical jump.[12] For example, correlations between the 40-yd sprint and the vertical jump of .625[13] and .48[40] have been found. However, the correlation between vertical jump and 40-yd sprint time is reduced to virtually zero ($r = -.05$) when body weight is considered as in calculating vertical jump power. The vertical jump was moderately correlated ($r = .49$) with the anaerobic 20-s Wingate Cycle Test in older persons.[10] Some investigators conclude that anaerobic tests are specific, not general, and anaerobic tests should not be universally applied to all aspects of anaerobic fitness.[39] McArdle and his colleagues further caution about a direct relationship of the vertical jump to phosphagenic capacity because no relationship has been established between jump-test scores and ATP-PC levels or depletion patterns. Although the calculated power from the Jump Test correlated well ($r = .83$) with the peak power of that derived from a computer-interfaced force plate, the Jump Test's *mean* power greatly underestimated the electronic *instantaneous* power.[24] Some researchers suggest that questions of validity using power formulas might be avoided by simply using the jump height, which correlates highly ($r = .92$) with peak power ($W \cdot kg^{-1}$) from a force platform.[15] Combining the results of the jump test with an analysis of a force curve from a force platform test may enhance the validity of the jump test.

Reliability

Reports on the test-retest reliability of the vertical jump have been high, ranging from a correlation of .93 when using the technique described in this text[20,28] to .985 when using a more restrictive jumping procedure.[21] Two investigators found a reliability correlation of .99 when testing university students.[12] Even when the test was administered to children, the test-retest reliabilities ranged from .90–.97.[34]

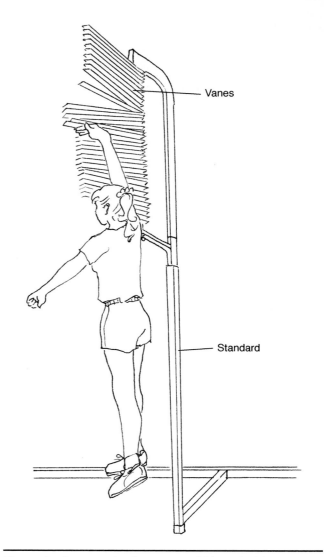

Figure 1 An example of a commercial jump test instrument (Vertek®).

measuring scale, but this is not preferred due to a greater likelihood of making visual errors when observing the jump mark. If the flat scale is used, then gymnast's chalk, chalk dust, or water (not saliva) on the jumper's fingers may be used to mark the peak jump of the performer.

The flat scale is not necessary if using a commercial jump scale (e.g., Vertek; Fig. 1). This standing scale resembles a volleyball standard and has red, white, and blue markers (vanes) spaced 0.5 in. apart; the red markers are spaced every 6.0 in., the blue ones every 1.0 in., and the white ones every 0.5 in. except where there is a red or a blue one. The jumper's hand causes the several vanes to swivel near the peak height of the jump. Thus, the highest vane that is moved represents the height of the jump.

Prior Exercise

Prior exercise need not be quite so extensive as that typically recommended for sprint running. However, a

"warmup" appears to enhance jumping performance.[17] About 5 to 10 min of loosening up and warming up, with the latter including a few vertical jumps at one-half to three-quarter effort should be sufficient.

Body Positions and Measurements

The jump distance is calculated from the two vertical measurements for the vertical jump test—the standing reach and the jump reach. These may be made in inches (in.) or centimeters (cm) to the closest one-half in. or 1 cm.[26]

Standing Reach

The standing reach (Fig. 2a) is measured as the jumper stands with the feet together and the dominant side against the wall or commercial apparatus (Vertek™). The jumper then reaches as high as possible with the dominant arm so that the palm of the hand is against the measurement scale[28] or the wall. If using the Vertek, adjust the standard so that the tip of the

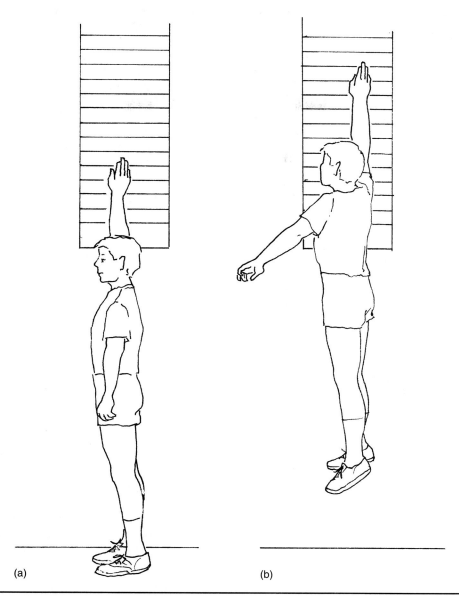

(a) (b)

Figure 2 The significant positions for the vertical jump: (a) the recorded standing-reach position and (b) the recorded jump position.

tallest finger during the reach is at the bottom surface of the lowest vane on the Vertek. The highest reach is observed and then recorded on Form VP 1. If the jumper cannot jump more than 24 in., then the Vertek standard can be adjusted so that the lowest vane is at the jumper's standing reach height. In this case, the standing height can be considered the zero point and can be recorded as such on Form VP 1.

Jumping Reach

After the standing reach is measured, the jumper moves the feet to a jumping position. The feet cannot change from this position prior to jumping nor are any preparatory movements permitted other than one quick dip (counter-movement) of the knees and one swing of the arms. The jump movement has been compared to the snatch or clean Olympic lifts.[18]

The performer makes the jump while touching or swatting the measurement scale or vanes at the peak of the jump (Fig. 2b). The chalk or water mark on the wall scale is observed by a technician who stands on a higher platform (e.g., a chair or a table) near eye level to the jump mark.

Three jump trials are usually given and the best trial used for group statistics. If a jumper continues to improve on the third trial, then subsequent trials can be given. However, comparisons are less valid because the norms were developed from only three trials. Due to the rapid recovery of the relatively small volume of phosphagens used for performing one vertical jump, the several seconds taken to observe and record the height of the jump is all that is needed for recovery between trials.

Jump Distance

The jump distance (D) is calculated by subtracting the standing reach height from the jumping reach height. For example, if a person's standing reach touches the measurement scale at 10 in., and the jumping height is 32 in., then the difference is 22 in. When converted to centimeters by dividing by 0.3937, the metric jump height becomes 56 cm to the closest whole centimeter, or 0.56 m. If using the commercial apparatus, technicians should calculate the number of inches (to closest 0.5 in.) to the highest vane that was moved. Because the Vertek standard was adjusted to zero, the highest touched vane represents the jump height, thus no subtraction is necessary.

Calculation of Power for the Vertical Jump Test

Mean power, not instantaneous power, can be estimated by knowing the work accomplished over a measured time period. The anaerobic power of this test may be derived without any calculations from the modified Lewis nomogram (Fig. 3). Equation 2 calculates the same power (P) value by considering the duration of the ascending phase of the flight, not the total thrust duration. In actuality, the flight time is derived from a constant based upon the rate of falling bodies.

$$P = 2.21 \times wt \times \sqrt{D} \qquad \text{Eq. 2}$$

where:

$\quad$ 2.21 = a constant; $\sqrt{4.9}$

$\quad\quad$ wt = body weight (kg) in jump clothes

$\quad\quad$ D = difference between standing reach and jump height (m)

For example, if a 67-kg person's difference in reach height and jump height was 20 inches (51 cm or 0.51 m), then the following calculation would provide the anaerobic power in kilogram meters per second ($kg \cdot m \cdot s^{-1}$):

$$P\left(kg \cdot m \cdot s^{-1}\right) = 2.21 \times 67 \text{ kg} \times \sqrt{0.51 \text{ m}}$$
$$= 148 \times 0.714$$
$$= 106$$

Because the International System of measuring units requires power units to be expressed in newton meters per second ($N \cdot m \cdot s^{-1}$) or watts (W), the rounded-conversions become:

$$1060 \text{ N} \cdot m \cdot s^{-1} \text{ and } 1060 \text{ W}.$$

An approximate estimate of anaerobic power may be made from the modified Lewis nomogram in Figure 3.[36] This is done by placing a straightedge on the Jump-Distance line (the difference between the reach height and the jump height in meters) and then pivoting the straightedge to the body weight (N). Where the straightedge crosses the Power line is the anaerobic power ($N \cdot m \cdot s^{-1}$ or W).

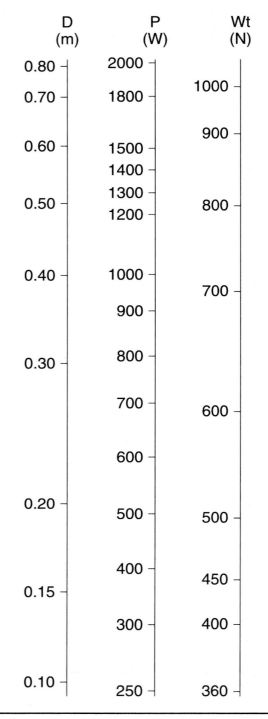

Figure 3 The Lewis nomogram for approximating the power (P; W) from the jump height difference (D; m) and body weight (Wt; N).

Results and Discussion

Two different aspects of power during the vertical jump can be predicted for college men and women athletes by using Equations 3 and 4.[30] One aspect—peak power (P_{pk})—reflects the highest power output during a single moment of the pushoff phase of the jump. The other

Table 1 Jump Height and Power on Various Vertical Jump Tests

Method of Testing	Jump Height		Power	
	in.	cm	W	$W \cdot kg^{-1}$
Unknown				
Michael Jordan[29]	41	104		
UCLA 1963–64 basketball team[46]	27–36	69–91		
Facing Wall, 2-Arm Reach				
Average college male	20	51		
Average college female[31]	13	33		
Method Described in this Text				
Highest P in CSUF laboratory[3]	33.5	85	2060	
Highest jump height at CSUF	39	99	1760	21.5
College football players[13]	20.9	53		
50th %ile 17-y-old boys[5]	19.5	50		
50th %ile 17-y-old girls[5]	13.0	33		
50th %ile 17–18-y-old boys[1]	20	51		
50th %ile 17–18-y-old girls[2]	13	33		
50th %ile 18–34-y-old men	16	41		
50th %ile 18–34-y-old women[28]	8	20		
Average male college students[12,20]	21.3; 21.6	54		
Active men college students[38]		53	1240	
Active women college students[38]		36	792	
Female college athletes[39]	15.7	40	877	13.8
Average female kinesiology major[3]			750	
Average male kinesiology major[3]			1340	
U.S. rugby team forwards[37]			1570	
CSUF baseball team	26	66	1500	18.1
Italian men's volleyball team[8]		44	1240	
Soldiers of India (38–43 y)[35]	12.5			

Table 2 Vertical Jump Scores of College Men and Women

	Height Difference					
Percentile	**Men**			**Women**		
	in.	cm	m	in.	cm	m
90	25	64	0.64	14	36	0.36
80	24	61	0.61	13	33	0.33
70	23	58	0.58	12	30	0.30
60	19	48	0.48	10	25	0.25
50	16	41	0.41	8	20	0.20
40	13	33	0.33	6	15	0.15
30	9	23	0.23	4	10	0.10
20	8	20	0.20	2	5	0.05
10	2	5	0.05	1	2.5	0.025

Modified from H. J. Montoye, *Living Fit*, page 53. Copyright © 1988 Benjamin/Cummings Publishing, Menlo Park, CA.

Table 3 Vertical Jump Height[a] in Finnish Men and Women ($n = 670$)

Age		Men			Women	
y	cm	SD	in.	cm	SD	in.
25	32.5	5.0	12.8	20.9	3.9	8.2
35	28.4	5.2	11.2	18.6	3.6	7.3
45	25.1	4.9	9.9	15.7	3.5	6.2
55	21.1	4.4	8.3	12.5	2.4	0.9

[a]Similar jump technique as in "*EP Lab*," but calculated from flight time of center of gravity as described in reference #7. Adapted from Table 2 on p. 891 of Kujala et al. (1994). Physical activity, $\dot{V}O_2$ max, and jumping height in an urban population. *Medicine and Science in Sports and Exercise, 26*, 889–895. © ACSM, 1994, Indianapolis, IN.

aspect—average power (P_{ave})—represents the average power output over the entire duration of the pushoff phase.

$$P_{pk} (W) = [78.5 \times VJ\ (cm)] + [60.6 \times M\ (kg)] - [15.3 \times ht\ (cm)] - 1308 \qquad \text{Eq. 3}$$

$$P_{ave} (W) = [41.4 \times VJ\ (cm)] + [31.2 \times M\ (kg)] - [13.9 \times ht\ (cm)] + 431 \qquad \text{Eq. 4}$$

where:

VJ = vertical jump; jump-reach minus standing-reach
M = body mass (wt)
ht = body stature; height

Vertical jump tests are often administered to track and field athletes and to basketball and volleyball players. Some of the high scores reported in the popular media (TV, radio, newspapers, and magazines) were not produced under the same procedures as the vertical jump described in this manual. For example, some measures were made while the jumper took two or three preparatory steps. In various scientific studies, some low vertical jump scores are the result of using a *more* restrictive method than the one presented here. For example, the jumper's reaching arm may have been restricted to remain in the elevated position during the preparatory and jump phases[21] or counter-movements were disallowed.[23] Counter-movements and arm swings combine to improve vertical jumps by more than 10%,[6,7] due to the contributions

of the stored elastic energy of the tendon-muscle complex and the neural facilitation of the stretch reflex. If timed optimally, the forward and upward thrusting of the arms enhances the momentum and, hence, the height of the jump.[44]

Some of the scores that have been accumulated under a variety of methods are presented in Table 1. It is not unusual for a heavier performer to have greater power than a lighter jumper even when the latter jumps higher. For example, the highest power value in our lab was 2060 W by a heavier person who jumped 85 cm, but the power of a lighter person was only 1760 despite jumping 99 cm.[3] Thus, a heavier person generates more power if jumping a given height.

The norms in Tables 2[42] and 3[33] are based upon larger samples but do not include power values. The values in Table 3 clearly show an age-related decline in jumping ability. For men and women, vertical jumps decrease about 4 and 3 cm, respectively, for every 10 y after the age of 25.[7,33] Power for the young adult population, expressed relatively as $W \cdot kg^{-1}$, may be estimated from Equation 5:[15]

$$\text{Power } (W \cdot kg^{-1}) = 1.37 + (0.893 \times cm) \qquad \text{Eq. 5}$$

where: cm = height jumped

References

1. AAHPER. (1966). *Skills test manual: Basketball for boys.* Washington, D.C.: AAHPER.
2. AAHPER. (1966). *Skills test manual: Basketball for girls.* Washington, D.C.: AAHPER.
3. Adams, G. M. (1992). Vertical jumps of college physical education majors. Unpublished raw data.
4. Bannister, E. W., & Mekjavic, I. B. (1987). *Experiments in human performance.* Philadelphia: W. B. Saunders.
5. Baumgartner, T. A., & Jackson, A. S. (1987). *Measurement for evaluation in physical education and exercise science.* Dubuque, IA: Wm. C. Brown.
6. Bosco, C., & Komi, P. V. (1979). Mechanical characteristics and fiber composition of human leg extensor muscles. *European Journal of Applied Physiology, 41,* 275–284.
7. Bosco, C., & Komi, P. V. (1980). Influence of aging on the mechanical behavior of leg extensor muscles. *European Journal of Applied Physiology, 45,* 209–219.
8. Bosco, C., Mognoni, P., & Luhtanen, P. (1983). Relationship between isokinetic performance and ballistic movement. *European Journal of Applied Physiology, 51,* 357–364.
9. Bosworth, J. M. (1964). *The effect of isometric training and rebound tumbling on performance in the vertical jump.* Master's thesis, Springfield College, MA.
10. Bowers, P., Coleman, A., & Oshiro, T. (1993). Measuring anaerobic power of aged men and women. *Sports Medicine, Training, and Rehabilitation, 4,* 304 (Abstract).
11. Clarke, H. H. (1957). Relationships of strength and anthropometric measures to physical performances involving the trunk and leg. *Research Quarterly, 28,* 223.
12. Considine, W. J., & Sullivan, W. J. (1973). Relationship of selected tests of leg strength and leg power on college men. *Research Quarterly, 44,* 404–416.
13. Costill, D. L., Miller, S. J., Myers, W. C., Kehoe, F. M., & Hoffman, W. M. (1968). Relationship among selected tests of explosive leg strength and power. *Research Quarterly, 39,* 785.
14. Cureton, T. K. (1941). Fitness of feet and legs. *Research Quarterly, 12,* 368.
15. Davies, C. T. M., & Young, K. (1984). Effects of external loading on short term power output in children and young male adults. *European Journal of Applied Physiology, 52,* 351–354.
16. deVries, H. A. (1971). *Laboratory experiments in physiology of exercise.* Dubuque, IA: Wm. C. Brown.
17. deVries, H. A., & Housh, T. J. (1994). *Physiology of exercise for physical education, athletics, and exercise science.* Dubuque, IA: Brown & Benchmark.
18. Garhammer, J., & Gregor, R. (1992). Propulsion forces as a function of intensity for weightlifting and vertical jumping. *Journal of Applied Sport Science Research, 6,* 129–134.
19. Genuario, S. E., & Dolgener, F. A. (1980). The relationship of isokinetic torque at two speeds to the vertical jump. *Research Quarterly for Exercise and Sport, 51,* 593–598.
20. Glencross, D. J. (1966). The nature of the vertical jump test and the standing broad jump. *Research Quarterly, 37,* 353–359.
21. Gray, R. K., Start, K. B., & Glencross, D. J. (1962). A test of leg power. *Research Quarterly, 33,* 44.
22. Hakkinen, K. (1991). Force production characteristics of leg extensor, trunk flexor and extensor muscles in male and female basketball players. *Journal of Sports Medicine and Physical Fitness, 31,* 325–331.
23. Harman, E. A., Rosenstein, M. T., Frykman, P. N., & Rosenstein, R. M. (1990). The effects of arms and countermovement on vertical jumping. *Medicine and Science in Sports and Exercise, 22,* 825–833.
24. Harman, E. A., Rosenstein, M. T., Frykman, P. N., Rosenstein, R. M., & Kraemer, W. J. (1989). Evaluation of the Lewis power output test. *Medicine and Science in Sports and Exercise, 21,* (Suppl.), Abstract #305, S51.
25. Harman, E. A., & Sharp, M. A. (1989). Prediction of power output during vertical jumps using body mass and flight time. *Medicine and Science in Sports and Exercise, 21* (Suppl. 2), Abstract #306, S51.
26. Henry, F. M. (1959). Influence of measurement error and intra-individual variation on the reliability of muscle strength and vertical jump tests. *Research Quarterly, 30,* 155.
27. Hortobagyi, T., Houmard, J. A., Stevenson, J. R., Fraser, D. D., Johns, R. A., & Israel, R. G. (1993). The effects of detraining on power athletes. *Medicine and Science in Sports and Exercise, 25,* 929–935.
28. Johnson, B. L., & Nelson, J. K. (1974). *Practical measurements for evaluation in physical education.* Minneapolis: Burgess.
29. Johnson, C. (1996, March). Bodies of evidence. *Outside,* 58–63.
30. Johnson, D. L., & Bahamonde, R. (1996). Power output estimate in university athletes. *Journal of Strength and Conditioning Research, 10,* 161–166.
31. Johnson, P. B., Updyke, W. F., Schaefer, M., & Stolberg, D. C. (1975). *Sport, exercise, and you.* New York: Holt, Rinehart, & Winston.
32. Kraemer, W. J., & Newton, R. U. (1994). Training for improved vertical jump. *Sports Science Exchange, 7*(6): 1–5. Gatorade Sports Science Institute.
33. Kujala, U. M., Viljanen, T., Taimela, S., & Viitasalo, J.T. (1994). Physical activity, $\dot{V}O_2$ max, and jumping height in an urban population. *Medicine and Science in Sports and Exercise, 26,* 889–895.

34. Latchaw, M. (1954). Measuring selected motor skills in fourth, fifth, and sixth grades. *Research Quarterly, 25,* 439.

35. Malhotra, M. S., Ramaswamy, S. S., Dua, G. L., & Sengupta, J. (1966). Physical work capacity as influenced by age. *Ergonomics, 9,* 305–316.

36. Mathews, D. K., & Fox, E. L. (1976). *The physiological basis of physical education and athletics.* Philadelphia: W. B. Saunders.

37. Maud, P. J., & Shultz, B. B. (1984). The U.S. National Rugby Team: A physiological and anthropometric assessment. *The Physician and Sportsmedicine,* (Sept.): 86–94, 99.

38. Maud, P. J., & Shultz, B. B. (1986). Gender comparisons in anaerobic power and anaerobic capacity tests. *British Journal of Sports Medicine, 20,* 51–54.

39. Mayhew, J. L., Bemben, M. G., Rohrs, D. M., & Bemben, D. A. (1994). Specificity among anaerobic power tests in college female athletes. *Journal of Strength and Conditioning Research, 8,* 43–47.

40. McArdle, W. D., Katch, F. I., & Katch, V. L. (1996). *Exercise physiology: Energy, nutrition, and human performance.* Baltimore: Williams & Wilkins.

41. Misner, J. E., Boileau, S. A., Plowman, S. A., Elmore, B. G., Gates, M. A., Gilbert, J. A., & Horswill, C. (1988). Leg power of female firefighter applicants. *Journal of Occupational Medicine, 30,* 433–437.

42. Montoye, H. J., Christian, J. L., Nagle, F. J., & Levin, S. M. (1988). *Living fit.* Menlo Park, CA: Benjamin/Cummings.

43. Sargent, D. A. (1921). The physical test of a man. *American Physical Education Review, 26,* 188.

44. Semenick, D. M., & Adams, K. O. (1987, June/July). The vertical jump: A kinesiological analysis with recommendations for strength and conditioning programming. *National Strength and Conditioning Association Journal, 8.*

45. Viitasalo, J. T. (1988). Evaluation of explosive strength for young and adult athletes. *Research Quarterly, 59,* 9–13.

46. Wooden, J. (1972). *They call me coach.* Waco, TX: Word Books.

Form *VP 1*

Individual Data for the Vertical Jump Test

Basic Data

Name [_____] Date [_____] Time [____] a.m. [____] p.m. [____]

Gender (M or F) [____] Age [____] y Ht (without shoes) [____] cm

Wt (in jump clothes) [____] kg [____] N

Jump Data[a]

Reach Position [____] in. (to closest 0.5 in.); ÷ 0.3937 = [____] (closest cm)

Jump Height
(Circle best trial) Trial #1 [____] in. [____] cm

Trial #2 [____] in. [____] cm

Trial #3 [____] in. [____] cm

Jump Ht minus Reach Ht [____] in. [____] cm [____] m

Power = 2.21 × [____] kg × $\sqrt{D}$ _____ m

= [____] × [____] m = [____] $kg \cdot m \cdot s^{-1}$; × 10 = [____] $N \cdot m \cdot s^{-1}$; W

P_{pk} (W) = 78.5 × VJ [____] cm + 60.6 × M [____] kg

− 15.3 × ht [____] cm − 1308

P_{ave} (W) = 41.4 × VJ [____] cm + 31.2 × M [____] kg

− 13.9 × ht [____] cm + 431

[a]Note: The height of the reach position does not need to be measured if it is simply used as a zero reference point.

Form *VP 2*

Group Data for Vertical Jump

MEN Initials	Jump Ht (m)	Power (W)	Relative Power (W·kg⁻¹)	WOMEN Initials	Jump Ht (m)	Power (W)	Relative Power (W·kg⁻¹)
1.				1.			
2.				2.			
3.				3.			
4.				4.			
5.				5.			
6.				6.			
7.				7.			
8.				8.			
9.				9.			
10.				10.			
11.				11.			
12.				12.			
13.				13.			
14.				14.			
15.				15.			
16.				16.			
M				*M*			

Chapter NC Anaerobic Cycling

The most popular anaerobic cycling test is the Wingate Anaerobic Test (WAnT), named after the university in Israel where it originated. The original test was designed for children but became popular for adults in the late 1970s.[5] It fulfilled the need for a precisely measured anaerobic power test. It may be used to test either arm or leg power but is most commonly used to test the legs.

This anaerobic test can determine the performer's **peak anaerobic power, average (mean) anaerobic power, total work,** and **fatigue index.** Peak power is based on the highest power level averaged over a 5-s period during the test, whereas mean power refers to the average power during the entire 30 s of the test. The total work represents the product of the number of pedal revolutions accomplished and the force or resistance level during the 30-s period. The fatigue index measures the rate of power decrease from the point of peak anaerobic power to the finish of the test.

Physiological Rationale for the Wingate Test

On the fitness continuum, this 30-s all-out effort test may be appropriately referred to as a power-endurance test because it is predominantly dependent upon the combination of the anaerobic pathway's powerful phosphagenic component and its enduring glycolytic component. Hence, the WAnT reflects both short-anaerobic fitness and long-anaerobic fitness, with the combination of the phosphagenic and glycolytic pathways representing estimates as much as 85% of the ATP production during the entire 30 s of the Wingate Cycle Test.[18]

The Wingate Cycle Test is truly a supramaximal test when maximal oxygen consumption serves as the maximal reference point, because the WAnT requires a power level that is usually two-to-four times greater than the participant's maximal oxygen consumption.[7] Thus, the physiological basis of the Wingate Test is best understood by focusing mainly on the contributions of the anaerobic pathway to the major components of the Wingate Test.

Peak Anaerobic Power (Pk-AnP)

The peak anaerobic power mostly reflects the participant's ability to use the phosphagenic system at a rapid rate because peak AnP is usually determined within the first 5[22] or 8 s of the Wingate test.[28] Although the phosphagenic system contributes only about 23% of the total ATP produced during the entire 30-s period of the WAnT when performed

by aerobically trained men,[46] it is likely that the phosphagenic percentage would be greater than this if only the first 10 s is examined in the average person. However, contrary to earlier reports,[33,34] even in the first 10 s, the glycolytic pathway makes a significant contribution based on lactate values after the 10-s period that may be four times the resting value.[27]

Mean Anaerobic Power (M-AnP) and Total Work

Mean anaerobic power often has been referred to as anaerobic capacity, but in deference to an originator of the test, Dr. Bar-Or,[7] and a logical rationale, the term mean anaerobic power is preferred. M-AnP reflects the ability to transform energy from a combination of the phosphagenic and anaerobic glycolytic pathways. Whereas the phosphagenic pathway likely contributes most to pk-AnP, the glycolytic pathway appears to contribute most to a performer's mean anaerobic power and total work in a 30-s time period. Despite contributing as much as 49% of all the ATP,[46] and, therefore, being the main contributor during the Wingate Test, the glycolytic capacity is not fully utilized due to the short (30-s) duration of the test.[25] Thus, some investigators suggest that the term anaerobic capacity may be misleading,[26] despite the report[6] of its correlation with maximal oxygen debt. The 30-s duration of the Wingate test is certainly shorter than the 40 s[33] or 2 min[38] that may be required to exhaust the anaerobic capacity or maximize the lactate production volume. However, it is possible that the maximal *rate,* not total amount, of lactate production, which indicates anaerobic power[37] or power-endurance, may occur sometime during the Wingate test. The anaerobic glycolytic production of ATP is evidenced by the moderate-to-high blood lactate values (ranging from 6 to 15 times the resting value) measured in Wingate-test performers by various investigators.[26,41,44,48,49,51]

The phosphagenic contribution to the entire 30 s of the test was substantiated by investigators[26] who found that female subjects reduced their phosphagen levels to 70% of their original adenosine triphosphate values and 40% of their original creatine phosphate values after performing the Wingate Test.

Although the aerobic source of energy accounts for a lesser amount than the combined anaerobic sources, it too contributes from 9% to 19%,[22,29] or 28%,[22,46] or as high as 40%,[38] depending upon assumptions regarding efficiency, oxygen consumption time delay, and oxygen stores.[22]

Accuracy of the Wingate Test

As with all exercise physiology tests, their accuracy is mainly dependent upon their validity and reliability.

Validity

There is no "gold standard" anaerobic performance test by which to compare the scores of the Wingate Test. It might be argued that for the Wingate Test to have physiological validity, the performers with the highest lactate values after the Wingate Test would be expected to have the highest glycolytic or anaerobic capacities. In a validation study,[49] only a moderate relationship ($r = 0.55$ and 0.60) was found between anaerobic capacity (W and W·kg^{-1}) and blood lactates; the relationship between anaerobic capacity and maximal oxygen debt was slightly lower. They concluded that the test's validity was tenuous. However, because of the contributions of the phosphagenic and oxidative systems, the Wingate's validity should not be dependent upon its ability to incur maximal lactates. For example, the physiological validity was supported by investigators who found a significant relationship between both the peak anaerobic power (pk-AnP for 5 s) and the total work versus the fast-twitch fiber area and percentage.[28]

Its performance validity was supported by the high relationship between pk-AnP and the time for the 50-m run ($r = -.91$),[28] and the vertical jump;[35] low to moderate correlations have been reported between mean AnP and 50-m time ($r = -.79$),[42] and between total work and the 300-m run ($r = -.64; -.83$).[11,45] Further evidence of the test's validity is provided by the higher power outputs found in more elite cyclists than less elite cyclists.[50] Strength, as measured by peak torque of hip and leg extension, appears to be highly correlated ($r = .91$) with mean anaerobic power of trained athletes.[1]

Reliability

It appears that anaerobic power tests are similar in day-to-day variability as aerobic tests, that is, about 5% to 6%.[14,52] The variability of the Wingate Test is partly attributed to its reliability. Reliability coefficients (test-retest comparisons) for maximal anaerobic power/capacity are very high, usually ranging from a low of .89 in elderly pulmonary patients[9] to as high as .95 to .98.[8,10,18,25,28] The retesting reliability of the fatigue index can range from low values near .43 to moderate values near .73.[52]

Therefore, because the Wingate Test is a maximal-effort exercise bout for 30 s, it relies principally upon the two anaerobic pathways, and secondarily upon the oxidative (aerobic) metabolic pathway to produce ATP.[24,46]

Method

The methodology for the Wingate Test includes a brief description of the equipment, such as ergometer, counter, and timer; it also includes a description of the test procedures and calculations.

Equipment

Ergometer

Although isokinetic ergometers have been used,[32] mechanically braked cycle ergometers, such as Monark™, Bodyguard™, and Fleisch™, usually are used to perform the WAnT. These ergometers utilize a constant force concept, meaning that the resistance does not change during the course of the test. Thus, the speed of pedaling determines the power in the mechanically braked ergometers, whereas the force produced on the pedals by the performer determines the power on the isokinetic ergometers.[8] Constant power ergometers do not facilitate Wingate testing because the power on these bikes does not change throughout the course of the test. Probably the best type of mechanically braked ergometer is one in which the force (kg; N) can be applied immediately and accurately. One such ergometer (e.g., Monark #814E) has a peg or basket-type device (0.5 kg) onto which the desired weights can be dropped,

thus eliminating the oscillation that occurs in the swinging force-pendulum of some ergometers. The most popular Monark cycle has a knob that the technician turns to the proper force setting.

The popularity of the WAnT has inspired various corporations (e.g., International Tapetronics, Sports Medicine Industries, Medical Graphics) to either modify or computerize ergometers (e.g., CardiO$_2$™; WATCycle™) so that their software facilitates the procedures and calculations required of the test. Some of these systems have inexpensive software, but complete packages of ergometer, computer, and software can be very expensive. If a laboratory is fortunate enough to have such systems then a separate revolutions counter and a timer are not needed. Sophisticated automation allows electromagnets to feed pedal counts into the port of a microcomputer that can calculate on-line all of the test indices.

Revolutions Counter

Ideally, the cycle ergometer should have a device that automatically counts the pedal revolutions. An inexpensive mechanical counter works by extending a lever out to the circuitous path of the pedal, whereby it is "tripped" with each pedal revolution. Also, more sophisticated electronic and magnetic counters can be assembled on the ergometer rather inexpensively. If the cycle ergometer does not have an automatic counter, then a technician must count and record the revolutions.

Timing Apparatus

At least three types of timers can be used to administer the Wingate Test: a laboratory set-timer, a stopwatch, or the

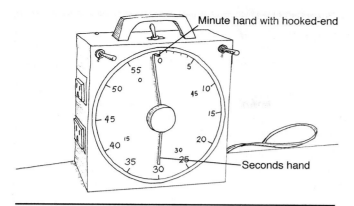

Figure 1 Laboratory set-clock (e.g., Gralab Universal Timer®).

timer attached to the ergometer. Any of these can monitor the 5-s time intervals and the total 30-s duration of the test.

The laboratory set-clock can be used to measure either elapsed time (i.e., continuous running time), or time remaining by setting it to buzz at the end of the test. Laboratory set-timers (e.g., Fig. 1) are preferable to wall clocks for either monitoring the time remaining, or the elapsed time, for any interval from 1 s to 60 min.

Elapsed time is the typical perception of time in an event. Thus, at the start and end of the WAnT, the timer displays zero and 30 s, respectively. The minute hand (hooked end) of the set-timer and its second hand make one counterclockwise revolution in 60 min and 60 s, respectively. Both hands of the elapsed timer are read on the inner circle of small numerals. The set-timer is set for elapsed time by moving both hands in a clockwise direction until they both rest on the small 0 (the same as the large 55).

Wall or built-in ergometer clocks may be used as elapsed timers. Also, the stopwatch mode on a wristwatch is an acceptable timer for the WAnT. Most laboratory facilities have wall clocks with second hands; however, these are recommended only if set-clocks are not available. Some ergometers have clocks built into the dashboard chassis. If stopwatches are used, technicians should secure them with a neck strap, just as one would treat an expensive camera.

Remaining time simply means that the timer displays 30 s at the start of the WAnT and zero seconds at the finish. The set-timer is set for remaining time by manually moving the minute hand in a clockwise direction to the outer-zero mark and the second hand to the outer-number 30; then the switch or knob is set to the buzzer label so that the sound occurs at the finish.

Weight Scale

An accurate platform beam scale or electronic digital scale may be used to measure the performer's body weight. Although body weight was not considered in the original Wingate test, it is now often used as the divisor to calculate the relative (e.g., $W \cdot kg^{-1}$) anaerobic power indices.[21]

Test Procedures

Teamwork among technicians is essential for the accurate administration of the WAnT; thus, the test procedures should be rehearsed prior to the actual test. Some of the factors to consider in the test procedures are (a) Preparation; (b) Wingate Test protocol, (c) force (load) selection, (d) timing/counting, and (e) calculations.

Preparation

Basic data, such as the performer's body weight, should be measured as described in Chapter UN. The performer's nude weight, or weight in scanty attire, or weight derived by subtracting the weight of the attire, should be recorded onto Form NC 1, along with the other basic data variables.

Meteorological data should be recorded on Form NC 1 even though environmental temperature, relative humidity, and the hydration of the performer do not affect the WAnT results.[16,25] High altitude, and its associated low barometric pressure, may be slightly influential as hypoxia was shown to affect marginally peak anaerobic power.[30]

Force (F) Setting. The body weight is not only necessary to derive relative power and work scores, but to prescribe the force (kg; N) setting on the arm or the cycle ergometer. The force selection varies with such factors as the general anaerobic fitness of the performer, gender, age, and the type of ergometer.[8] Obtaining the optimal force for each person would require testing that person several times. Thus, for practical reasons, equations are presented that may approximate the optimal force setting for a person. For leg ergometry by nonsedentary adult women and men on Monark™ and Bodyguard™ cycles[a], Equations 1 and 2 are recommended.[7,17,52] For anaerobically fit males and females, Equation 3 is recommended, whereby the force setting may range from 9.0%[47] or 9.4%[43] or 9.5%[50] to 10%[7,47] of body weight. For sedentary persons, or children and older adults, the traditional equations can be used for leg (Eq. 4) and arm[b] (Eq. 5) ergometry, respectively.[5,18,28,39]

Nonsedentary Adult Women:

$$\text{Leg Force } (\sim N^c) = \text{body wt (kg)} \times 0.86 \qquad \text{Eq. 1}$$

---

[a]For Fleisch ergometers, leg and arm ergometry uses 0.45 and 0.30, respectively. This is because the Fleisch flywheel goes 10 m per pedal revolution, not 6 m as the Monark; thus, the values represent 60% of the others.

[b]Monark arm ergometers have wheel perimeters of 1 m; the wheel covers a distance of 2.5 m per pedal revolution.

[c]The wavy approximate sign ($\sim$) indicates that kg is being converted to N by the rounded-off value of 1 kg = 10 N, not the exact value 1 kg = 9.80665 N. These forces can be expressed also in work units as joules per pedal revolution per kg body weight. The original prescribed force (Eq. 2) is equivalent to 4.4 $J \cdot rev^{-1} \cdot kg^{-1}$; eq. 1 = 5.59 $J \cdot rev^{-1} \cdot kg^{-1}$. If using a basket-loading ergometer, the basket itself represents 0.5 kg or 5 N. An example of $J \cdot rev^{-1} \cdot kg^{-1}$ for a 75.5 kg person is: If the F = 7.1 kg (or $\sim$71 N) and one revolution = 6 m, then 6 m $\times$ 71 N = 426 J; then dividing by 75.5 kg body weight = 5.53 $J \cdot rev^{-1} \cdot kg^{-1}$.

Nonsedentary Adult Men:

$$\text{Leg Force } (\sim N) = \text{body wt (kg)} \times 0.90 \qquad \text{Eq. 2}$$

Anaerobically Fit Persons (Athletes):

$$\text{Leg Force } (\sim N) = \text{body wt (kg)} \times 0.90 \text{ to } 1.0 \qquad \text{Eq. 3}$$

Children, Older Adults, and Sedentary Persons:

$$\text{Leg-Force } (\sim N) = \text{body wt (kg)} \times 0.75 \qquad \text{Eq. 4}$$

$$\text{Arm-Force } (\sim N) = \text{body wt (kg)} \times 0.5 \qquad \text{Eq. 5}$$

For example, if the body weight of a sedentary person is 67.7 kg, then the load (F) setting for leg ergometry is calculated as

$$F (\sim N) = 67.7 \times 0.75 = 50.7 = 51 \text{ N (or 5.1 kg)}$$

Whereas the leg-force setting in non-anaerobically fit persons (Eq. 4) represents about 7.5% of kilogram body weight, the force setting in Equation 1 represents 9.0% to 10% body weight. Force settings between 8.5% to 9.5% of kilogram body weight are likely to elicit greater anaerobic indices for young men[12,43] and female softball players.[47] However, it appears that resistance settings greater than 10% of body weight do not enhance Wingate scores.[15] Although nothing short of having to perform two trials at different force settings to rectify it, the force necessary to yield optimal peak power in the WAnT is greater than the force necessary to yield optimal mean power.[17,43]

Seat Height. After the performer's force setting is recorded onto Form NC 1, the technician should adjust the seat height so that the performer's knee is slightly bent when the ball of the foot is on the pedal. Most cycle ergometers have seat posts labeled with heights, which then can be recorded onto the performer's data collection form.

Wingate Test Protocol

The Wingate protocol (Table 1) has five distinct time periods: (1) prior exercise, (2) recovery interval, (3) acceleration period, (4) Wingate Test,[6,8] and (5) cool-down period.

As with the other anaerobic tests, **prior exercise** is recommended for both safety (e.g., ischemic prevention)[3,4] and performance reasons. The warmup includes 5 min of low-intensity pedaling at about 50 to 60 rpm, interspersed by four to five all-out sprints of 4- to 6-s duration; the sprints should progressively increase in resistance (force) so that by the fourth or fifth sprint the prescribed resistance for the Wingate Test is reached.[8,23]

The **recovery interval** between the end of the prior exercise and the beginning of the Wingate Test should not be less than 2 min after the prior exercise, nor more than 5 min after the warmup portion of the prior exercise. The 2-min minimum provides some time for the performer's recovery from any possible fatigue that may have occurred during the warmup, and allows both performer and technicians to collect their thoughts about the ensuing test. The 5-min maximum still retains muscle temperature and blood flow to a significant extent. The activity during the recovery in-

Table 1 Wingate Test Protocol		
Period	**Time Length**	**Activity**
Prior Exercise	5 min	Cycle at low intensity; intersperse with 4–5 sprints of 4–6 s at prescribed force (F).
Recovery Interval	2–5 min	Rest or cycle slowly against minimal F.
Acceleration Period	6–15 s	1st phase: Cycle for 5–10 s at one-third prescribed F at 20–50 rpm. 2nd phase: Cycle 1–5 s against approach to prescribed F at near-maximal rpm.
Wingate Test	30 s	Cycle at highest rpm possible against prescribed F.
Cool-Down Period	2–3 min	Cycling at low to moderate aerobic power level (e.g., 25–100 W).

terval may consist of simply resting while seated on the bike or pedaling at a minimal resistance (e.g., 1 kg or 10 N at an rpm between 10 and 20; about 10–20 W).

The **acceleration period** consists of two brief phases beginning immediately after the recovery interval. In the first phase, the performer pedals at about 20 to 50 rpm for about 5 to 10 s at a resistance which is about one-third of that prescribed from one of the chosen equations. In the second phase, the performer increases the rpm to a near-maximal rate while the technician loads the prescribed force (F) setting immediately, if using a basket-loaded ergometer, or within 3, 4, or 5 s if using a pendulum-loaded ergometer. The total acceleration period, therefore, may last for as little as 6 s or as long as 15 s.

The actual **Wingate Test duration** of all-out cycling is 30 s. It begins at the end of the acceleration period and divides the 30-s period into six continuous time intervals of 5 s each. The performer continuously tries to obtain the highest number of revolutions during each 5-s interval. For example, the performer does not pace the effort so that the last 5-s interval contains as many revolutions as the previous 5-s intervals. Thus, the test can be described as a rush to the peak power and a fading to the lowest power.

The **cool-down** period lasts for 2 to 3 min[8] and consists of pedaling at a low to moderate power level on the cycle ergometer immediately after the Wingate Test. Thus, the force setting can be set between 5 and 20 N, and the revolutions at 50 rpm to produce between 25 and 100 W. If, for some reason a repeat test on the same person and on the same day is necessary, then about 10 minutes of recovery is recommended.[2,20]

Timer, Force-Setter, Revolutions Counter, and Recorder

One technician is needed to serve as the timer for the Wingate protocol time periods, especially the 5-s intervals and the duration of the test. At least three other technicians and the performer must pay close attention to the timer in order to perform their roles effectively. These other technicians may be called the force-setter, the revolutions-counter, and the recorder. After coordinating the Wingate protocol periods for prior exercise, recovery interval, and the acceleration period, the timer officially begins the test itself as soon as the force-setter finishes setting the prescribed resistance. The force-setter yells, "Start!" or "Go!" when the prescribed load is set. The timer begins the clock, and the performer begins pedalling as fast as possible for a 30-s period while remaining seated on the bike during this time. The timer shouts the time every 5 s, while the force-setter maintains the prescribed setting on the bike ergometer. The counter shouts the number of pedal revolutions for the respective 5-s intervals by observing the number of times the left or right pedal makes a complete rotation from the original pedal position at the "GO" signal. The counter gives the whole, not fractional, number of revolutions for each 5-s interval. For example, when the timer yells "five seconds," if the pedal is at half of a complete rotation after having made 10 complete revolutions, the counter tells the recorder "ten," not "ten and a half." The counter then counts the completion of that half-rotation as a whole revolution for the next 5-s interval. Usually, the count starts over at "one," but sometimes the number can be continued, for example, as "eleven."

The recorder records each 5-s value onto Form NC 1. At the end of 30 s the timer yells, "End!" or "Stop!" or the buzzer of the laboratory set-timer signals the end of the test. At this time, the force-setter lowers the force setting to a cool-down recovery setting (usually between 10 and 20 N; 1–2 kg) while the performer continues pedalling comfortably at about 50 rpm for 2 to 3 min.

It should be evident why sophisticated computers can enhance the accuracy of the WAnT by precisely recording the exact pedal position at the exact time. If an inexpensive automatic counter is attached to the ergometer, then the counter technician can simply record the observed number at the Start or Go command of the timer and the subsequent numbers at 5-s intervals.

Summary of Preparation and Procedural Steps

Preparation

1. Body weight is measured and recorded as described in Chapter UN.
2. The force (resistance) is prescribed using the appropriate equation (1–5).
3. Ergometer seat is adjusted so that performer has slight bend at knee.
4. The technician tells the performer that the test requires an all-out effort but is a brief test.
5. The Wingate protocol for (1) prior exercise; (2) recovery interval; and (3) acceleration period is followed according to Table 1.

Procedures

1. The force-setter dictates the start of the WAnT by applying the prescribed force.

2. The timer shouts "GO!" or "Start!"; the performer pedals at an all-out rate.
3. The revolutions-counter mentally notes the position of the performer's pedal at the timer's "GO" signal and starts counting pedal revolutions.
4. The timer shouts the elapsed time every five seconds: "5," "10," etc.
5. The counter tells the recorder how many revolutions occurred during each 5-s interval during the 30-s period; the recorder records these values on Form NC 1.
6. The force-setter ensures that the prescribed force is sustained throughout the 30-s test.
7. Technicians motivate the performer throughout the test.
8. At the 30th second the force-setter lowers the resistance to about 10–20 N (1–2 kg) as the performer pedals at about 50 rpm for 2–3 min.
9. Calculations are made to derive the peak anaerobic power, total work, mean anaerobic power, and fatigue index.

Calculations

Although data collection and calculations can be performed by a computer interfaced with the appropriate hardware and software,[40] the calculations described here are performed without such means. Calculations are made to derive such indices of the WAnT as: (1) peak anaerobic power (pk-AnP) expressed in watt (W) and relative watts (W·kg^{-1}); (2) total work (w) expressed in joules (J) or kilojoules (kJ) and relative joules (J·kg^{-1}); (3) mean anaerobic power (M-AnP) expressed the same as pk-AnP; and (4) fatigue index (FI) expressed as a percentage (%).

Peak Anaerobic Power (Pk-AnP). Peak anaerobic power should be expressed in the scientifically accepted unit of watts. To facilitate this, it is probably best to use the newton (N) unit as the expression for force (F), the newton meter (N·m) or joule (J) as the expression for work (w), and the newton meter per minute or per second (n·m·min^{-1}; N·m·s^{-1}) because of the relative ease in converting them to watts. Although automated systems can derive the peak power for a specific second, the hand-calculated method derives the average peak power for a 5-s interval (N·m-5 s). Thus, Equation 6 is used, based on the law that power is the rate of work (P = w·t^{-1}). The work component in Equation 6 is represented by the first part of the equation whereby the force (F) setting (N) is multiplied by the distance traveled in 5 s, which is the product of the highest number of revolutions (Rmax) among the 5-s intervals (usually the first or second 5-s interval) and six—the rounded-off distance in meters that the Monark cycle's wheel^{d} travels for each pedal revo-

---

^{d}The precise circumference of the Monark cycle's flywheel is 1.62 m, and travels 6 m for every pedal revolution. Monark arm ergometers have wheel perimeters of 1 m; the wheel covers a distance of 2.5 m per pedal revolution. Fleisch ergometer's wheels travel 10 m per pedal revolution. The Bodyguard™ ergometer's flywheel is only 0.73 m in circumference;[19] one pedal revolution = 8.2 revolutions of the Bodyguard's flywheel, thus achieving an effective distance of 300 m at 50 rpm (0.73 × 8.2 × 50) in 1 min.

lution. The product of these two products is then divided by the time component, 5 s.

$$\text{Power} = \text{work} / \text{time}$$
$$\text{Force} \quad \text{Distance}$$
$$\text{Pk-AnP (N·m·s}^{-1}\text{; W)} = [N \times (Rmax \times 6)] / 5 \quad \text{Eq. 6}$$

For example, if a person's highest 5-s interval was 12 revolutions at a force setting of 45 N on a Monark cycle ergometer in which the wheel's perimeter travels 6 m per pedal revolution, then a Pk-AnP of 648 W would be calculated from Equation 6 as follows:

$$\text{Pk-AnP (N·m·s}^{-1}\text{; W)} = [45 \text{ N} \times (12 \text{ Rmax} \times 6 \text{ m})] / 5$$
$$= (45 \text{ N} \times 72 \text{ m}) / 5$$
$$= 3240 \text{ N·m} / 5$$
$$= 648$$

Relative Peak Anaerobic Power (rel-pk-AnP). Because relative anaerobic power is often more important than absolute power,[21] Wingate scores that are expressed in watts are often divided by body weight (Eqs. 7 and 9). Thus, the score to indicate relative (rel) pk-AnP is expressed in units of W·kg^{-1}.

$$\text{rel-pk-AnP (W·kg}^{-1}\text{)} = W/kg \quad \text{Eq. 7}$$

If the person in our previous example weighed 60 kg, then rel-pk-AnP is calculated simply by dividing the respective watts by the 60-kg body weight. Thus, the rel-pk-AnP of 10.8 W·kg^{-1} is found by dividing 648 W by 60 kg.

Total Work (w). Total work is based upon the total number of revolutions at the end of the 30 s. If an automated counter was reset to zero at the start of the test, then the counter's display at the end of 30 s is the total number of revolutions. But if the counter was not reset to zero, then the number on the counter at the start of the test must be subtracted from the final 30-s total. If the revolutions were counted by a technician's observation, then the total number of revolutions is the sum of the six 5-s revolutions. Equation 8 uses the same principle as the work portion of Equation 6 except that the number of revolutions in 30 s replaces the number in 5 s.

$$\text{w (N·m; J)} = N \times (R \text{ in } 30 \text{ s} \times 6 \text{ m}) \quad \text{Eq. 8}$$

Using the same person as an example, if a total of 52 revolutions in the 30-s period were made, then total work would be calculated from Equation 8 as follows:

$$\text{w (N·m; J)} = 45 \text{ N} \times 52 \text{ R in } 30 \text{ s} \times 6 \text{ m}$$
$$= 14,040 \text{ N·m} = 14,040 \text{ J} = 14.04 \text{ kJ}$$

Relative Total Work (rel-w). Relative total work (J·kg^{-1}) can be normalized for weight by dividing the total work by body weight as dictated by Equation 9.

$$\text{rel-w} = w \text{ (J)} \div \text{body wt (kg)} \quad \text{Eq. 9}$$

For example, that same 60-kg person accomplishing 14,040 J in 30 s would have a relative total work of 234 J·kg^{-1} based on the following calculation:

$$\text{rel-w} = 14,040 \text{ J} \div 60 \text{ kg}$$
$$= 234 \text{ (J·kg}^{-1}\text{)}$$

Mean Anaerobic Power (M-AnP). The average anaerobic power (W) during the test is calculated from Equation 10 simply by dividing the total work (J) by 30 s.

$$\text{M-AnP (W; J·s}^{-1}\text{)} = \text{total w (J)} / 30 \text{ s} \quad \text{Eq. 10}$$

For example, the person accomplishing 14,040 J in 30 s would have a M-AnP of 468 W based on the following calculation:

$$\text{M-AnP (W; J·s}^{-1}\text{)} = 14,040 \text{ J} / 30 \text{ s}$$
$$= 468 \text{ J·s}^{-1} = 468 \text{ W}$$

Relative Mean Anaerobic Power (rel-M-AnP). The relative mean anaerobic power (W·kg^{-1}) is found by dividing the M-AnP (W) by the body weight (kg) as in Equation 11.

$$\text{rel-M-AnP (W·kg}^{-1}\text{)} = \text{M-AnP (W)} / \text{body wt (kg)} \quad \text{Eq. 11}$$

For example, the 60-kg person with a M-AnP of 468 W would have a rel-M-AnP of 7.8 W·kg^{-1} based on the following calculation:

$$\text{rel-M-AnP (W·kg}^{-1}\text{)} = 468 \text{ W} / 60 \text{ kg}$$
$$= 7.8 \text{ W·kg}^{-1}$$

Fatigue Index (FI). The fatigue index indicates the degree of decrease in power from the pk-AnP to the lowest AnP. The higher the person's percentage value the greater is the decrease. The power output may decline due to fatigue by 40%[22] or more from the first 5-s period to the last 5-s period. Equation 12 shows that FI (%) is calculated by dividing the difference between the pk-AnP (W) and the lowest AnP (W) by the pk-AnP, and then multiplying by 100 to get a percentage. Usually the lowest AnP is calculated from the last 5-s interval because it has the lowest number of revolutions.

$$\text{FI (\%)} = [(\text{pk-AnP} - \text{lowest AnP}) / \text{pk-AnP}] \times 100 \quad \text{Eq. 12}$$

For example, if the pk-AnP is 648 W and the lowest AnP is 300 W, then the FI % is 54% based on the following calculation:

$$\text{FI (\%)} = [(648 \text{ W} - 300 \text{ W}) / 648] \times 100$$
$$= (348 \text{ W} / 648 \text{ W}) \times 100$$
$$= 54\%$$

Hence, this person's power declined by 54% from the pk-AnP to the lowest AnP.

Summary of Calculations. Although these calculations and indices can be quite intimidating at first, they can serve

Table 2 Comparative Scores for the Wingate Bike Test

Group	F-Set	Pk-AnP	Rel-Pk-AnP	Total w	M-AnP	Rel-M-AnP
Males	%wt	W	W·kg^{-1}	kJ	W	W·kg^{-1}
Normals						
18–29 y[23]	7.5	540	8.2	13.5	450	7.0
25–34 y	7.5	700	9.2	16.2	540	7.2
35–44 y	7.5	660	8.6			
18–28 y[35]	7.5				563	7.3
Athletes[28]	7.5		11.8			
Cyclists[50]						
Category II–IV	9.5	963	13.3		783	10.8
Ice Hockey[39]	7.5			15.6		
Volleyball Olympians[49]	10.0			23.9	797	9.1
Sprinters[45]	9.0		14.2	23.9		
Nondesignated[22]	9.5	1064		25		
Females						
PE Majors[25]	~7.7	561	9.0		453	7.2
Softball Players[47]	7; 8		9.1; 9.6			
	9; 10		10.8; 11.1			

as another way to become familiar with a few physical principles and the common terms and expressions used by exercise physiologists. It can be helpful to visualize a person's WAnT performance by plotting the power values (vertical axis) for the six 5-s time intervals (horizontal axis) using the graph on Form NC 2.

Results and Discussion

High scores on the WAnT are meant to indicate high anaerobic fitness. Some of those anaerobic factors reportedly[52] associated with higher scores are (1) greater capacity to produce lactic acid; (2) greater stores of the phosphagens; (3) greater buffering capacity; and (4) a combination of greater motivation and greater tolerance of discomfort. As mentioned previously in the introduction to this test, however, aerobic metabolism, thus aerobic fitness, plays a small but significant part in this 30-s exercise bout.

Although it would be impossible for persons to maintain their peak or mean Wingate anaerobic power for an entire minute, these anaerobic indices make for an interesting comparison with minute-based power levels that are frequently prescribed for aerobic cycle ergometry. For example, 200 W might be considered a heavy aerobic intensity for typical males, whereas their mean anaerobic powers of 700 W[13] from the WAnT would not be unusual.

The scores presented in Table 2 are for comparative purposes. They should not be used to classify people because they are not based upon large representative samples nor equal force settings. Also, some studies may have used toe stirrups, which may increase peak and mean anaerobic power by 5–12%.[31] When comparing genders, there are large differences between average men and women when peak and mean anaerobic power are expressed in absolute

terms, but these differences are minimized when expressed in relative terms of body weight or fat-free mass.[35] Scores for male children and adolescents are available,[23] as are those for the men's U.S. Olympic volleyball team.[49] The Olympians were tested with the force setting at 10%, instead of 7.5%, of the body weight. The Olympians averaged 46.5 pedal revolutions in the 30-s period. By varying the force setting for the female softball players, higher peak powers were elicited for the higher settings (9% and 10% of body weight) than for the lower ones (7% and 8%).[47] Some values in the table are based upon a force setting of 9.5% body weight.[22] The percentiles listed in Tables 3, 4, and 5 are based on men and women between the ages of 18 and 28 y.[36] The average men's and women's peak anaerobic powers are about 700 W and 454 W, respectively; their relative peak anaerobic powers are about 9.2 W·kg^{-1} and 7.6 W·kg^{-1}, respectively. The mean anaerobic powers are about 563 W and 381 W, respectively; their relative mean anaerobic powers are about 7.3 W·kg^{-1} and 6.3 W·kg^{-1}, respectively.

Anaerobic power and work values in a wide age-range of adults are scarce in the literature. However, the values from one group of investigators[32] may be helpful despite their use of an isokinetic cycle ergometer, which makes comparisons with the traditional mechanically braked ergometer's scores less valid. Their participants, aged 15–71 y, pedalled with maximal effort for 30 s at a constant 60 rpm. The torque exerted on the pedals, which allowed the calculation of peak power, mean power, and total work, showed a 6% decrease in these indices for each age decade, but not for the fatigue index. (The participants' peak and mean powers were also related to lean thigh volume). As with the norms in Tables 3 and 4, the values in this wider age group demonstrated that the women's anaerobic indices were about two-thirds of the men's values (see Fig. 2).

Table 3 Percentile (%ile) Norms for Pk-AnP (W) and Rel-Pk-AnP (W·kg⁻¹) for the Wingate Test in Physically Active Men ($n = 62$) and Women ($n = 68$) Ages 18–28 y

%ile Rank	Pk-Anaerobic Power (W)		Relative-Pk-AnP (W·kg⁻¹)	
	Men (W)	Women (W)	Men (W·kg⁻¹)	Women (W·kg⁻¹)
95	867	602	11.1	9.3
90	822	560	10.9	9.0
85	807	530	10.6	8.9
80	777	527	10.4	8.8
75	768	518	10.4	8.6
70	757	505	10.2	8.5
65	744	493	10.0	8.3
60	721	480	9.8	8.1
55	706	464	9.5	7.8
50	689	449	9.2	7.6
45	678	447	9.0	7.2
40	671	432	8.9	7.0
35	662	418	8.6	7.0
30	656	399	8.5	6.9
25	646	396	8.3	6.8
20	618	376	8.2	6.6
15	594	362	7.4	6.4
10	570	353	7.1	6.0
5	530	329	6.6	5.7
M	699.5	454.5	9.18	7.61
SD	94.7	81.3	1.43	1.24
Minimum	500	239	5.3	4.6
Maximum	927	623	11.9	10.64

From P. J. Maud and B. B. Schultz, *Research Quarterly for Exercise and Sport, 60*(2), p. 147, 1989. Copyright © 1989 AAHPERD, 1900 Association Dr., Reston, VA 22091.

Table 4 Percentile (%ile) Norms for M-AnP (W) and Rel-M-AnP (W·kg⁻¹) for the Wingate Test in Physically Active Men ($n = 60$) and Women ($n = 69$) Ages 18–28 y

%ile Rank	M-Anaerobic Power (W)		Relative-M-AnP (W·kg⁻¹)	
	Men (W)	Women (W)	Men (W·kg⁻¹)	Women (W·kg⁻¹)
95	677	483	8.63	7.5
90	662	470	8.24	7.3
85	631	437	8.09	7.1
80	618	419	8.01	7.0
75	604	414	7.96	6.9
70	600	410	7.91	6.8
65	592	402	7.70	6.7
60	577	391	7.59	6.6
55	575	386	7.46	6.5
50	565	381	7.44	6.4
45	553	377	7.26	6.2
40	548	367	7.14	6.15
35	535	361	7.08	6.13
30	530	353	7.00	6.0
25	521	347	6.79	5.9
20	496	337	6.59	5.7
15	485	320	6.39	5.6
10	471	306	5.98	5.3
5	453	287	5.56	5.1
M	562.7	381	7.28	6.35
SD	66.5	56.4	0.88	0.73
Minimum	441	235	4.6	4.5
Maximum	711	529	9.1	8.1

From P. J. Maud and B. B. Schultz, *Research Quarterly for Exercise and Sport, 60*(2), p. 146, 1989. Copyright © 1989 AAHPERD, 1900 Association Dr., Reston, VA 22091.

Table 5 Percentiles (%ile) for Fatigue Index of the Wingate Test in Physically Active Men ($n = 52$) and Women ($n = 50$) Ages 18–28 y

%ile	Fatigue Index (%)	
	Men (%)	Women (%)
95	55	48
90	52	47
85	47	44
80	46.7	43.6
75	45	42
70	43	40
65	42	39
60	40	38
55	39	38
50	38	35
45	37	34
40	35	33.7
35	34	31
30	31	29
25	30	28
20	29.5	26
15	27	25
10	23	25
5	21	20
M	37.7	35.0
SD	9.9	8.3
Minimum	15	18
Maximum	58	49

From P. J. Maud and B. B. Schultz, *Research Quarterly for Exercise and Sport, 60*(2), p. 148, 1989. Copyright © 1989 AAHPERD, 1900 Association Dr., Reston, VA 22091.

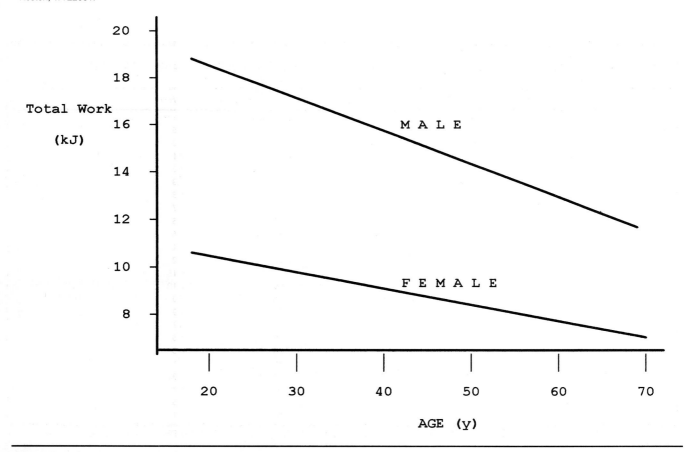

Figure 2 The relationship between age and total work (kJ) in males and females 15 to 70 y of age. Modified from Makrides, L., Heigenhauser, G. J. F., McCartney, N., & Jones, N. L. (1985). Maximal short term exercise capacity in healthy subjects aged 15–70 years. *Clinical Science, 69,* 200.

References

1. Abler, P., Foster, C., Thompson, N. N., Crowe, M., Alt, K., Brophy, A., & Palin, W. D. (1986). Determinants of anaerobic muscular performance. *Medicine and Science in Sports and Exercise, 18,* Abstract #3, S1.

2. Ainsworth, B. E., Serfass, R. C., & Leon, A. S. (1993). Effects of recovery duration and blood lactate level on power output during cycling. *Canadian Journal of Applied Physiology, 18,* 19–30.

3. Barnard, R. J. (1975). Warm-up is important for the heart. *Sports Medicine Bulletin, 10*(1): 6.

4. Barnard, R. J., Gardner, G. W., Diaco, N. V., MacAlpin, R. N., & Kattus, A. A. (1973). Cardiovascular responses to sudden strenuous exercise—heart rate, blood pressure, and ECG. *Journal of Applied Physiology, 34,* 833–837.

5. Bar-Or, O. (1978). A new anaerobic capacity test: Characteristics applications. Proceedings of the 21st World Congress in Sports Medicine at Brasilia.

6. Bar-Or, O. (1981). Le test anaerobie de Wingate. *Symbiosis, 13,* 157–172.

7. Bar-Or, O. (1987). The Wingate Anaerobic Test: An update on methodology, reliability, and validity. *Sports Medicine, 4,* 381–394.

8. Bar-Or, O. (1994). *Testing of anaerobic performance by the Wingate Anaerobic Test.* Bloomington, IL: ERS Tech, Inc.

9. Bar-Or, O., Berman, L., & Salsberg, A. (1992). An abbreviated Wingate anaerobic test for women and men of advanced age, *Medicine and Science in Sports and Exercise, 24,* Abstract, S22.

10. Bar-Or, O., Dotan, R., & Inbar, O. (1977). A 30-second all-out ergometric test: Its reliability and validity for anaerobic capacity. *Israel Journal of Medical Science, 13,* Abstract, 326.

11. Bar-Or, O., & Inbar, O. (1978). Relationships among anaerobic capacity, sprint and middle distance running of school children. In R. J. Shephard & H. Lavallee (Eds.), *Physical fitness assessment—Principles, practice and application,* 142–147. Springfield, IL: Charles C Thomas.

12. Beld, K., Skinner, J. S., & Tran, Z. V. (1989). Load optimization for peak and mean power output on the Wingate Anaerobic Test. *Medicine and Science in Sports and Exercise, 21* (Suppl., 2), Abstract #164, S28.

13. Bulbulian, R., Jeong, J.-W., & Murphy, M. (1996). Comparison of anaerobic components of the Wingate and Critical Poser tests in males and females. *Medicine and Science in Sports and Exercise, 28,* 1336–1341.

14. Coggan, A. R., & Costill, D. L. (1983). Day-to-day variability of three bicycle ergometer tests of anaerobic power. *Medicine and Science in Sports and Exercise, 15,* Abstract #1, 141.

15. Davy, K., Pizza, F., Guastella, P., McGuire, J., & Wygand, J. (1989). Optimal loading of Wingate power testing in conditioned athletes. *Medicine and Science in Sports and Exercise, 21* (Suppl., 2), Abstract #160, S27.

16. Dotan, R., & Bar-Or, O. (1980). Climatic heat stress and performance in the Wingate anaerobic test. *European Journal of Applied Physiology, 44,* 237–243.

17. Dotan, R., & Bar-Or, O. (1983). Load optimization for the Wingate anaerobic test. *European Journal of Applied Physiology, 51,* 409–417.

18. Evans, J. A., & Quinney, H. A. (1981). Determination of resistance settings for anaerobic power testing. *Canadian Journal of Applied Sport Science, 6,* 53–56.

19. Gledhill, N., & Jamnik, R. (1995). Determining power outputs for cycle ergometers with different sized flywheels. *Medicine and Science in Sports and Exercise, 27,* 134–135.

20. Hebestreit, H., Mimura, K., & Bar-Or, O. (1993). Recovery of anaerobic muscle power following 30 s supramaximal exercise: Comparison between boys and men. *Journal of Applied Physiology, 74,* 2875–2880.

21. Henrich, T. W., Hasson, S. M., Gadberry, W. G., Fang, F., & Barnes, W. S. (1986). The relationship between absolute and relative leg power. *Medicine and Science in Sports and Exercise, 18* (2), Abstract, S6–7.

22. Hill, D. W., & Smith, J. C. (1992). Calculation of aerobic contribution during high intensity exercise. *Research Quarterly for Exercise and Sport, 63,* 85–88.

23. Inbar, O., & Bar-Or, O. (1986). Anaerobic characteristics in male children and adolescents. *Medicine and Science in Sports and Exercise, 18,* 264–269.

24. Inbar, O., Dotan, R., & Bar-Or, O. (1976). Aerobic and anaerobic component of a thirty-second supramaximal cycling test. *Medicine and Science in Sports, 8,* 51.

25. Jacobs, I. (1980). The effects of thermal dehydration on performance of the Wingate Anaerobic Test. *International Journal of Sports Medicine, 1,* 21–24.

26. Jacobs, I., Bar-Or, O., Karlsson, J., Dotan, R., Tesch, P., Kaiser, P., & Inbar, O. (1982). Changes in muscle metabolites in females with 30-s exhaustive exercise. *Medicine and Science in Sports and Exercise, 14*(6) 457–460.

27. Jacobs, I., Tesch, P. A., Bar-Or, O., Karlsson, J., & Dotan, R. (1983). Lactate in human skeletal muscle after 10 and 30 s of supramaximal exercise. *Journal of Applied Physiology: Respiratory, Environmental, Exercise Physiology, 55,* 365–367.

28. Kaczkowski, W., Montgomery, D. L., Taylor, A. W., & Klissourous, V. (1982). The relationship between muscle fiber composition and maximal anaerobic power and capacity. *Journal of Sports Medicine and Physical Fitness, 22,* 407–413.

29. Kavanagh, M. F., & Jacobs, I. (1988). Breath-by-breath oxygen consumption during performance of the Wingate Test. *Canadian Journal of Sport Sciences, 13,* 91–93.

30. Kavanagh, M. F., Jacobs, I., Pope, J., Symons, D., & Hermiston, A. (1986). The effects of hypoxia on performance of the Wingate Anaerobic Power Test (WAnT). *Canadian Journal of Applied Sport Sciences, 11,* Abstract 22P.

31. LaVoie, N. F., Dallaire, J., Brayne, S., & Barrett, D. (1984). Anaerobic testing using the Wingate and Evans-Quinney protocols with and without toe stirrups. *Canadian Journal of Applied Sport Sciences, 9,* 1–5.

32. Makrides, L., Heigenhauser, G. J. F., McCartney, N., & Jones, N. L. (1985). Maximal short term exercise capacity in healthy subjects aged 15–70 years. *Clinical Science, 69,* 197–205.

33. Margaria, R., Cerretelli, P., & Mangili, F. (1964). Balance and kinetics of anaerobic energy release during strenuous exercise in man. *Journal of Applied Physiology, 19,* 623–628.

34. Margaria, R., Oliva, D., DiPrampero, P. E., & Cerretelli, P. (1969). Energy utilization in intermittent exercise of supramaximal intensity. *Journal of Applied Physiology, 26,* 752–756.

35. Maud, P. J., & Schultz, B. B. (1986). Gender comparisons in anaerobic power and capacity tests. *British Journal of Sports Medicine, 20,* 51–54.

36. Maud, P. J., & Schultz, B. B. (1989). Norms for the Wingate Anaerobic Test with comparison to another similar test. *Research Quarterly for Exercise and Sport, 60*(2), 144–151.

37. Medbo, J. I., & Burgers, S. (1990). Effect of training on the anaerobic capacity. *Medicine and Science in Sports and Exercise, 22,* 501–507.

38. Medbo, J. I., Mohn, A. C., Tabata, I., Bahr, R., Vaage, O., & Sejersted, O. M. (1989). Anaerobic capacity determined by maximal accumulated O_2 deficit. *Journal of Applied Physiology, 64,* 50–60.

39. Montgomery, D. L. (1982). The effect of added weight on ice hockey performance. *The Physician and Sportsmedicine* (Nov.): 91–95, 99.

40. Nicklin, R. C., O'Bryant, H. S., Zehnbauer, T. M., & Collins, M. A.. (1990). A computerized method for assessing anaerobic power and work capacity using maximal cycle ergometry. *Journal of Applied Sports Science Research, 4,* 135–140.

41. Pate, R. R., Goodyear, L., Dover, V., Dorociak, J., & McDaniel, J. (1983). Maximal oxygen deficit: A test of anaerobic capacity. *Medicine and Science in Sports and Exercise, 15*(2): Abstract, 121–122.

42. Patton, J. F., & Duggan, A. (1987). An evaluation of tests of anaerobic power. *Aviation, Space, and Environmental Medicine, 58,* 237–242.

43. Patton, J. F., Murphy, M. M., & Frederick, F. A. (1985). Maximal power outputs during the Wingate anaerobic test. *International Journal of Sports Medicine, 6,* 82–85.

44. Perez, H. R., Ywgand, J. W., Kowalski, A., Smith, T. K., & Otto, R. M. (1986). A comparison of the Wingate Power Test to bicycle time trial performance. *Medicine and Science in Sports and Exercise, 18* (Suppl., 2), Abstract #1, S1.

45. Scott, C. B., Roby, F. B., Lohman, T. G., & Bunt, J. C. (1991). The maximally accumulated oxygen deficit as an indicator of anaerobic capacity. *Medicine and Science in Sports and Exercise, 23,* 618–624.

46. Serresse, O., Lortie, G., Bouchard, C., & Boulay, M. R. (1988). Estimation of the contribution of the various energy systems during maximal work of short duration. *International Journal of Sports Medicine, 9,* 456–460.

47. Shaw, K., Davy, K., Coleman, C., & Kamimukai, C. (1988). Optimal resistance loading of the Wingate Power Test in female softball players. *Medicine and Science in Sports and Exercise, 20* (Suppl., 2), Abstract #105, S18.

48. Song, T. K., Serresse, O., Ama, P., Theriault, G., Boulay, M. R., & Bouchard, C. (1988). Effects of three anaerobic tests on venous blood values. *Medicine and Science in Sports and Exercise, 20* (Suppl., 2), Abstract #229, S39.

49. Tamayo, M., Sucec, A., Phillips, W., Laubach, L., Frey, M., & Buono, M. (1984). The Wingate anaerobic power test, peak blood lactate, and maximal oxygen debt for elite male volleyball players: A validation study. *Medicine and Science in Sports and Exercise, 16* (2): Abstract #10, 126.

50. Tanaka, H., Bassett, D. R., Swensen, T. C., & Sampredo, R. M. (1993). Aerobic and anaerobic power characteristics of competitive cyclists in the United States Cycling Federation. *International Journal of Sports Medicine, 14,* 334–338.

51. Thompson, N. N., Foster, C., Crowe, M., Rogowski, B., & Kaplan, K. (1986). Serial responses of anaerobic muscular performance in competitive athletes. *Medicine and Science in Sports and Exercise, 18* (Suppl.), Abstract, S1.

52. Vandewalle, H., Peres, G., & Monod, H. (1987). Standard anaerobic exercise tests. *Sports Medicine, 4,* 268–289.

Form *NC 1*

Individual Data for Wingate Cycle Test

Name: TOYA HART Date: 10-4-99 Age: 22 y

Gender (M or F): F Ht. 69 in. 175 cm

Body Wt 64 kg × 0.075 = Prescribed Force (F) Setting 4.8 kg; × 10 = 48 N Seat Ht. [ ]

Toe Clips: Yes ✓ No [ ] T 21 °C RH 64 % P_B 750 torr

Technicians' Initials: Force-Setter [ ] Timer [ ] Counter [ ]

Time Interval (5 s)	0–5	5–10	10–15	15–20	20–25	25–30	Total
Pedal Revolutions (Rmax; circle highest)	7	10	9	9	7	7	49

Calculations:

Peak-AnP (W) = (Rmax [ ] in 5 s × 6 m^a × F [ ] N) ÷ 5

= [ ] N · m-5 s ÷ 5

= [ ] W

Rel Peak-AnP (W·kg^{-1}) = [ ] W/ [ ] kg body wt

= [ ] W·kg^{-1}

Total work (N·m-30 s) = [ ] Total R in 30 s × 6 m × [ ] N

= [ ] N·m-30 s; = [ ] J = [ ] kJ

Mean-AnP (W) = [ ] J-30 s ÷ 30 = [ ] J·s^{-1} or W

Rel-M-AnP (W·kg^{-1}) = [ ] W/ [ ] kg body wt = [ ] W·kg^{-1}

^{a}2.5 m if Monark™ arm ergometer

FI% = [([ ] W_{pk} − [ ] W_{low}) ÷ [ ] W_{pk}] × 100

= ([ ] W ÷ [ ] W) × 100

= [ ] %

Form **NC 2**

Individual Power Output at 5-s Intervals During 30-s Bout

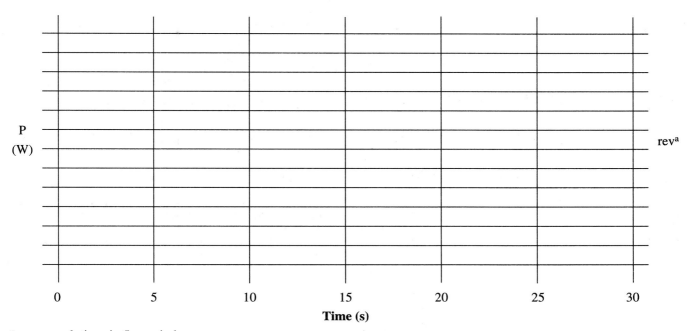

P
(W)

rev^a

Time (s)

^{a}rev = revolutions in 5-s period

Form NC 3

Group Data for Wingate Cycle Test

Initials	Pk-AnP	Rel-Pk-AnP	Total w	M-AnP	Rel-M-AnP	FI
Men	W	$W \cdot kg^{-1}$	kJ	W	$W \cdot kg^{-1}$	%
1.						
2.						
3.						
4.						
5.						
6.						
7.						
8.						
9.						
10.						
M						
Women	W	$W \cdot kg^{-1}$	kJ	W	$W \cdot kg^{-1}$	%
1.						
2.						
3.						
4.						
5.						
6.						
7.						
8.						
9.						
10.						
M						

Chapter NS Anaerobic Stepping

The anaerobic field/lab step test may be categorized as a long-anaerobic test because the test duration is 60 s; long-anaerobic activity was defined earlier as all-out events lasting from a minimum of 10 to 30 s to a maximum of 60 to 90 s. Thus, the performance of the anaerobic step test is primarily dependent on the glycolytic pathway (lactate system) of metabolism; secondly, on the phosphagenic system; and thirdly, on the oxidative system. Maximal efforts involving large muscle groups of one-minute duration require metabolic contributions of about 30–35% aerobic and 65–70% anaerobic.[1] The highest lactate values occur "in well-trained athletes at the end of competitive events of 1–2 minutes duration."[1] Blood lactates in elite athletes engaging in all-out efforts of long-anaerobic activities have been reported as high as 17 times (16.7 mmol·L^{-1}) the resting value.[3] Thus, the anaerobic step test is expected to elicit moderately high lactate values because of its duration of 1 min.

However, because only one leg is used predominantly during the Anaerobic Step Test, the lactate values are less than maximal. Thus, despite presumably high lactate levels in the local muscle mass of the dominant leg, the lactate levels are diluted in the general circulation because of the smaller muscle mass compared to two-legged exercise. Indeed, the postanaerobic step test values of finger-pricked blood lactate were about six times greater (~6 mmol·L^{-1}) than resting values (~1 mmol·L^{-1}).[8]

Method

The Method section in the description of most exercise physiology tests includes descriptions of equipment, preparations, procedures, and calculations.

Equipment

The equipment for the Anaerobic Step Test is very inexpensive. It requires only a bench (step), a watch with a seconds indicator, a calculator, and an accurate body weight scale. The step or bench is lower than the 18-inch height used by the investigators in the original study[2] who adopted the same height as used for the Skubic and Hodgkins[6] aerobic step test. The height of 40 cm (15.75 in.) is the same as that used by males who perform the Forestry Aerobic Step Test.

A watch with a seconds indicator (digital or sweep) can be used for timing the test. Laboratory set-clocks are

Accuracy

Validity

The number of steps performed by ninth-grade girls in the earlier version of the Anaerobic Step Test was found to be highly correlated ($r = -.824$) with the time for the 600-yd run.[2] In the earlier test, however, they were allowed to change support legs during the test; this would lead, presumably, to higher anaerobic scores. Anaerobic Step Test capacity/power (W) in one minute for NCAA basketball players increased during their preseason training.[9] This shows that the Anaerobic Step Test is sensitive to the effects of heavy anaerobic training. There appears to be a strong relationship ($r = .87$) between the anaerobic power of the anaerobic step test and lean body mass; there is a moderate relationship ($r = .61$) between the anaerobic step test score and dominant-leg strength.[4]

Reliability

The test-retest reliability of the Anaerobic Step Test is high ($r > .90$) based upon two tests each administered no more than 1 week apart to thirty university students.[8]

excellent for this test because a buzzer may be sounded at the end of the test. A basic pocket calculator is convenient for making all of the calculations for the Anaerobic Step Test. An accurate platform scale should be used to weigh the performer in stepping attire.

Preparation

In preparation for the Anaerobic Step Test, the stepper should follow the basic plan of the prior exercise regimen outlined in Table 1. The prior exercise also serves to familiarize the stepper with the proper stepping technique. The performer should avoid becoming fatigued at any time during the prior exercise.

Procedures

The Anaerobic Step Test is a modification of three other step tests—the Forestry[5] and Skubic and Hodgkins[6] *aerobic* step tests, and an earlier *anaerobic* step test.[2] There are four major differences between the anaerobic step test and the aerobic step tests—one concerned with the position of the stepper, another concerned with cadence, another with

Table 1 Prior Exercise Prescription for the Anaerobic Step Test

Time (min)	Activity
0:00–2:00	Walk in place at a moderate rate; lift thighs to 90°
2:00–3:00	Loosen up (stretch): (1) Groin; (2) Quadriceps; (3) Calf
3:00–5:00	Step up and down on step, stool, or bench at a moderate pace (~15–20 steps per minute)
5:00–7:00	Relief Interval: Mild walking in place or loosening up

the primary leg, and, finally, another concerned with calculation of power or capacity. Also, the newer anaerobic step test provides more information than the older anaerobic step test, because body weight is used to calculate anaerobic power.

Stepping Technique

The stepping technique is different from any of the common aerobic stepping techniques. The technique for the Anaerobic Step Test places a greater emphasis on one leg than the other. The stepper's initial position is that of standing alongside the bench, not in front of it. The preferred (dominant, or support leg) rests on the top of the step (bench) in preparation for the start of the test (Fig. 1a). The other leg, called the free leg, need not touch the bench when the test leg lifts the body (Fig. 1b).

During the test, each step raises the body to the top of the step with the one test leg. The free leg dangles in a straight position during the ascent, and the heel reaches the height of the bench. The foot of the free leg can push off when it contacts the floor. The legs and the back must be straightened with each step. In fact, the back should start in a straight position and never be changed throughout the test. The arms may be used for balance but cannot be pumped vigorously during the test. Ideally, the arms should maintain a penguinlike position.

The cadence for the test is at a 1-2 count; 1 is up and 2 is down. This, of course, is different from the typical 4-count cadence of aerobic step tests. An additional difference is that the performer goes as fast as possible at a pace designed to give a maximum number of steps during the one-minute time period. Thus, the stepper should barely be able to perform another step at the end of one minute.

Measurements

Measurements are made on only three items: (a) the weight of the performer, (b) the performer's number of steps, and (c) the duration of the test.

Body Weight. The performer should be weighed to the closest tenth of a kilogram in the same clothes and shoes that are worn for the step test. The weight is important because it will be entered as newtons into the calculations for anaerobic power.

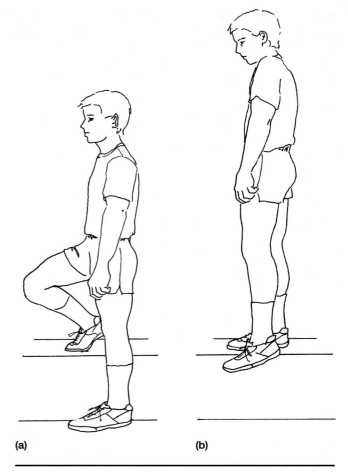

(a)   (b)

Figure 1 The positions for the Anaerobic Step Test: (a) The starting position with the body alongside the bench; (b) The "up" position.

Number of Steps. A step is counted for each time the stepper's support leg is straightened and then returned to the starting position. Steps are not counted if the support leg does not straighten or if the back is bent. Technicians count aloud in order to give immediate feedback to the participant. The counting should be as follows: "up-1, up-2, up-3, up-4, up-5," etc. Thus, a full step is considered to be a return to the starting position (down) after the ascent. The technician records the number of steps fully completed in 60 s onto Form NS 1.

Duration. The duration of the test is the same for everyone—1 min. The time begins with the first upward movement of the stepper. The technician should call out the time every 15 s, or the timer can be visible for the stepper. The laboratory set-clock can be set to buzz at the end of the test.

Recovery from the Anaerobic Step Test

The performer's support leg is likely to be very weak at the end of this test, perhaps, causing a few "buckled" walking steps. The quadriceps of the test leg and the calf of the free leg are the most likely muscle groups to become sore within 12 hours. In order to prevent or minimize delayed onset muscle soreness (DOMS), static stretching exercises should be repeated periodically after the test throughout the day. Based on the enhanced subsequent performance of 60-s events and lactate removal, active recovery such as walking, mild jogging, or walking-in-place, is recommended immediately after the test.[10]

A summary of the procedures is as follows:

1. Weigh the performer in stepping attire.
2. Convert the weight to newtons (10 × kg) and record onto Form NS 1.
3. Performer stands alongside the bench with foot of support leg on bench.
4. The time begins when the performer starts.
5. The technician counts aloud the number of correct steps.
6. The technician reminds the performer to keep back straight and arms in penguinlike position.
7. A technician states the time every 15 s.
8. At the end of 1 min, the last complete step is noted.
9. The performer is thanked for his/her cooperation and effort.
10. The technicians encourage the performer to actively recover immediately, and to stretch muscles periodically throughout the day.

Calculations

In the first edition of *Exercise Physiology Laboratory Manual,* two components of the Anaerobic Step Test were discussed: (1) peak anaerobic power and (2) anaerobic capacity. However, because the norms were based on the subjects' pacing themselves during the entire 60 s of the test, in contrast to the immediate all-out effort of the Wingate Test, it is more valid to eliminate the peak anaerobic power portion. Also, the term *anaerobic capacity* may be considered anaerobic power because of the 1-min time period of the test.

By using Equation 1, anaerobic power (AnP) is calculated from the work accomplished in a 1-min time period. This represents a person's capacity for work or mean power in 1 min, hence the unit of measure watts (W). Eccentric exercise (negative work) is accounted for by the 1.33 factor of bench stepping (see Chapter TE). There is no need to calculate the backward and forward component of work because there is very little, if any, such motion in this step test. There may be a slight lateral movement in some fatigued performers.

$$AnP\ (W) = ({}^+w \times 1.33) \div t \qquad \text{Eq. 1}$$

where:

$${}^+w = \text{positive work (Force} \times \text{Distance) in 1 min}$$
$$\text{force} = \text{body wt in N}$$
$$\text{distance} = \text{height of step (0.40 m)} \times \text{steps in 1 min}$$
$$1.33 = \text{factor to convert } {}^+w \text{ to total work}$$
$$t = 60\ s$$

Table 2 Comparative Anaerobic Powers (AnP;W) for the Anaerobic Step Test

Group	Anaerobic Power (W) Mean	Highest
Active College Students (2nd trial)[8]		
Men: ($n = 14$)	454	583
Women: ($n = 11$)	338	457
Pro Football Players[7]	626 ($SD = 108$)	810
Active Adults[4]		
Men: ($n = 130$; 17–30 y)	460 ($SD = 90$)	
Women: ($n = 70$; 18–30 y)	307 ($SD = 61$)	
NCAA Basketball Players[9]	576 ($SD = 53$)	

Table 3 Norms for Anaerobic Step Test in Active Men ($n = 130$) and Women ($n = 70$) between 18–30 y

Percentile	Men's Power (W)	Women's Power (W)
99	730	490
95	608	407
90	584	391
85	554	370
80	536	358
75	520	348
70	507	339
65	495	331
60	483	322
55	472	315
50	460	307
45	448	299
40	438	292
35	425	283
30	413	275
25	400	266
20	384	258
15	366	244
10	336	223
5	312	207

Source: M. Petersen, p. 22, 1989.

For example, if a 68-kg (680-N) person stepped fifty times in the 60-s period, then the following calculation would produce the anaerobic power:

$$AnP\ (W) = (680\ N \times 0.40 \times 50 \times 1.33) \div 60$$
$$= 18,088 \div 60$$
$$= 301\ W$$

Results and Discussion

The anaerobic powers of self-selected adults between the ages of 17 and 30 y ($M = 23$ y) attending a fitness center were 460 W for men and 307 W for women.[4] (See Tables 2 and 3.) After preseason training,[9] NCAA basketball players averaged 576 W.[a] Comparisons of anaerobic power may be

---

[a]The publication's value expresses the power in kg·m·min⁻¹, but W was intended.

made with fifteen off-season players on an NFL professional football team, but in their test no restrictions were placed on their arm movements, and they stood facing the step bench.[7]

References

1. Astrand, P. O., & Rodahl, K. (1977). *Textbook of work physiology.* NY: McGraw-Hill.
2. Manahan, J. E., & Gutin, B. (1971). The one-minute step test as a measure of 600-yard run performance. *Research Quarterly, 42,* 173–177.
3. Parkhouse, W. S., & McKenzie, D. C. (1983). Anaerobic capacity assessment of elite athletes. *Medicine and Science in Sports and Exercise, 15* (Suppl. 2), Abstract, 142.
4. Petersen, M. (1989). *AnP norms and the relationship between anaerobic power versus leg strength and lean body mass.* Master's thesis, California State University, Fullerton.
5. Sharkey, B. J. (1984). *Physiology of fitness.* Champaign, IL: Human Kinetics.
6. Skubic, V., & Hodgkins, J. (1963). Cardiovascular efficiency tests for girls and women. *Research Quarterly, 34,* 191–198.
7. Smith, C. D. (1987). *The effect of offseason training on anaerobic power training in pro football players.* Master's project, California State University, Fullerton.
8. Stojanovski, J. (1989). *The reliability and validity of the AnP step test.* Master's project, California State University, Fullerton.
9. Tavino, L. P., Bowers, C. J., & Archer, C. B. (1995). Effects of basketball on aerobic capacity, anaerobic capacity, and body composition of male college players. *Journal of Strength and Conditioning Research, 9,* 75–77.
10. Weltman, A., Stamford, B. A., Moffatt, R. J., & Katch, V. L. (1977). Exercise recovery, lactate removal, and repeated high-intensity exercise performance. *Research Quarterly, 48,* 786–796.

Form NS 1

Individual Data Form for the Anaerobic Step Test

Name [_____] Date [_____] Age [____] y

Gender (M or F) [____] Ht [____] cm Wt (in stepping attire) [____] kg [____] N

Number (#) of complete steps in 1 min [____]

Percentile (18–30 y) [____] %ile
(Table 3)

AnP (W) = ([____] N × 0.40 × [____] Steps × 1.33) ÷ 60

= [____] ÷ 60

= [____] W

Form NS 2

Group Data for Anaerobic Step Test

MEN

Initials	Power (AnP; W)
1.	
2.	
3.	
4.	
5.	
6.	
7.	
8.	
9.	
10.	
11.	
12.	
13.	
14.	
15.	
16.	
17.	
M	

WOMEN

Initials	Power (AnP; W)
1.	
2.	
3.	
4.	
5.	
6.	
7.	
8.	
9.	
10.	
11.	
12.	
13.	
14.	
15.	
16.	
17.	
M	

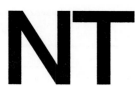

Anaerobic Treadmill Tests

The treadmill tests presented here are laboratory tests, not field or field/lab tests, because of the bulk and expense of a treadmill capable of moving a belt to 8 mph (9.6 km·h^{-1}) up a 20% slope. Additionally, the treadmill tests do not lend themselves to simultaneous testing of many people, for obvious reasons. However, the physiological sophistication of these treadmill tests is as simple as most field tests.

Various versions of Anaerobic Treadmill (An-TM) Tests exist. For most college-aged men, the two tests described here may be classified as long-anaerobic tests because they usually elicit maximal effort durations between 30 and 90 s. For most women, the faster of the two treadmill tests is more appropriately classified as a short-anaerobic test because of the difficulty in running at 8 mph up a 20% slope for longer than 30 s. The slightly different expected durations of the two treadmill tests may be used to categorize them as a *fast (F) test*—faster speed, shorter duration, and a *slow (S) test*—slower speed, longer duration.

Physiological Rationale for the An-TM Tests

These two tests certainly are supramaximal tests when maximal oxygen consumption is used as the reference point. An all-out treadmill sprint that lasts from 54 to 105 s represents about 125% of a runner's aerobic capacity, and produces a pH of about 6.88 in the gastrocnemius and vastus lateralis muscles.[4] Because performance in the An-TM fast test never exceeds 100 s, and performance in the slow test usually is less than 100 s, it is clear that these two tests represent oxygen consumptions exceeding 125% of maximal. The slow test, especially, would be expected to incur higher lactic acid values due to the longer time to accumulate lactic acid during glycolytic anaerobism. The derived anaerobic contribution to an exhaustive treadmill run, at a steady pace of 12.9 mph (345 m·min^{-1}) to 14.4 mph (386 m·min^{-1}) for about 60 s at a 5% slope, ranges from about 64–72% with the higher value elicited by trained sprinters. The contribution of the glycolytic pathway for this 60-s run was greater than that of the phosphagenic portion of the anaerobic pathway.[13]

The slow Anaerobic Treadmill Test was used to test the anaerobic capacity of dinghy (sailboat) sailors,[9] whereas the shorter and faster Anaerobic Treadmill Test was used to test hockey forwards,[6] 800-m runners,[8] elite soccer players,[11] and alpine ski racers.[2] Using heart rate as a familiar variable by which to substantiate the high inten-

Accuracy of Anaerobic Treadmill Tests

Validity

The anaerobic capacities of college-aged participants related well ($r = -.82$) with their performance in a 329-m run.[13] A more intense treadmill test (e.g., 10 mph at 20% slope) may be a more valid measure of anaerobic performance in elite athletes.[10] However, a slower speed and lesser slope may enhance distinctions among college women.

Reliability

The test-retest reliability coefficient of the fast treadmill test ranges from .76 to .91,[3] or up to .94.[10] More studies on the validity and reliability of these tests are needed.

sity of such anaerobic power treadmill tests, males had peak heart rates that averaged 192 b·min^{-1} when running for about 93 s (±29 s) at 16 km·h^{-1} on an 8% slope.[7]

Method

High-intensity efforts on a treadmill often are induced by increasing both the speed and slope of the treadmill. It is best to use a combination of these, because if only one is used, the subject may be limited by a singular contributing factor to long anaerobic power. For example, if only a fast speed at a level slope is used, slow runners might find themselves trailing off the back of the treadmill; if only a steep slope at a slow speed is used, those with inferior leg strength may succumb to premature leg fatigue. Thus, these anaerobic tests for long anaerobic power use a combination of slope and speed to accommodate the supramaximal efforts of many people.

Equipment

Treadmill

Obviously a treadmill is the major piece of equipment for the An-TM tests. Theoretically, it is possible to use the slope of a road if it has the prescribed slope as that of the tests described here. However, roads at 20% slope are rarely found; for example, interstate highway regulators discourage the construction of roads with more than a

Table 1 Protocols for the Long Anaerobic-Slow (S) and Fast (F) Treadmill Tests

Period	Time (min)	Activity
Prior Exercise and Familiarization	0:00–10:00	(1) Jog in place; (2) Slow jogging; (3) Short runs on level TM, progressing to very brief bouts at test speed
Relief Interval	10:00–11:00	Slow walking or walking in place

Treadmill Test	Slope (%)	Speed
Slow	20	6 mph (9.6 km·h^{-1}; 160 m·min^{-1}; 2.67 m·s^{-1}; 10 min per mile pace)
Fast	20	8 mph (12.8 km·h^{-1}; 215 m·min^{-1}; 3.58 m·s^{-1}; 7.5 min per mile pace)
Cool-Down	0:00–5:00	Gradually slower jogging and walking; stretching

6% slope. Good treadmills are very expensive, especially research-precision ones. Treadmills with front and side handrails are required for the anaerobic TM tests. A harness attached from the subject to the rail or ceiling is ideal for maximizing safety and uninhibited all-out efforts.

Timer

A seconds-watch, not necessarily one that is capable of measuring tenths of a second, is needed to measure the duration of the performance to the closest second.

Treadmill Protocol

The protocol for the treadmill tests should include a prior exercise and familiarization period, along with a cool-down period (Table 1). The prior exercise should consist of a warmup and loosening-up regimen that mimics the movements of running and stretches the running muscles. The warmup should not cause fatigue; some investigators[5,6] did not allow a warmup for the runners in their research studies.

The Fast (F) Test should be performed first if both tests are given within 1 hour. This is because recovery from this shorter test is quicker than that of the Slow (S) Treadmill Test. However, it is probably wiser to do the two tests on separate days so that the Slow Test can be administered first. This gives the performers and technicians some input into the runners' capabilities for the more intimidating Fast Test. For example, if runners in the longer test cannot continue longer than 30 s, they may not be able to run without the use of the handrails at the least, and only a few seconds at the most, on the faster treadmill test. For these latter performers, the speed of the fast test might be reduced from 8 mph to 7 mph and noted on Form NT 1. One or two trials may be run for each performer, depending upon the fatigue of the performer and the administrative considerations of the lab director.

The cool-down period should be done off the treadmill, and begin with fast walking and gradually slower walking for a combined time of about 3–5 min.

Procedures

As with all test procedures, technicians must be concerned with the safety and psychological well-being of the partici-

pants prior to and during the treadmill test. As with all tests, basic data should be recorded, but meteorological data are not necessary under standard laboratory conditions for the anaerobic treadmill tests. The key measurement for these tests is the total time that the performer can continue running at the given speed.

Safety

These treadmill tests can induce more psychological distress than any tests described in this manual. A fast-moving treadmill belt can be intimidating, even to experienced subjects. Thus, the technician's sensitivity to the performers' fears should include a sincere effort to familiarize them with the safe and proper technique of using the handrails to get on and off the fast-moving treadmill belt. Subjects should be given time to practice this procedure. The key to the runners' mental security is their contact with the handrails. If a person is too fearful to let go of the handrail, then the test should be modified to a speed that the performer selects. The technician in control of the treadmill should be prepared to stop the treadmill as soon as the runner touches the handrails in preparation of exiting, while a spotter at the rear end of the treadmill should be prepared to support the runner if necessary.

Measurements

Except for the basic data, there is only one measurement—the time (to the closest second) spent at the prescribed speed on the treadmill. The timer starts the clock as soon as the performer, while running, releases the handrails. The timer stops the watch when the runner takes hold of the handrails in preparation to exiting from the treadmill belt. If two trials are given, the better time is used for statistical purposes. In summary, the checklist of procedures is as follows:

1. Record the performer's weight in running attire onto Form NT 1.
2. The runner follows an appropriate prior exercise regimen.
3. The runner practices getting on and off the treadmill.
4. A technician (*protocoller*) places the treadmill at the prescribed speed (slow = 6 mph or 2.67 m·s; fast = 8 mph or 3.58 m·s) and slope (20%).

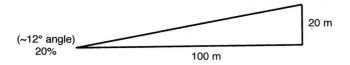

Figure 1 An example of a treadmill sloped at 20% (~12°).

5. With hands on the rails, the performer either straddles or stands alongside the treadmill.
6. With hands still holding onto the rails, the performer steps onto the moving treadmill belt.
7. A technician (timer) starts the watch as soon as the runner's hands release the handrail.
8. The timer stops the seconds-watch as soon as the runner touches the handrails.
9. Also at this time, the protocoller stops the treadmill.
10. The time is recorded to the closest second on Form NT 1.
11. The performer cools down (see Table 1).

Calculations

The calculation of anaerobic work capacity may be made from the time spent on the treadmill, the slope and speed of the treadmill, and the weight of the runner. The percent grade or slope is defined as the distance of the vertical rise (D_v) per 100 horizontal meters. Running up a 20% slope simply means that for every 100 meters traveled horizontally there will be a vertical rise of 20 m (see Fig. 1). Sometimes the slope is expressed in degrees, but the value is not the same as the percent value. The degree value is always less than the percent value.

Equation 1 for calculating the work on a treadmill is similar to the work equation in Chapter TE except that the vertical distance factor has been emphasized by the subscript v:

$$w = F \times D_v \qquad \text{Eq. 1}$$

where: w = work in N·m or J
   F = force (weight of performer) in N; ($N = 10 \times kg$)
   D_v = vertical distance in m

The vertical distance (D_v) is found by dividing the % slope by 100 and then multiplying by the horizontal distance (D_h), as in Equation 2.

$$D_v = (\% \text{ slope}/100) \times D_h \qquad \text{Eq. 2}$$

The horizontal distance is found by multiplying the speed by the total time, as in Equation 3.

$$D_h = \text{mph or km·h}^{-1} \text{ or m·min}^{-1} \qquad \text{Eq. 3}$$
$$\text{or m·s}^{-1} \times t \text{ (h; min; s)}$$

where t = time in decimal h or min or whole seconds.

Table 2 Comparative Scores for the Anaerobic Treadmill Tests

Reference	Group	Time (s)
	Slow Test	
#1 ($n = 30$)	Male PE Majors	72 ($R = 49–153$)
($n = 21$)	Female PE Majors	38 ($R = 20–54$)
#9	Dinghy Sailors	65; $SD = 16$
	Fast Test	
#1 ($n = 36$)	Male PE Majors	33 ($R = 18–47$)
($n = 7$)	Female PE Majors	11 ($R = 8–19$)
#2 ($n = 10$)	National Alpine Skiers	77
($n = 22$)	Less Elite Club Skiers	56
#5 ($n = 8$)	Normal Males	
	Pretraining:	52; $SD = 13$
	Post-training:	64
#6 ($n = 11$)	College Hockey Forwards	54; $SD = 15$
#8 ($n = 6$)	Elite 800-m Runners	114
#10 ($n = 6$)	Elite Athletes	82; $SD = 20$
#11	Olympic Soccer Players	92; $SD = 10$ ($R = 68–102$)
#12 (7 mph)	Female Basketball Players	39; $SEM = 2.2$

For anaerobic treadmill tests it is simpler to convert mph to m·min^{-1} or m·s^{-1} by using the approximate conversion factors:

$$1 \text{ mph} = 27 \text{ m·min}^{-1} = 0.45 \text{ m·s}^{-1}$$

The calculation of work for a 68-kg person running at a 20% grade and 8 mph (12.8 km·h^{-1} or 215 m·min^{-1} or 3.58 m·s^{-1}) for 60 s (1.0 min) is made as follows:

$$
\begin{aligned}
w &= F \times D_v \\
&= 680 \text{ N} \times (0.20 \times 215 \text{ m·min}^{-1}) \times 1.0 \text{ min} \\
&\quad \text{or } 680 \text{ N} \times (0.20 \times 3.58 \text{ m·s}^{-1}) \times 60 \text{ s} \\
&= 680 \text{ N} \times 43 \text{ m·min}^{-1} \times 1.0 \text{ min} \\
&\quad \text{or } 680 \text{ N} \times 0.716 \text{ m·s}^{-1} \times 60 \text{ s} \\
&= 29{,}240 \text{ N·m or J; or } 29.2 \text{ kJ}
\end{aligned}
$$

Results and Discussion

Norms, especially expressed in total work units, are needed for these treadmill tests. Those presented in Table 2 are not *true* norms due to the small samples from the typical population and the lack of true work units. Thus they are presented for comparative, not classification, purposes.

References

1. Adams, G. M. (1992). Anaerobic treadmill tests in college physical education majors. Unpublished raw data.
2. Brown, S. L., & Wilkinson, J. G. (1983). Characteristics of national, divisional, and club male Alpine ski racers. *Medicine and Science in Sports and Exercise, 15,* 491–495.

3. Bouchard, C., Taylor, A. W., Simoneau, J. A., & Dulac, S. (1991). Testing anaerobic power and capacity. In J. D. MacDougall, H. A. Wenger, & H. J. Green (Eds.), *Physiological testing of the high performance athlete.* Champaign, IL: Human Kinetics.

4. Costill, D. L., Barnett, A., Sharp, R., Fink, W. J., & Katz, A. (1983). Leg muscle pH following sprint running. *Medicine and Science in Sports and Exercise, 16,* 325–329.

5. Cunningham, D. A., & Faulkner, J. A. (1969). The effect of training on aerobic and anaerobic metabolism during a short exhaustive run. *Medicine and Science in Sports and Exercise, 1,* 65–69.

6. Houston, M. E., & Green, H. J. (1976). Physiological and anthropometric characteristics of elite Canadian ice hockey players. *Journal of Sportsmedicine and Physical Fitness, 16,* 123–128.

7. Mackova, E. V., Melichna, J., Vondra, K., Jurimae, T., Tomas, P., & Novak, J. (1985). The relationship between anaerobic performance and muscle metabolic capacity and fibre distribution. *European Journal of Applied Physiology, 54,* 413–415.

8. McKenzie, D. C., Parkhouse, W. S., & Hearst, W. D. (1982). Anaerobic performance characteristics of elite Canadian 800 meter runners. *Canadian Journal of Applied Sport Science, 7,* 158–160.

9. Niinimaa, V., Wright, G., Shephard, R. J., & Clarke, J. (1977). Characteristics of the successful dinghy sailor. *Journal of Sportsmedicine and Physical Fitness, 17,* 83–96.

10. Parkhouse, W. S., & McKenzie, D. C. (1983). Anaerobic capacity assessment of elite athletes. *Medicine and Science in Sports and Exercise, 15,* Abstract, 142.

11. Rhodes, E. C., Mosber, R. E., McKenzie, D. C., Franks, J. M., Potts, J. E., & Wenger, H. A. (1986). Physiological profiles of the Canadian Olympic Soccer Team. *Canadian Journal of Applied Sport Sciences, 11,* 31–36.

12. Rlezebos, M. L., Paterson, D. H., Hall, C. R., & Yuhasz, S. (1983). Relationship of selected variables to performance in women's basketball. *Canadian Journal of Applied Sport Sciences, 8,* 34–40.

13. Thomson, J. M., & Garvie, K. J. (1981). A laboratory method for determination of anaerobic energy expenditure during sprinting. *Canadian Journal of Applied Sport Science, 6,* 21–26.

Form NT 1

Individual Data for Treadmill Anaerobic Tests

Name [   ] Date [   ] Time [   ] a.m. [   ] p.m. [   ]

Age [   ] y   Gender (M or F) [   ]   Ht [   ] cm   Wt [   ] kg [   ] N

Slow-Test Time (6 mph)

Trial 1 [   ] s (closest s)

Trial 2 [   ] s (Optional)

Fast-Test Time (8 mph)

[   ] s

[   ] s (Optional)

Modified (7 mph)

[   ] s

[   ] s (Optional)

Slow-Test Work (N·m; J): w = F × D_v

D_v = 20% slope/100 × D_h; D_h = 2.67 m·s^{-1} × [   ] s = [   ] m

   = 0.2 × [   ] m = [   ] m

w = F [   ] N × D_v [   ] m = [   ] N·m; J ÷ 1000 = [   ] kJ

Fast-Test Work (N·m; J): w = F × D_v

D_v = 20% slope/100 × D_h; D_h = 3.58 m·s^{-1} × [   ] s = [   ] m

   = 0.2 × [   ] m = [   ] m

w = F [   ] N × D_v [   ] m = [   ] N·m; J ÷ 1000 = [   ] kJ

Modified-Test Work (N·m; J): w = F × D_v

D_v = 20% slope/100 × D_h; D_h = 3.15 m·s^{-1} × [   ] s = [   ] m

   = 0.2 × [   ] m = [   ] m

w = F [   ] N × D_v [   ] m = [   ] N·m; J ÷ 1000 = [   ] kJ

Form NT 2

Group Data for Anaerobic TM Tests

MEN Initials	Time (s) Slow Test (6 mph)	Fast Test (8 mph)	WOMEN Initials	Time (s) Slow Test (6 mph)	Fast Test (8 mph)
1.			1.		
2.			2.		
3.			3.		
4.			4.		
5.			5.		
6.			6.		
7.			7.		
8.			8.		
9.			9.		
10.			10.		
11.			11.		
12.			12.		
13.			13.		
14.			14.		
15.			15.		
16.			16.		
17.			17.		
18.			18.		
19.			19.		
20.			20.		
M			M		

Chapter AR Aerobic Running and Walking

Aerobic tests measure aerobic power, a term that is often used synonymously with *cardiovascular endurance.* Aerobic power is of primary importance in performing exercise that continues beyond 3 min. Thus, most aerobic tests do not require short explosive bouts of exercise, but usually require submaximal bouts of exercise varying in duration. For example, some step tests may conclude in 3 min, whereas some, such as the Texas Steady-State Run test, may take 30 min.[11] Valid estimates of aerobic power ($\dot{V}O_2$max) for low to moderately fit persons are available that require no exercise testing. These usually consider such factors as gender, age, percent fat (or body mass index), and a questionnaire that allows a rating for habitual physical activity (e.g., PA-R).[2,37,38] Physical activity questionnaires may also help to ensure that any kind of exercise testing is safe for the participant. For example, the Physical Activity Readiness Questionnaire (PAR-Q) asks seven questions pertaining to (1) doctor's assessment of your heart condition and physical activity; (2) chest pain at exercise; (3) chest pain during the last month without exercising; (4) balance and dizziness; (5) bone or joint problems; (6) prescription drugs; and (7) participant's opinion of his/her possible problems associated with exercise.[56]

The importance of aerobic fitness is accentuated by the reported association of low cardiovascular (aerobic) endurance fitness and increased coronary heart disease risk factors.[23] The existing norms for the run/walk tests allow us to classify the aerobic fitness level of individuals and to enhance the individuality of a possible exercise prescription.

This chapter includes a discussion of three popular field tests—the 1.5-Mile/12-Minute Test, the AAHPERD Run Test, and the Rockport Walk Test. These are good examples of field tests due to the use of minimal equipment, their application to large groups, and their ease of administration. Aerobic run/walk tests are the most common field tests of cardiorespiratory fitness.[24] They should not be considered as tests to replace the direct measure of oxygen consumption in research studies. A portion of this chapter includes a discussion of some physiological measures that can be estimated or measured while performing the aerobic run tests.

The 12-Minute Test was developed from Balke's[10] original 15-Minute Run Test by Dr. Kenneth Cooper. Cooper's Test includes the 12-minute and 1.5-mile versions. The 1.5-Mile/12-Minute Test is widely accepted by some authoritative organizations. For instance, it is a test

Table 1 Suitability of Different Versions of Aerobic Run/Walk Tests

Age (y) and Fitness Status	Aerobic Run/Walk Test
All ages if apparently healthy and habitual exerciser	1.5-Mile Run for Time or 12-Min Run for Distance (Cooper's Test)
All ages if apparently healthy (no medical exam required)	Rockport Walk Test
College age or 13–17 y	1.5-Mile/12-Min or 1.0-Mile/9-Min Run (AAHPERD Test)
	George-Fisher Jogging Test
5–12 y	1.0-Mile Run for Time or 9-Min Run for Distance (AAHPERD Test)

routinely administered by the U.S. Navy, U.S. Air Force, and the American Alliance of Health, Physical Education, Recreation, and Dance (AAHPERD).

The AAHPERD Run Test includes both versions of Cooper's Test, in addition to the 1.0-Mile and 9-Minute Run Tests[3] (Table 1). The short versions of the AAHPERD Run Tests are recommended for children between the ages of 5 and 12 y, whereas 13- to 17-y-olds and college students have the option of performing either of the four versions of the AAHPERD Aerobic Run Test.

Tests that prescribe walking may be most prudent for middle-age and older adults because walking is a moderate exercise that is more friendly to the joints. The American College of Sports Medicine does not feel a need to recommend a medical examination for apparently healthy older adults prior to performing tests of moderate exercise.[6] The Rockport 1.0-Mile Walk Test predicts aerobic fitness for ages ranging from 30 to 69 y.[41] This test incorporates the time to finish the walk and such factors as exercise heart rate, body weight, age, and gender into an equation to predict aerobic fitness. A similar test, the George-Fisher Jogging Test, utilizes the principles from the Rockport Test, but applies them more specifically to physically fit college-age persons.[32,33]

Purpose of the Aerobic Run/Walk Tests

The purpose of Aerobic Run Tests as performed in *Exercise Physiology Laboratory* is slightly different from what Dr. Cooper originally intended for the general public. He was concerned with measuring aerobic power (cardiovascular endurance) in addition to stimulating the populace to exercise.

Accuracy of the Aerobic Run/Walk Tests

Validity

Validation of the 12-Minute Test is usually done by comparing the 12-min distance with maximal oxygen consumption ($\dot{V}O_2$max), a measure of aerobic power. The correlation coefficients were very high (r = .897 and .91) when testing young Air Force servicemen[20] and females,[34] respectively. Thus the greater the distance run in 12 min by the participants, the greater their maximal oxygen consumption as measured under laboratory conditions. Validity coefficients have been reported to range from as low as .28 to as high as .94[52] with a standard error of estimate (*SEE*) around 10%.[62] Shorter runs, such as the 1.0-Mile and the 9-Minute Tests, are valid measures of aerobic power, especially in children.[39]

A graphic generalization (Fig. 1) of Cooper's data depicts the high validity of the 12-Minute Test. The criterion test ($\dot{V}O_2$max) on the horizontal axis is plotted against the predictive test (12-min distance) on the vertical axis, showing that those persons with the highest laboratory-tested $\dot{V}O_2$max run the farthest in 12 min.

Again using $\dot{V}O_2$max as the criterion, the validity of the Rockport Walk Test was .92 in ages 30–69 y with an *SEE* of 0.355 L/min.[40] However, these values were based on electronically monitored pulse rates during field testing; thus, accurate pulse taking should be emphasized in order to obtain similar accuracy. Reported correlations for different ages and genders are .89 and .74 for 65 to 69 y-old men and women, respectively;[31] and .79 for 30–39 y-old women.[62] Although the Rockport Test underestimates $\dot{V}O_2$max considerably in sedentary older persons,[31,49,57] it appears to be a valid test for older women (*M* = 73.5 y) accustomed to walking.[57] It may overestimate maximal oxygen consumption in college students.[28] On some occasions it might be advantageous to perform the Rockport Test on a treadmill; in such cases, Nieman[47] reported that the treadmill gives similar results.[58]

Reliability

The reliability of a test may be thought of as its repeatability or consistency. One reviewer of the 12-Minute Test reported test-retest reliability correlation coefficients around .90.[26]

Although the Rockport 1-mile Walk Test appears to be a reliable test, even for older women,[49] there appears to be a learning effect from the first trial through the third trial.[31]

It would be difficult to control all of the variables that influence the validity and reliability of the Aerobic Run/Walk Tests; if it were possible, these field tests would qualify as field/lab tests. In general, these tests are most accurate if the environment is comfortable, if the participant is motivated and runs or walks at a steady pace, and if the technicians measure and record accurate distances or times.

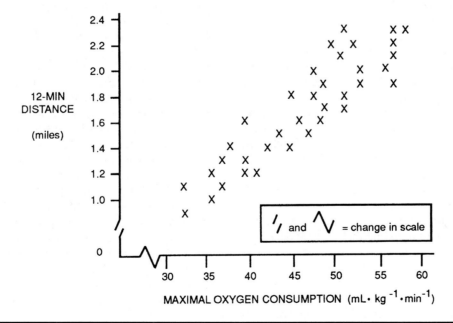

Figure 1 The direct (positive; linear) relationship between the distance run in 12 minutes and maximal oxygen consumption.

Our laboratory objectives also include Cooper's objectives, but add objectives related to the physiological effects of running and walking, and to the administrative aspects of the tests.

Physiological Rationale for the Aerobic Run/Walk Tests

Oxidative metabolism predominates for events that last for about 3 or more min. Oxygen is transported first by the respiratory (pulmonary) system to the cardiovascular system, and then from there to the contracting muscles. The muscles consume the oxygen in order to provide sufficient amounts of adenosine triphosphate (ATP) for the myosin filaments to pull the actin filaments; the pulling within the muscles causes muscle action. Without a sufficient amount of oxygen, there is not enough ATP produced to sustain muscular action beyond a few minutes. Thus, other factors being equal, the runner who can supply the highest rate of oxygen to the muscles will be able to continue aerobic exercise at a faster speed.

Method

The method section includes descriptions of the (1) facility and equipment; (2) procedures; and (3) calculations.

Facility and Equipment

Facility

The facility requires a level terrain that has accurately measured distances. Many new track facilities are ovals of 400 meters, which means that each lap on the metric track is 2.5 yd shorter than the older 440 yd American ovals (Fig. 2). This means that if performing on a metric track, the runner or walker must go 10 yd (9 m) beyond 4 laps for the 1.0-mile test, and 15 yd (14 m) beyond for the 1.5-mile test. The straightaways and the turns of a quarter-mile (440 yd) track are all 110 yards. Thus any distance halfway between this interval is 55 yd. Also, keep in mind that the 400-m or 440-yd distance for one lap only applies to the inside lane (about 1 ft from the curb). If you are performing the Rockport Walk Test, a treadmill is optional.[47,58]

Runners of the 9- and 12-Minute Tests may be troubled by estimating the distance of their run. Ideally, the distances should be estimated as closely as possible in order to accommodate the available norms (e.g., the nearest 10 yd or 9 m for AAHPERD 9-Minute Test). The norms in Table 4 are presented in about 175-yd increments.[4] When distances are estimated and rounded off, fitness differences may become obscured.

Equipment

The only piece of equipment that is absolutely necessary to conduct the Aerobic Run/Walk Tests is a watch with a sec-

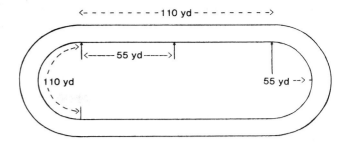

Figure 2 Layout of a quarter-mile (440-yd) track. The straightaways and turns are 110 yards each; thus the midpoints between these are 55 yards each.

onds indicator. For greater accuracy in measuring heart rate for the Rockport Test, electronic monitoring using miniature transmitters and receivers (e.g., Polar™) are practical[43] and inexpensive (about $100). These monitors have a transmitting device and chest electrodes built into the chest strap. A receiver, which also serves other functions, digitally displays the updated heart rate every five seconds. The runner or walker wears the strap and the "wristwatch" receiver; or the technician, within five feet of the participant, can hold the receiver ("wristwatch").

Large groups may be tested easily on these tests. At the "Go!" signal all participants begin running or walking, and the timer starts the clock. At the end of either the prescribed time or the prescribed distance, the timer yells out the times so that the participants or recorders can write down their times or distances.

Procedures for the Aerobic Run/Walk Tests

The primary measurement for both the 1.5-Mile Run and the 1.0-Mile Run is time in minutes and seconds. Based on performance time, each participant's aerobic fitness category, percentile, or maximal oxygen consumption ($\dot{V}O_2$max) may be estimated. Knowledge of the $\dot{V}O_2$max is vital in understanding the physiological basis of aerobic fitness.

The estimated maximal oxygen consumption ($ml \cdot kg^{-1} \cdot min^{-1}$) is needed in order to categorize performers of the 12-min distance run or the Rockport Walk Test. Performers in the 12-min distance run can obtain their $\dot{V}O_2$max values from Table 6[60] or the transposition of Cooper's[18,20] original equation (Eq. 1). The Rockport walkers obtain their values from Equation 2. Charts depicting the fitness levels for Rockport Walk performers are available from The Rockport Company™ and can be found in various sources.[36]

Procedural Steps for the 1.0- or 1.5-Mile Run Tests

1. Participants run on a level terrain for the prescribed distance of one mile (1609 m; 1.6 km) or 1.5 miles (2414 m; 2.4 km).
2. The timers record the participants' times to the closest second onto Form AR 1.

Table 2 1.5-Mile Times and Fitness Categories for Moderately-Fit College Males and Females 17 to 35 Years

Fitness Category	Time (min:s)	Time (min:s)
	Ages 17–25	Ages 26–35
Superior		
Females	<10:30	<11:30
Males	<8:30	<9:30
Excellent		
Females	10:30–11:49	11:30–12:49
Males	8:30–9:29	9:30–10:29
Good		
Females	11:50–13:09	12:50–14:09
Males	9:30–10:29	10:30–11:29
Moderate		
Females	13:10–14:29	14:10–15:29
Males	10:30–11:29	11:30–12:29
Fair		
Females	14:30–15:49	15:30–16:49
Males	11:30–12:29	12:30–13:29
Poor		
Females	>15:49	>16:49
Males	>12:29	>13:29

Source: Draper & Jones, (1990). *JOPERD,* AAHPERD, Reston, VA.

3. The fitness level is determined by consulting Tables 2 or 3 for the 1.5-mile run, and Table 4 for the 1.0-mile run.
4. For the 1.5-Mile Test, the $\dot{V}O_2max$ is estimated by consulting Table 5 or using Equation 1,[17] which gives slightly higher values than those in the table.

$$\dot{V}O_2max\ (ml\cdot kg^{-1}\cdot min^{-1}) = (483 \div t) + 3.5 \qquad Eq.\ 1$$

where: t = time to the closest 0.1 min; e.g., 30/60 = 0.5 min
3.5 = resting metabolism in $ml\cdot kg^{-1}\cdot min^{-1}$; one MET

Sample Calculation: If a performer runs 1.5 miles in 13:30, then the calculation proceeds as follows:

$$\dot{V}O_2max\ (ml\cdot kg^{-1}\cdot min^{-1}) = (483 \div 13.5) + 3.5$$
$$= 35.8 + 3.5 = 39.3$$

Procedural Steps for the 9- or 12-Min Run Tests

1. Participants run for the prescribed time (9 or 12 min).
2. Runners and their assistants estimate the distance to the closest 10 yd or 9 m.
3. The fitness level for the 9-min test is determined by consulting Table 4.
4. The fitness level for the 12-min test requires first an estimation of $\dot{V}O_2max$ by consulting Table 6 or using Equation 2 (men and women).
5. $\dot{V}O_2max$ is calculated by inserting the distance (closest 100th of a mile) into Equation 2.

$$\dot{V}O_2max\ (ml\cdot kg^{-1}\cdot min^{-1}) = (D\ in\ miles - 0.3138)$$
$$\div 0.0278 \qquad Eq.2$$

For example, if the distance in 12 min was 1.25 miles, then the maximal oxygen consumption can be calculated as follows:

$$\dot{V}O_2max\ (ml\cdot kg^{-1}\cdot min^{-1}) = (1.25 - 0.3138) \div 0.0278$$
$$= 0.936 \div 0.0278$$
$$= 33.7\ ml\cdot kg^{-1}\cdot min^{-1}$$

6. The fitness category may be found by referring to Table 7 (males) and Table 8 (females).[53]

Procedural Steps for the Rockport Walk Test

1. Technicians weigh the participants as described in Chapter UN.
2. Participants walk as fast as possible for one mile on any level terrain.
3. Heart rates (HR) are taken by technicians or the participants by pulse palpation or electronic monitoring for 10 or 15 s immediately upon crossing the 1-mile mark.
4. Multiply the 10-s value by six, or the 15-s value by four, and record the product onto Form AR 1.
5. Timers record the participants' times to the closest second and later convert them to the nearest hundredth minute onto Form AR 1. For example, if the participant finishes in 13:30, then the recorded time is converted to the nearest hundredth minute by dividing the seconds—30, by 60. Thus the time is 13.50 min.
6. Calculate $\dot{V}O_2max$ $(ml\cdot kg^{-1}\cdot min^{-1})$ according to Equation 3:

$$\dot{V}O_2max\ (ml\cdot kg^{-1}\cdot min^{-1}) = 132.85 - (0.0769 \times lb\ wt) \qquad Eq.\ 3$$
$$- (0.3877 \times age) + (6.315 \times gender)$$
$$- (3.2649 \times t\ in\ 100th\ of\ min) - (0.1565 \times HR\ in\ b\cdot min^{-1})$$

where: gender = 0 for women, and 1 for male

Example of calculating $\dot{V}O_2max$ $(ml\cdot kg^{-1}\cdot min^{-1})$:

Age = 30 y   Wt = 150 lb   time (t) to walk 1 mile = 13.50
Gender = male   HR = 145 b · min^{-1}
$$\dot{V}O_2max\ (ml\cdot kg^{-1}\cdot min^{-1}) = 132.85 - (0.0769 \times 150\ lb)$$
$$- (0.3877 \times 30\ y) + (6.315 \times 1) - (3.2649 \times 13.50)$$
$$- (0.1565 \times 145\ b\cdot min^{-1})$$
$$= 132.85 - 11.535 - 11.631 + 6.315 - 44.076 - 22.693$$
$$= 49.23$$

7. Charts depicting the fitness levels for Rockport Walk performers are available from The Rockport Company™ and can be found in various sources.[36] If these are not easily obtained, fitness levels are presented in Tables 7 and 8[53].

Table 3 Aerobic Fitness vs. 1.5-Mile Times for Men (M) and Women (W) Ages 13–60+ Years

Fitness Level		13–19	20–29	Age (y) 30–39 1.5-Mile Time (min:s)	40–49	50–59	60+
Very Poor	M	>15:30	>16:00	>16:30	>17:30	>19:00	>20:00
	W	>18:30	>19:00	>19:30	>20:00	>20:30	>21:00
Poor	M	12:11–15:30	14:01–16:00	14:44–16:30	15:36–17:30	17:01–19:00	19:01–20:00
	W	16:55–18:30	18:31–19:00	19:01–19:30	19:31–20:00	20:01–20:30	20:31–21:00
Fair	M	10:49–12:10	12:01–14:00	12:31–14:45	13:01–15:35	14:31–17:00	16:16–19:00
	W	14:31–16:54	15:55–18:30	16:31–19:00	17:31–19:30	19:01–20:00	19:31–20:30
Good	M	9:41–10:48	10:46–12:00	11:01–12:30	11:31–13:00	12:31–14:30	14:00–16:15
	W	12:30–14:30	13:31–15:54	14:31–16:30	15:56–17:30	16:31–19:00	17:31–19:30
Excellent	M	8:37– 9:40	9:45–10:45	10:00–11:00	10:30–11:30	11:00–12:30	11:15–13:59
	W	11:50–12:29	12:30–13:30	13:00–14:30	13:45–15:55	14:30–16:30	16:30–17:30
Superior	M	<8:37	<9:45	<10:00	<10:30	<11:00	<11:15
	W	<11:50	<12:30	<13:00	<13:45	<14:30	<16:30

Source: Adapted from Table 14 with permission from Kusinitz, I., & Fine, M. (1991). *Your guide to getting fit.* Mountain View, CA: Mayfield Publishing.

Table 4 AAHPERD Percentile (%ile) Norms for the 1-Mile and 9-Min Run

College Men				College Women		
Percentile (%ile)	1-Mile Run (min:s)	9-Min (yd)	Distance (m)	1-Mile Run (min:s)	9-Min (yd)	Distance (m)
99th	5:06	3035	2775	6:04	2640	2414
75th	6:12	2349	2148	8:15	1870	1710
50th	6:49	2200	2012	9:22	1755	1605
25th	7:32	1945	1779	10:41	1460	1335
5th	9:47	1652	1511	12:43	1101	1007

Reprinted by permission of the American Association for Health, Physical Education, Recreation and Dance, 1900 Association Dr., Reston, VA 22091.

Table 5 1.5-Mile Time and Maximal Oxygen Consumption ($\dot{V}O_2max$)

1.5-Mile Time (min:s)	$\dot{V}O_2max$ (ml·kg⁻¹·min⁻¹)	1.5-Mile Time (min:s)	$\dot{V}O_2max$ (ml·kg⁻¹·min⁻¹)
<7:31	75	12:31–13:00	39
7:31–8:00	72	13:01–13:30	37
8:01–8:30	67	13:31–14:00	36
8:31–9:00	62	14:01–14:30	34
9:01–9:30	58	14:31–15:00	33
9:31–10:00	55	15:01–15:30	31
10:01–10:30	52	15:31–16:00	30
10:31–11:00	49	16:01–16:30	28
11:01–11:30	46	16:31–17:00	27
11:31–12:00	44	17:01–17:30	26
12:01–12:30	41	17:31–18:00	25

From Wilmore and Bergfeld, "A Comparison of Sports: Physiological and Medical Aspects," Table 24–6, p. 363, 1979, in *Sports Medicine and Physiology,* edited by R. H. Strauss. Copyright © 1979 W. B. Saunders Company, Philadelphia, PA.

Table 6 The Relationship Between Maximal Oxygen Consumption and 12-Min Distance

Distance miles	¼-Mile Laps	Distance m	$\dot{V}O_2max$ $ml\cdot kg^{-1}\cdot min^{-1}$	Distance miles	¼-Mile Laps	Distance m	$\dot{V}O_2max$ $ml\cdot kg^{-1}\cdot min^{-1}$
<1.0	<4	<1609	25.0	1.500	6	2414	42.6
1.000	4	1609	25.0	1.530	...	2462	43.8
1.030	...	1658	26.0	1.565	6.25	2519	45.0
1.065	4.25	1714	27.0	1.590	...	2559	46.0
1.090	...	1754	28.2	1.625	6.5	2615	47.2
1.125	4.5	1811	29.0	1.650	...	2655	48.0
1.150	...	1851	30.2	1.687	6.75	2715	49.2
1.187	4.75	1910	31.6	1.720	...	2768	50.2
1.220	...	1963	32.8	1.750	7	2816	51.6
1.250	5	2012	33.8	1.780	...	2865	52.6
1.280	...	2060	34.8	1.817	7.25	2924	53.8
1.317	5.25	2120	36.2	1.840	...	2961	54.8
1.340	...	2157	37.0	1.875	7.5	3018	56.0
1.375	5.5	2213	38.2	1.900	...	3058	57.0
1.400	...	2253	39.2	1.937	7.75	3117	58.2
1.437	5.75	2313	40.4	1.970	...	3170	59.2
1.470	...	2366	41.6	2.000	8	3219	60.2

Adapted from J. H. Wilmore & D. L. Costill, *Training for Sport and Activity,* 3d ed. Copyright © 1988 Wm. C. Brown Communications, Inc., Dubuque, Iowa. All Rights Reserved. Reprinted by permission.

Table 7 Aerobic Fitness Categories for Men Ages 18 to 75 Years

Age (y)				Fitness Category[a] Maximal Oxygen Consumption ($ml\cdot kg^{-1}\cdot min^{-1}$)				
	Excel	V Good	Good	Ave	Fair	Poor	V Poor	
18–20	>63	62–57	56–51	50–46	45–39	38–33	<33	
21–25	>62	62–56	55–51	50–45	44–38	37–32	<32	
26–30	>59	59–55	54–48	47–42	41–36	35–30	<30	
31–35	>56	56–52	51–47	46–40	39–35	34–29	<29	
36–40	>54	54–49	48–45	44–38	37–33	32–28	<28	
41–45	>51	51–47	46–42	41–36	35–31	30–26	<26	
46–50	>49	49–45	44–40	39–35	34–30	29–25	<25	
51–55	>46	46–42	41–37	36–33	32–28	27–24	<24	
56–60	>44	44–39	38–35	34–31	30–26	25–22	<22	
61–65	>41	41–37	36–33	32–29	28–25	24–21	<21	
66–70	>38	38–35	34–31	30–27	26–24	23–19	<19	
71–75	>35	35–32	31–28	27–24	23–21	20–17	<17	

[a]Note: Excel = excellent; V = very; ave = average.
Reading error in transition ±1–2 $ml\cdot kg^{-1}\cdot min^{-1}$
Table derived from graphs in Shvartz, E., & Reibold, R. C. (1990). Aerobic fitness norms for males and females aged 6 to 75 years: A review. *Aviation, Space, and Environmental Medicine, 61,* 3–11.

Results and Discussion

This section includes comments and tables to help interpret the results of the Aerobic Run/Walk Tests. Thus norms are included, along with some physiological measures that are associated with the test. Data collection forms at the end of the chapter allow us to compile the statistics, which, in turn, allow us to make a concluding statement.

The Surgeon General's Report on Physical Activity and Health reinforces the message that inactivity is a serious health threat.[13,54] The interpretation of the aerobic fitness norms should consider such factors as (1) differences in body composition, (2) running economy (efficiency), and (3) fractional utilization (%) of maximal oxygen con-

sumption, that is, the ability to run or walk continuously at a high percentage of maximal oxygen consumption.

Norms for 1.5-Mile Time

Norms are usually categorized into different levels of fitness ranging from poor (low) to superior (high). The norms in Table 2 are based on over 1500 moderately-fit college students.[29] The six fitness categories represent a bell curve with three areas delineated by three standard deviations (*SD*) above and below the mean. Thus the good, excellent, and superior categories are in the area within 1, 2, and 3 *SD* from the mean. The investigators present a convincing

Table 8 Aerobic Fitness Categories for Women Ages 18 to 75 Years

| Age (y) | Excel | V Good | Fitness Category[a] Maximal Oxygen Consumption ($ml \cdot kg^{-1} \cdot min^{-1}$) | | | | |
			Good	Ave	Fair	Poor	V Poor
18–20	>53	53–48	47–43	42–38	37–33	32–28	<28
21–25	>50	50–46	45–42	41–36	35–32	31–27	<27
26–30	>48	48–44	43–40	39–35	34–31	30–26	<26
31–35	>46	46–42	41–37	36–33	32–29	28–25	<25
36–40	>43	43–39	38–35	34–31	30–27	26–23	<23
41–45	>40	40–36	35–33	32–29	28–26	25–22	<22
46–50	>37	37–35	34–31	30–27	26–24	23–20	<20
51–55	>36	36–32	31–28	27–25	26–24	23–20	<20
56–60	>33	33–30	29–26	25–23	22–20	19–17	<17
61–65	>30	30–27	26–24	23–21	20–18	17–15	<15
66–70	>27	27–25	24–22	21–19	18–16	15–14	<14
71–75	>25	25–23	22–20	19–17	16–15	14–13	<13

[a]Note: Excel = excellent; V = very; ave = average.
Reading error in transition ±1–2 $ml \cdot kg^{-1} \cdot min^{-1}$
Table derived from graphs in Shvartz, E., & Reibold, R. C. (1990). Aerobic fitness norms for males and females aged 6 to 75 years: A review. *Aviation, Space, and Environmental Medicine, 61*, 3–11.

argument for replacing the former Cooper norms (e.g., Table 3), which have much easier criteria, with their more recent norms in Table 2 that reflect a more active population, especially for women.

The traditional norms are based on data collected in the 1970s.[21] The values between *fair* and *good* fitness categories in Table 3[42] are considered *average* for men and women from ages thirteen to over fifty years. In order to qualify for the *good* fitness category, men and women between twenty and twenty-nine years of age must run 1.5 miles in less than 12:01 and 15:55, respectively; this compares to the newer more stringent "good" category criteria of 10:30 and in Table 2 13:10 that were derived from testing moderately fit college men and women 25 y of age.

Norms for the 12-Minute Distance Test

Fitness categories for men and women ages six to seventy-five years may be derived by using Table 6 or Equation 2 in conjunction with Tables 7 (males) and 8 (females).[1,53]

Norms for the AAHPERD Health-Related Test

Table 4 presents the norms for college men and women performing the AAHPERD 1-Mile Run Test or 9-Minute Test.[4] There are no age distinctions because of the similarity of scores for the typical college-age range. The norms are presented as percentiles (%ile) for each gender. Percentile values are simple and practical. For example, if a 21-y-old man ran 1 mile in 6 min 49 s (6:49), he would be at the 50th percentile, meaning that he runs the mile faster than 50% of all college-aged men from whom these norms were extracted. Some authorities suggest criterion norms (standards) with the *minimal acceptable* percentile as the 25th and the *minimal goal* percentile as the 50th.[12] Decisively superior scores might be those above the 80th per-

centile. The AAHPERD 9-Minute Test recommends that distances be estimated to the closest 10 yd (11 m) in order to interpret the test to the closest percentile when using their original percentile table.[3]

Interpretation of Norms

Running 1.5 miles in less than 12 min is consistent with a maximal oxygen consumption above 43 $ml \cdot kg^{-1} \cdot min^{-1}$ (Table 5). Two reviewers[25] stated that Cooper[19] suggested a $\dot{V}O_2max$ of 42 $ml \cdot kg^{-1} \cdot min^{-1}$ as being consistent with good health and functional capacity for daily living in men, and that only 35 $ml \cdot kg^{-1} \cdot min^{-1}$ was necessary in women due to their greater essential fat and lower blood hemoglobin concentration. These criteria values were adopted also by FITNESSGRAM of the Institute for Aerobics Research (1987) and represent the means of young adults,[8,61] and are associated with a reduced risk of all-cause mortality.[13]

The *AAHPERD Physical Best* criterion-referenced standards for the 1-Mile Run are 50 and 43 $ml \cdot kg^{-1} \cdot min^{-1}$ for 20-y old men and women, respectively.[5] Thus, they are 8 $ml \cdot kg^{-1} \cdot min^{-1},$ or one standard deviation, higher than Cooper's criteria. Cooper's criteria seem applicable to middle-aged persons, whereas the AAHPERD criteria are applicable to young adults.[25]

Summary of the Aerobic Run Tests

Five versions of walk/run tests were presented as aerobic field tests of fitness. The 1.5-Mile Test, 12-Minute Test, 1.0-Mile Test, 9-Minute Test, and Rockport Test are all *field tests* because they require accessible facilities, minimal equipment, simple procedures, and may be administered to many persons simultaneously. They are aerobic fitness tests because they measure performance in large-muscle, rhythmic, continuous activities. They are physiologically meaningful because they allow the estimation of aerobic power in units of maximal oxygen consumption, an indicator of cardiovascular endurance. Norms are available that allow participants to be categorized according to their fitness level.

Optional Physiological Measures for the Run/Walk Tests

Some physiological variables that lend themselves to simple measurement before, during, and after the run tests are (a) heart rate, (b) respiratory frequency and depth of breathing, (c) the rate of perceived exertion, (d) perspiration, and (e) subjective muscle responses.

Heart Rate

The recording of heart rate can provide insights into such factors as (a) the degree of anxiety preceding the run test (the anticipatory effect), (b) the degree of effort and motivation during the test, and (c) the fitness comparisons among individuals and also in the same individual when repeating the test.

In order to measure heart rate accurately, electronic monitoring or the best palpatory site should be selected. Additionally, the timing and counting technique should be mastered.

Palpation

The feeling of a pulse or vibration is called palpation. Pulses are generated by the whiplike action of the aorta artery, whereas the vibration pulse (apical beat) is generated by the left ventricle hitting against the chest wall (precordium) near the fifth rib. The arterial pulses that may be felt most easily are the radial, carotid, and temporal. The apical beat can be quite prominent in lean persons immediately after exercise. It can be palpated by the entire hand held as in the pledge of allegiance over the left side of the chest.

Counting Technique

A stopwatch or digital watch should be used to count the number of pulses or beats in 10 or 15 s. If a partner is timing, then the voice command should be one-syllable words such as *Count* and *Stop*. The heart rate in beats per minute ($b \cdot min^{-1}$) is obtained, of course, by multiplying the 10-s count by six or the 15-s count by four. The heart rate that serves to represent the exercise heart rate is taken immediately after exercise. Thus, as soon as the run test is completed, the subject should palpate the pulse or beat within 5 s. To avoid pooling of blood in the lower extremities, the performer should walk slowly or in place while taking the heart rate. The subject should tell the partner the number of beats in 10 or 15 s so that the partner can record it on Form AR 2. Students are encouraged to practice the palpation and counting of heart rate before collecting the actual walk/run-test data.

Heart Rate (HR) Data Prior to the Run Test (Preexercise)

Form AR 2 can be used to record your **resting heart rate (HR)** under two conditions: (1) In the standing position under relaxed conditions in the laboratory before arrival at the test field (or track); and (2) In the standing position at the starting line immediately prior to the Go! signal for the run test. If a warmup does not precede the measurement of the latter heart rate, it may be designated as the anticipatory (or excitatory) heart rate.

Exercise Heart Rate

The exercise and post exercise (recovery) heart rates are also recorded onto Form AR 2. As mentioned previously, the 15-s count is started before 5 s has elapsed in postexercise. The number of beats is recorded by the same partner who recorded the run time or distance.

The heart rate from the 5th to 20th s postexercise is approximately 90% of the actual peak exercise rate.[45] Equation 4 shows that the 15-s count is first multiplied by four, then the product is multiplied by 1.10 in order to account for the slight decrease during the 15+ s it took to measure it.

$$\text{Exercise HR } (b \cdot min^{-1}) = (4 \times 15\text{-s count}) \times 1.10 \qquad \text{Eq. 4}$$

For example, if the 15-s count is 40 beats, then multiplying this by 4 gives the product, 160; 160 multiplied by the constant, 1.10, gives a value of 176 $b \cdot min^{-1}$.

Recovery Heart Rate

In *absolute* terms, the heart rates of most run-test participants at the fifth minute into recovery are often at least 50 beats less than their peak exercise heart rates. For example, if a person's heart rate upon crossing the finish line for the 1.5-mile run is 190 $b \cdot min^{-1}$, then it is likely that the 5-min recovery heart rate will be less than 140 $b \cdot min^{-1}$.

Heart Rate and Motivation

An approximate indication of motivation during the Aerobic Run Tests may be made by comparing the finish-line heart rate with the known or predicted maximal heart rate of the participant. Those who are closer to their maximal heart rate are considered to have given a greater effort. This should be interpreted cautiously, however, if using *predicted* maximal heart rates because of the 10-beat variation in age-group maximal heart rates.[9]

Maximal heart rate is best determined by monitoring the electrocardiogram at the exhaustive point of a progressive exercise test. An approximate estimate of maximal heart rate (HRmax) is made by subtracting age (y) from 220 (Eq. 5). Higher maximal heart rates may exist in women, thus some reviewers recommend subtracting the woman's age from 226.[30]

$$\text{HRmax } (b \cdot min^{-1}) = 220 - age \text{ (y)} \qquad \text{Eq. 5}$$

Respiration During the Run Test

Both the cardiovascular and respiratory systems play prominent roles during the performance of aerobic run tests. Previously, the heart rate's role in the cardiovascular system was examined. Now, breathing frequency and breathing depth are examined as respiratory variables during the run/walk tests. Prior to these tests, however, students should practice observing breathing frequency and depth by recording on Form AR 2 the values at rest and while jogging in place for 3 min.

Breathing Frequency (f)

The rate of breathing, of course, increases as the intensity of exercise increases. Breathing frequency can be influenced voluntarily, but this influence during exercise is minimized. The expected breathing frequencies will range from about 25 to 45 breaths per min ($br \cdot min^{-1}$) for most persons during the run tests. Breaths should be counted for one minute during the fifth or sixth minute in order to assure that steady state has been attained.

Depth of Breathing (tidal volume; V_T or TV)

The size of each breath is called the tidal volume. Under laboratory conditions it is measured in liters or milliliters by special respiratory instruments. Although subject to considerable error, an approximation of tidal volume can be made by subjectively comparing the tidal volume during the run/walk test with that at rest. Thus the runner simply judges how much greater the depth of the exercise breath is than the resting breath; the depth of the exercise breath is an estimated multiple of the resting value. In many cases, the multiple will be between three and five.

Subjective Responses to the Run/Walk Tests

Exercise physiology students can apply their newly acquired knowledge by being aware of various physiological symptoms as they perform their daily routines or, as in this case, as they perform the run/walk tests. Thus it is not always necessary to have instruments by which to measure these symptoms or responses. Subjective responses are those that are estimated by the participant; they may include thermal, muscular, and psychological responses. Each timer/recorder should remind his or her running partner to verbally express the state of these factors as they occur or at designated times during the run.

Thermal Response—Perspiration

The sweating response is influenced not only by exercise but also by such factors as the environmental temperature, relative humidity, convection (breezes), clothing, and state of hydration. Students are encouraged to make a mental note as to the chronology of sweating, that is, the time of onset for sweating and the length of time it continued. The site of perspiration should be noted also.

Muscle Response

Obviously, the muscles are responsible for the movement of the limbs in running during these tests. Muscles may be perceived to alter their state of smoothness (efficiency) or tightness at various times throughout the test due to such factors as warmup, fatigue, and psychological factors (perception). It is also possible that uncommon episodes such as cramps and side stitch may occur along with the expected muscle fatigue.

Rating of Perceived Exertion (RPE)

The rating of perceived exertion[14,15,16] integrates a variety of strain signals into a general whole sensation. Thus, signals coming from the body as a whole—cardiovascular, respiratory, muscular, and nervous systems—provide the performer with a perception of the intensity of exertion. The original Borg RPE category scale ranges from the lowest degree of exertion, 6, to the highest degree, 20; thus, it is sometimes referred to as the Borg 15-category RPE scale. Odd numbers are given anchor descriptions such as *very, very light* for 7, and *very, very hard* for 19. For example, 7 describes the exertion while pedaling a bike slowly at zero resistance, and 19 describes the most physically exhaustive exercise ever encountered by the performer.[50]

The original RPE scale, based on the linear relationship between RPE, power output, and heart rate,[48] was revised with ratio properties based on the nonlinear (exponential or power function) properties of psychophysical and some physiological variables, such as blood lactate and ventilation.[7] For example, the original Borg RPE scale (6–20) would not indicate that lactate is really increasing about three times more at the top (16–17) of the scale than at the bottom. Thus, Borg's newer scale sets the semantic descriptions (e.g., weak, moderate, and strong) to a positively accelerating function.[48] This newer category-ratio (CR-10) scale may be more suitable for determining subjective symptoms associated with breathing, aches, and pains; it also has a high correlation with lactate.[16,55] One researcher suggests that heart rates between 110–150 $b \cdot min^{-1}$ would elicit in most people RPE values between 3 ("moderate") and 5 ("strong"; "hard").[47] CR-10 ratings between 4 and 7 correspond to exercise intensities between 50 and 85% of maximal oxygen consumption,[11] whereas the original RPE scale's ratings between 11 and 16 represent about 50 to 75% of maximal.[6] Either scale is recommended for the run tests and can be used to prescribe and monitor exercise training programs.[27,35]

All run/walk performers must be oriented in RPE terminology (Table 9) in order to use the RPE scale effectively. The performers should read the instructions while in the laboratory prior to testing. Again, someone should read the instructions aloud just prior to the Go! signal for the run test. Specific instructions for the CR-10 scale are found in other sources,[7,11] but are similar to those for the original

Table 9 The Rating of Perceived Exertion

The 15 Category Scale (6–20)[a]	The Category Ratio (CR-10) Scale[b]
6	0 Nothing at all
7 Very very light	0.5 Very, very (extremely) weak; (just noticeable)
8	1 Very weak
9 Very light	2 Weak (light)
10	3 Moderate
11 Light	4 Somewhat strong
12	5 Strong (heavy)
13 Somewhat heavy (hard)	6
14	7 Very strong
15 Heavy (Hard)	8
16	9
17 Very heavy (hard)	10 Very, very (extremely) strong (almost maximal)
18	10+ Maximal (strongest ever)
19 Very very heavy (hard)	
20	

[a]From Borg, *Scandinavian Journal of Rehabilitative Medicine, 2,* Table 1, p. 93, 1970.
[b]From G. Borg, "Psychophysical Bases of Perceived Exertion" in *Medicine and Science in Sports and Exercise, 14*(5), 377–381, Table 2, p. 380, 1982. Copyright © 1982 Williams & Wilkins Publishers. Reprinted by permission of Lea & Febiger.

RPE scale.[46] The instructions are read aloud to the performer as follows:

> You are now going to take part in a work test. We want you to try to estimate how hard you feel the exercise is; that is, we want you to rate the degree of perceived exertion you feel. By perceived exertion we mean the total amount of exertion and physical fatigue, combining all sensations and feelings of physical stress, effort and fatigue. Don't concern yourself with any one factor such as leg pain, shortness of breath, or exercise intensity, but try to concentrate on your total, inner feeling of exertion. Try to estimate as honestly and objectively as possible. Don't underestimate the degree of exertion you feel, but don't overestimate it either. Just try to estimate as accurately as possible.

As an optional RPE method the category 6–20 scale may be differentiated into three distinctive categories:[44] (1) local; (2) central, and (3) overall. The local category represents the participant's rating of strain in the exercising muscles and joints; the central rating reflects ventilatory strain; and the overall rating integrates local and central factors.

References

1. Adams, G. M. (1994). *Exercise physiology laboratory manual.* Dubuque, IA: Brown & Benchmark.
2. Ainsworth, B. E., Richardson, M. T., Jacobs, D. R., & Leon, A. S. (1992). Prediction of cardiorespiratory fitness using physical activity questionnaire data. *Medicine, Exercise, Nutrition Health, 1,* 75–82.
3. American Alliance for Health, Physical Education, Recreation, and Dance. (1980). *Health related physical fitness test manual.* Washington, D.C.: Author.
4. American Alliance for Health, Physical Education, Recreation, and Dance. (1985). *Norms for college students.* Washington, D.C.: Author.
5. American Alliance for Health, Physical Education, Recreation, and Dance. (1988). *Physical best.* Reston, VA: AAHPERD.
6. American College of Sports Medicine. (1991). *Guidelines for exercise testing and prescription.* Philadelphia: Lea & Febiger.
7. American College of Sports Medicine. (1995). *ACSM's Guidelines for exercise testing and prescription.* Philadelphia: Williams & Wilkins.
8. American Heart Association. (1972). *Exercise testing and training of apparently healthy individuals: A handbook for physicians.* New York: American Heart Association.
9. Astrand, P. O., & Rodahl, K. (1977). *Textbook of work physiology.* New York: McGraw-Hill.
10. Balke, B. (1963). *A simple field test for the assessment of physical fitness.* (CARI Report 63-18). Oklahoma City: Civil Aeromedical Research Institute, Federal Aviation Agency.
11. Baumgartner, T. A., & Jackson, A. S. (1991). *Measurement for evaluation in physical education and exercise science.* Dubuque, IA: Wm. C. Brown.
12. Blair, S. N., Falls, H. B., & Pate, R. R. (1983). A new physical fitness test. *The Physician and Sportsmedicine* (April): 87–91, 94–95.
13. Blair, S. N., Kohl, H. W., Paffenbarger, R. S., Clark, D. H., Cooper, K. H., & Gibbons, L. W. (1989). Physical fitness and all-cause mortality. A prospective study of healthy men and women. *Journal of American Medical Association, 262,* 2395–2401.
14. Borg, G. A. V. (1962). *Physical performance and perceived exertion.* Lund, Sweden: Gleerup.
15. Borg, G. A. V. (1970). Perceived exertion as an indicator of somatic stress. *Scandinavian Journal of Rehabilitative Medicine, 2,* 92–98.
16. Borg, G. (1982). Psychophysical bases of perceived exertion. *Medicine and Science in Sports and Exercise, 14,* 377–381.
17. Brooks, G. A., Fahey, T. D., & White, T. P. (1996). *Exercise physiology: Human bioenergetics and its applications.* Mountain View, CA: Mayfield Publishing.
18. Cooper, K. H. (1968). A means of assessing maximal oxygen intake. *Journal of the American Medical Association, 203,* 135–138.
19. Cooper, K. H. (1968b). *Aerobics.* New York: M. Evans & Bantam Books.
20. Cooper, K. H. (1968c). Testing and developing cardiovascular fitness within the United States Air

Force. *Journal of Occupational Medicine, 10,* 636–639.

21. Cooper, K. H. (1970). *The new aerobics.* New York: Bantam Books.

22. Cooper, K. H. (1982). *The aerobics program for total well-being.* New York: M. Evans & Co.

23. Cooper, K. H., Pollock, M. L., Martin, R. P., White, S. R., Linnerud, A. C., & Jackson, A. (1976). Physical fitness levels vs. selected coronary risk factors. *Journal of American Medical Association, 236,* 166–169.

24. Cureton, K. J. (1987). Commentary on children and fitness: A public health perspective. *Research Quarterly for Exercise and Sport, 58,* 315–320.

25. Cureton, K. J., & Warren, G. L. (1990). Criterion-referenced standards for youth health-related fitness tests: A tutorial. *Research Quarterly for Exercise and Sport, 61,* 7–19.

26. deVries, H. A., & Housh, T. J. (1994). *Physiology of exercise.* Dubuque, IA: Brown & Benchmark.

27. Dishman, R. K., Patton, R. W., Smith, J., Weinberg, R., & Jackson, A. (1987). Using perceived exertion to prescribe and monitor exercise training heart rate. *International Journal of Sports Medicine, 8,* 208–213.

28. Dolgener, F. A., Hensley, L. D., Marsh, J. J., & Fjelstul, J. K. (1994). Validation of the Rockport Fitness Walking Test in college males and females. *Research Quarterly for Exercise and Sport, 65,* 152–158.

29. Draper, D. O., & Jones, G. L. (1990, September). The 1.5 mile run revisited—-An update in women's times. *JOPERD,* 78–80.

30. Edington, D. W., & Cunningham, L. (1975). *Biological awareness.* Englewood Cliffs, NJ: Prentice-Hall.

31. Fenstermaker, K. L., Plowman, S. A., & Looney, M. A. (1992). Validation of the Rockport Fitness Walking Test in females 65 years and older. *Research Quarterly for Exercise and Sport, 63,* 322–327.

32. George, J. D., Fisher, A. G., & Vehrs, P. R. (1994). *Laboratory experiences in exercise science.* Boston: Jones and Bartlett.

33. George, J. D., Vehrs, P. R., Allsen, P. E., Fellingham, G. W., & Fisher, A. G. (1993). $\dot{V}O_2max$ estimation from a submaximal 1-mile track jog for fit college-age individuals. *Medicine and Science in Sports and Exercise, 25,* 401–406.

34. Getchell, L. H., Kirkendall, D., & Robbins, G. (1977). Prediction of maximal oxygen uptake in young adult women joggers. *Research Quarterly, 48,* 61–67.

35. Glass, S. C., Knowlton, R. G., & Becque, M. D. (1992). Accuracy of RPE from graded exercise to establish exercise training intensity. *Medicine and Science in Sports and Exercise, 24,* 1303–1307.

36. Hastad, D. N., & Lacy, A. C. (1994). *Measurement and evaluation in physical education and exercise science.* Scottsdale, AZ: Gorsuch Scarisbrick, Publishers.

37. Heil, D. P., Freedson, P. S., Ahlquist, L. E., Price, J., & Rippe, J. M. (1995). Nonexercise regression models to estimate peak oxygen consumption. *Medicine and Science in Sports and Exercise, 27,* 599–606.

38. Jackson, A. S., Blair, S. N., Mahar, M. T., Wier, L. T., Ross, R. M., & Stuteville, J. E. (1990). Prediction of functional aerobic capacity without exercise testing. *Medicine and Science in Sports and Exercise, 22,* 863–870.

39. Jackson, A. S., & Coleman, A. E. (1976). Validation of distance run tests for elementary school children. *Research Quarterly, 47,* 86–94.

40. Kline, G. M., Porcari, J. P., Freedson, P. S., Ward, A., Ross, J., Wilke, S., & Rippe, J. (1987). Does aerobic capacity affect the validity of the one-mile walk $\dot{V}O_2max$ prediction? *Medicine and Science in Sports and Exercise, 19,* Abstract #172, S29.

41. Kline, G. M., Porcari, J. P., Hintermeister, R., Freedson, P. S., Ward, A., McCarron, R. F., Ross, J., & Rippe, J. (1987). Estimation of $\dot{V}O_2max$ from a one-mile track walk, gender, age, and body weight. *Medicine and Science in Sports and Exercise, 19,* 253–259.

42. Kusinitz, I., & Fine, M. (1991). *Your guide to getting fit.* Mountain View, CA: Mayfield Publishing.

43. Leger, L., & Thivierge, M. (1988). Heart rate monitors: Validity, stability, and functionality. *The Physician and Sportsmedicine, 16*(5): 143–151.

44. Maresh, C. M., Deschenes, M. R., Seip, R. L., Armstrong, L. E., Robertson, K. L., & Noble, B. J. (1993). Perceived exertion during hypobaric hypoxia in low- and moderate-altitude natives. *Medicine and Science in Sports and Exercise, 25,* 945–951.

45. McArdle, W. D., Zwiren, L., & Magel, J. R. (1969). Validity of postexercise heart rate as a means of estimating heart rate during work of varying intensities. *Research Quarterly, 40,* 523–529.

46. Morgan, W. P. (1981). Psychophysiology of self-awareness during vigorous physical activity. *Research Quarterly for Exercise and Sport, 52,* 385–427.

47. Nieman, D. C. (1995). *Fitness and sports medicine.* Palo Alto, CA: Bull Publishing.

48. Noble, B. J., Borg, G. A. V., Jacobs, I., Ceci, R., & Kaiser, P. (1983). A category-ratio perceived exertion scale: Relationship to blood and muscle lactates and heart rate. *Medicine and Science in Sports and Exercise, 15,* 523–528.

49. O'Hanley, S., Ward, A., Zwiren, L., McCarron, R., Ross, J., & Rippe, J. M. (1987). Validation of a one-mile walk test in 70–79 year olds. *Medicine and Science in Sports and Exercise, 19,* Abstract #167, S28.

50. Perkins, K. A., Sexton, J. E., Solberg-Kassel, R. D., & Epsteing, L.H. (1991). Effects of nicotine on perceived exertion during low-intensity activity. *Medicine and Science in Sports and Exercise, 23,* 1283–1288.

51. The Rockport Walking Institute. (1986). *Rockport fitness walking test.* Marlboro, MA: The Rockport Company.

52. Safrit, M. J., Hooper, L. M., Ehlert, S. A., Costa, M. G., & Patterson, P. (1988). The validity generalization of distance run tests. *Canadian Journal of Sport Science, 13,* 188–196.

53. Shvartz, E., & Reibold, R. C. (1990). Aerobic fitness norms for males and females aged 6 to 75 years: A review. *Aviation, Space, and Environmental Medicine, 61,* 3–11.

54. Simons-Morton, B. G., O'Hara, N. M., Simons-Morton, D. G., & Parcel, G. S. (1987). Children and fitness: A public health perspective. *Research Quarterly for Exercise and Sport, 58,* 295–302.

55. Sylven, C., Borg, G., Holmgren, A., & Astrom, H. (1991). Psychophysical power functions of exercise limiting symptoms in coronary heart disease. *Medicine and Science in Sports and Exercise, 23,* 1050–1054.

56. Thomas, S., Reading, J., & Shephard, R. J. (1992). Revision of the Physical Activity Readiness Questionnaire (PAR-Q). *Canadian Journal of Sport Science, 17,* 338–345.

57. Warren, B. J., Dotson, R. G., Nieman, D. C., & Butterworth, D. E. (1993). Validation of a 1-Mile Walk Test in elderly women. *Journal of Aging and Physical Activity, 1,* 3–21.

58. Widrick, J., Ward, A., Ebbeling, C., Clemente, E., Rippe, J. M. (1992). Treadmill validation of an overground walking test to predict peak oxygen consumption. *European Journal of Applied Physiology, 64,* 304–308.

59. Wilmore, J. H., & Bergfeld, J. A. (1979). A comparison of sports: Physiological and medical aspects. In R. H. Strauss (Ed.), *Sports Medicine and Physiology,* 353–372. Philadelphia: W. B. Saunders.

60. Wilmore, J. H., & Costill, D. L. (1988). *Training for sport and activity.* Dubuque, IA: Wm. C. Brown.

61. Zuti, W. B., & Corbin, B. (1977). Physical fitness norms for college students. *Research Quarterly, 48,* 499–503.

62. Zwiren, L. D., Freedson, P. S., Ward, A., Wilke, S., & Rippe, J. M. (1991). Estimation of $\dot{V}O_2$max: A comparative analysis of five exercise tests. *Research Quarterly for Exercise and Sport, 62,* 73–78.

Form *AR 1*

Individual Run/Walk Test Form

Name [   ] Date [   ] Time [   ] a.m. [   ] p.m.

Age [   ] y   Gender (M or F) [   ]   Ht [   ] cm   Wt [   ] kg; × 2.2 = [   ] lb

Environmental T [   ] °C   RH [   ] % P_B [   ] torr

Altitude: (Circle the appropriate description from each category)

| m: | <1515 | 1515–1818 | 1819–2121 | 2122–2424 | >2424 |
| ft: | <5000 | 5000–5900 | 6000–6900 | 7000–8000 | >8000 |

Smog Stages: none   light   1st   2nd   3rd

Wind: none   low   moderate   gusty (>2 m · s^{-1}; >4.5 mph)

Run Test (check): 1.5 Mile (2414 m) [   ]   12 Min [   ]   1.0 Mile (1609 m) [   ]   9 Min [   ]

Type of Course (check): 1/4-Mile Track (440-yd) [   ]   400-m Track (437-yd) [   ]   Other [   ]

Time (min:s): 1.5-Mile [   ]   1.0-Mile [   ]   HR [   ] b·min^{-1}

12-Min Test Distance (1/4-Mile Track):

Number of Laps (closest 0.1) [   ]; × 0.25 mile = [   ] mile

12-Min Test Distance (400-m Track):

Number of Laps (closest 0.1) [   ]; × 400 m = [   ] m; ÷ 1609 = [   ] (to closest 0.1 mile)

9-Min Test Distance (1/4-Mile Track):

Number of Whole Laps [   ]; × 440 = [   ] yd; + Portion of incomplete lap [   ] (closest 10 yd)

= [   ] yd

400-m Track: [   ] m; × 1.0936 = [   ] yd; ÷ by 1760 = [   ] mi

Fitness Category or Percentile: [   ]

Rockport $\dot{V}O_2$max (ml·kg^{-1}·min^{-1}) = 132.85 − (0.0769 × [   ] lb) − (0.3877 × [   ] y)

+ (6.315 × 0 or 1) − (3.2649 × [   ] min) − (0.1565 × [   ] b·min^{-1})

Form AR 2

Individual Physiological Data Form for Run Test

Estimated Maximal Oxygen Consumption ($\dot{V}O_2$max 12-Min Test)

Predicted $\dot{V}O_2$max = (D [____] mi − 0.3138)/0.0278

($ml \cdot kg^{-1} \cdot min^{-1}$)

= [____] /0.0278 = [____] $ml \cdot kg^{-1} \cdot min^{-1}$

Heart Rate (HR; $b \cdot min^{-1}$)

Practice at rest (15-s count): Radial [____] Carotid [____] Apical [____]

Practice after 2-min jog in place: 15-s count [____] × 4 × 1.10 = [____] $b \cdot min^{-1}$

Rest	Preexercise	Exercise	Recovery
(Standing)	(Standing at start)	(Immediate Post-Run Test)	(5th min)
[____]	[____]	15-s count [____] × 4 × 1.10 = [____]	[____]

Predicted Maximal HR = 220 − age [____] y = [____] $b \cdot min^{-1}$

Absolute Recover HR = Ex HR [____] − 5th min Recovery HR [____] = [____] $b \cdot min^{-1}$

Breathing Frequency (f; $b \cdot min^{-1}$)   Tidal Volume (V_T; Multiple of Rest)

Rest	Jog in place	Run Test	Jog in place	Run Test
(Standing)	(2nd–3rd min)	(5–6th min)	(2nd–3rd min)	(5–6th min)
[____]	[____]	[____]	[____]	[____]

Rating of Perceived Exertion (RPE; 6–20 or 1.0–10.0⁺):

During the last min or last lap of test [____] 6–20 scale; [____] 1–10 scale

Perspiration:

Time of onset [____] (closest min)   Body site: [____]

Muscles: (check if any of the following were present during test)

Tightness [____]   Side stitch [____]   Cramp [____]

Form AR 3

Group Data Form for Run/Walk Tests

Initials Men	1.5-Mile		12-Min		1-Mile	9-Min	1-Mile Walk	
	min:s	$\dot{V}O_2$	miles	$\dot{V}O_2$	min:s	yd; m	min:s	$\dot{V}O_2$
1.								
2.								
3.								
4.								
5.								
6.								
7.								
8.								
9.								
10.								
M								

Initials Women	1.5-Mile		12-Min		1-Mile	9-Min	1-Mile Walk	
	min:s	$\dot{V}O_2$	miles	$\dot{V}O_2$	min:s	yd; m	min:s	$\dot{V}O_2$
1.								
2.								
3.								
4.								
5.								
6.								
7.								
8.								
9.								
10.								
M								

Chapter 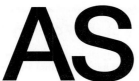 Aerobic Stepping

Field/lab tests may be administered under field or laboratory conditions. Aerobic step tests may be classified as field/lab tests if they are designed to be submaximal tests that predict aerobic fitness; they may be categorized as laboratory tests if they are used as the exercise mode during the direct measurement of oxygen consumption or for clinical evaluation of a physiological system such as the cardiovascular (e.g., ECG) or respiratory systems. They usually require more stringent controls and more complex measurements (e.g., heart rate) than the typical field test. Step tests are simple. Their portability, for example, is demonstrated by the ease with which an appropriately dimensioned box-step can be easily carried from one environmental site to another. In general, they are safe, convenient, inexpensive, and uncomplicated tests. Most step tests, including heart rate measurement, can be completed in less than 6 min. The Forestry Step Test will be discussed as an example of the more than thirty step tests that have been used to measure aerobic fitness.

Forestry Step Test

The Forestry Step Test is important because of its universal applicability, its ability to assess aerobic fitness, and its simplicity. For exercise physiology laboratory students the test also serves to teach some basic physiological principles along with some basic laboratory techniques.

The Forestry Step Test was designed as a screening test for safety and emergency personnel (e.g., forestry firefighters, police, lifeguards).[16] The screening test prevents the employers for these physically demanding occupations from recruiting unfit persons. For instance, all federal, and many state, agencies have adopted a maximal oxygen consumption standard for firefighters based on their performance on the Forestry Step Test.

The Forestry Step Test[16] is a modification of the original Harvard Test[4] and the modified Harvard Test.[13] Although exercise physiologists may differ in their choice of descriptive terms for classifying the intensity of exercise, the terms often chosen are "light, moderate, heavy, and severe"[7] (see Table 1). For most young adults, the exercise intensity for the Forestry Step Test is between moderate and heavy (W).[6] The test also fits into the moderate-to-heavy category based upon an arbitrarily chosen range of heart rates between 120–160 beats per minute[7] and based

Table 1 Classification of Exercise Intensity by Power (W), Heart Rate (b · min⁻¹), and MET Level

Power	Exercise Intensity Classification		
	Light–Moderate W	Moderate–Heavy W	Heavy–Severe W
Men	100	100–200	200
Women	75	75–150	150
	$b \cdot min^{-1}$	$b \cdot min^{-1}$	$b \cdot min^{-1}$
Heart Rate	<120	120–160	>160
MET	<4	4–8	>8

on typical MET values of 6.9 (25 $ml \cdot kg^{-1} \cdot min^{-1}$) and 8.3 (~29 $ml \cdot kg^{-1} \cdot min^{-1}$) for women's and men's Forestry step heights.[1]

Although the test was originally designed for forestry firefighters, it is applicable for most apparently healthy persons. The moderate exercise intensity required for this test should enable most persons to complete the prescribed duration of the test (5 min). The intensity is probably high enough to raise the heart rates of fit persons above those rates that might possibly be influenced by emotional factors. However, the test may be too severe for persons of extremely low fitness and for many persons over sixty years of age.

In addition to its ability to classify the fitness status of its participants, this test also provides an indirect measure of maximal oxygen consumption. By relating this predicted value of maximal oxygen consumption to the requirements of certain occupations, it is possible to predict the job suitability of either the candidate or a present employee.

Because the final score derived from the Forestry Step Test is a maximal oxygen consumption value, the score may be related to norms for maximal oxygen consumption that have been adjusted according to age categories for aerobic fitness (Table 8). Although there are age and gender modifications for the fitness categories of this test, it is recommended that they be disregarded if the primary purpose of the test is to screen persons for occupational suitability.

Recent amendments to the federal Age Discrimination in Employment Act, which made the hiring or firing of persons based on gender or age illegal, have allowed state and local governments to require mandatory retirement of police and fire personnel. Despite these amendments, most police and fire departments rely on fitness tests, such as the Forestry Test, for new recruits and periodic testing of current personnel. In other words, selecting and maintaining personnel is based upon *performance* qualifications, not age per se.

In addition to classifying the fitness level, this test may be used to develop a prescription for exercise. Periodic testing of the exercise participant will allow for evaluation of both the prescription and the participant.

Purposes of the Forestry Step Test

The purposes of the Forestry Step Test are related to its importance. The primary purpose is to measure the aerobic (cardiovascular endurance) fitness of persons. Secondly, the test may be used to screen potential employees for their physical aptitude in an occupation. Thirdly, because of its portability, the test may evaluate individuals under a variety of environmental conditions (e.g., heat or altitude).

Physiological Rationale

All tests in exercise physiology should be based upon a valid physiological rationale. The physiological rationale for the Forestry Step Test focuses upon the relationships between oxygen consumption, heart rate, and exercise. The prediction of maximal oxygen consumption is based on the direct linear (positive) relationship between oxygen consumption and exercise. Dr. Sharkey's original objective was to develop a simple test that would predict the success of wilderness firefighters. He found that direct field measurements of wilderness fire-fighting tasks averaged 22.5 ml·kg^{-1}·min^{-1}.[16] Given the intermittent nature of fire-fighting tasks, Sharkey reasoned that a physically fit individual could sustain work rates not more than 50% of capacity over an 8-hour period. Therefore, he concluded that a maximum aerobic capacity of at least 45 ml·kg^{-1}·min^{-1} would be required. This criterion has been adopted by the U.S. Forest Service.[21]

As with oxygen consumption, heart rate is linearly and positively related to exercise. This also means that heart rate and oxygen consumption are directly related. Heart rates are not measured *during* the Forestry Test but at *recovery* from the stepping exercise. Therefore, it is important that the recovery heart rate be relatively indicative of the exercise heart rate. There appears to be ample evidence to support a high relationship between exercise recovery heart rate and the actual exercise heart rate.[12,14,19]

The fitness of a person is related to both maximal oxygen consumption and submaximal heart rate response. Low recovery heart rates reflect a low stress level by the performer, whereas high rates reflect a high stress level. This cardiovascular stress, as reflected by recovery heart rate, indicates the degree of aerobic fitness of the individual. Obviously, low stresses (or heart rates) at any given exercise

---

Accuracy of the Forestry Step Test

Obviously, predictive tests such as the aerobic run tests and the step tests are not as valid as making actual measurements of maximal oxygen consumption. The validity correlations based on the relationship between various step test scores and directly measured $\dot{V}O_2$max are reported to range from .46 to .66.[11] In general, step tests have standard errors of estimate (*SEE*) ranging from about 12%–15%.[6] This means that the predicted score may overestimate or underestimate the directly measured maximal oxygen consumption in two-thirds of the population by as much as 12%–15%; thus, the error in one-third of the population is even larger. If an error of 12% is assumed, and an individual's directly measured maximal oxygen consumption is 50 ml·kg^{-1}·min^{-1}, then the estimated values from the step test would likely fall between 44 and 56 "ml's" [calculated as: 50 ml ± (0.12 × 50)]. A significant part of the error in predicting $\dot{V}O_2$max from submaximal step testing is due to the within-subject variation in oxygen demand when tested on different days.[20] This may also contribute to the daily variation of heart rate at submaximal exercise, which is reported to vary by about 5 b·min^{-1}.[12] An additional error may be attributed to habituation, whereby performers improve their stepping efficiency as a result of the first or second test.[18] Finally, as with all heart-rate based fitness tests, the differences in maximal heart rates contribute to the standard error of prediction. Although the length of the performer's legs (or stature) is sometimes presumed to affect the results of stepping, there has been only weak,[20] or U-shaped,[15] or no relationship.[5] One general guideline is that if the top of the bench is no higher than the performer's knee, there is no disadvantage in the efficiency of stepping.

(step test) level equate with higher predicted maximal oxygen consumption values, which indicate a higher aerobic fitness level.

Method

Some of the factors described for the Forestry Test under the heading *Method* are: (a) equipment, (b) preparation, and (c) testing.

Equipment

The recommended pieces of equipment are presented in Table 2. Besides the obvious pieces of equipment, such as the step apparatus and a timing device for measuring the duration of the test and the performer's heart rate, instruments to measure the performer's stature and weight, and the environment's meteorological condition are also necessary. Some of these meteorological instruments may be expensive, such as a single unit that combines automated wet/dry, bulb/globe thermometers with an anemometer for measuring wind speed. Also, laboratories should have a good barometer for measuring the barometric pressure. Environmental temperature (T) and relative humidity (RH) are especially important meteorological readings for step tests

Table 2 Equipment for Forestry Step Test

Type of Measure	Type of Instrument
Meteorological	
Environmental Temperature (°C)	Dry bulb; wet bulb;[a] globe[a]
Relative Humidity (RH%)	Hygrometer;[a] sling psychrometer[a]
Barometric Pressure (torr)	Mercury barometer;[a] aneroid[a]
Basic Data	
Weight (kg)	Platform scale
Stature (cm; m)	Anthropometer; stadiometer
Ergometric	
Step Ergometer (cm; m)	Bench, stool, box, or bleacher/stadium step
	Men: 40 cm (15.75 in.) Women: 33 cm (13 in.)
Timing	
Minutes; seconds (min:s)	Laboratory timer;[a] stopwatch; watch; clock
Metronome	Mechanical or electronic; audio recording of cadence

[a]Optional instruments for more controlled testing

performed in the field or in laboratories without thermostatic control. Both temperature and humidity will influence heart rate when they are outside a certain range. For example, the norms for the Forestry Step Test are based upon environmental temperatures between 20–26.3°C (68–79°F).[17] Relative humidity may be calculated from an inexpensive sling psychrometer's wet and dry bulb temperatures or may be measured directly from a hygrometer.

The ergometric equipment—the step itself—is simple, inexpensive, and often portable. Step benches may be built to accommodate one person or groups of persons. Sometimes sturdy benches may be elevated to the prescribed height by simply inserting appropriately sized blocks under the supports of the bench. The commercially available StairMaster® 4000 is an example of an electronically programmed step ergometer.[10]

A field test, such as the Forestry Step Test may be converted into a laboratory test by controlling meteorological variables and by enhancing the sophistication of the physiological measurements. For example, greater sophistication occurs when replacing finger palpation of pulse rate with electrocardiograph monitoring of heart rate.

Preparation

Administration of any step test requires appropriate preparations on the part of both the participant and the technician. The preparation of the participant for this test applies to most field/lab tests, with a prior exercise regimen added for anaerobic tests and some other aerobic tests. The participant should follow these guidelines:

1. Relax five minutes immediately preceding the test. The subject should not have performed fatiguing exercise within two hours of the test. *No* warmup is permitted prior to the test; loosening up (stretching), however, is permitted.

Calibration for the Step Test

Calibration of some instruments does not have to be repeated on every test occasion. For example, after the initial verification of the step ergometer's height, it may never need to be measured again. The calibration of the platform scale was discussed in Chapter UN. The metronome should be checked for accuracy by counting the number of beats for 1 min at the prescribed test setting. For example, the setting for the Forestry Step Test is 90 beats per min. Thus, when starting a watch with a second hand simultaneously with a beat (sound) on the metronome and then counting the next beat as one, the 90th beat should occur at the end of 1 min.

2. Take no stimulants (tobacco, "uppers," coffee, tea, colas, chocolate, etc.) or depressants (alcohol, "downers") 4–24 hours preceding the test; the variable length of time is dependent upon the strength and amount of the particular drug dosage.

3. No heavy meal within three hours of the test;[2] on the other hand, the subject should not be hungry (e.g., not >5 hours without food).

4. Be euhydrated, meaning normal hydration, which is neither dehydrated nor superhydrated.

5. Wear lightweight shoes and lightweight/loose clothing (preferably tennis shoes and shorts). An exception to this might be if the objective is to determine the stress response under occupational or athletic conditions (e.g., firefighters, cross-country skiers, etc.).

6. Have no distension of the urinary bladder.[8]

The technician's preparations for many lab/field tests usually consider three major factors: (1) calibration, (2) the gathering of basic and meteorological data, and (3) the orientation of the participant to the testing procedure.

Basic and meteorological data are important in interpreting the test. For example, a very small stature or excess weight of a performer may influence the efficiency of stepping. The weight of the performer includes the exercise clothes and shoes.[17] Contrary to most normative data, this clothed weight should be used to calculate the relative maximal oxygen consumption ($\dot{V}O_2max$ divided by body weight).

If a fan is used during the test, it should be noted on the test form. A good fan might allow an additional 2°C to the upper limit of temperature for any exercise tests in the laboratory.[3]

Orientation makes the performer aware of the purpose of the test. Secondly, it provides instructions and information that may satisfy legal or ethical requirements for informed consent. Thirdly, it may enhance the accuracy and validity of the test.

The technician emphasizes the importance of keeping proper cadence and of straightening the back and legs at the top of the step (Fig. 1). The cadence may be kept with the aid of the metronome which is set to 90 steps per minute in

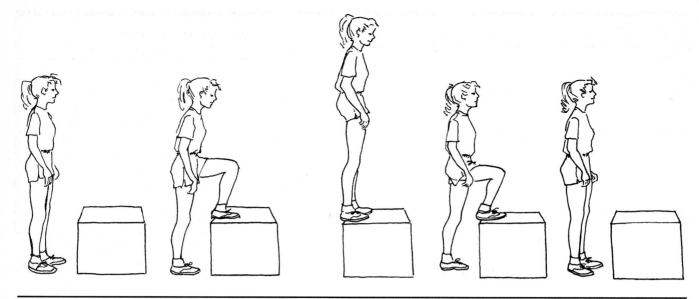

Figure 1 The 4-count stepping technique for the step-test subject.

order to produce the prescribed step rate of 22.5 per minute for the Forestry Step Test. The four-count cadence is as follows:

"Up-one": One foot goes to top of step
"Up-two": The other foot follows to top of step
"Down-one": One foot descends to floor
"Down-two": The other foot follows to floor

The performer's leading foot (first foot on step) may be changed a few times during the test. The technician reminds the subject to sit down on the bench immediately following the test. Upon being seated, both the performer and technician palpate the subject's pulse at predesignated sites. It is a good idea to practice heartbeat palpation prior to the test. The pulse may be palpated at various sites.

The technician's preparatory steps for many field/lab tests are as follows:

1. Calibrate the instruments prior to on-site orientation of the performer.
2. Set metronome to proper cadence; Forestry Step Test = 90 beats per min.
3. Record meteorological data:
   a. Environmental temperature (°C)
   b. Relative humidity (%RH)
   c. Barometric pressure (P_B; torr)
4. State the purpose of the test to the participant, e.g., " . . . to record postexercise heart rate in order to estimate your aerobic fitness."
5. Question the participant regarding drugs, physical activity, meal time, or any possible medical factors that might contraindicate (argue against) exercise testing at the present time.
6. Record basic data—date, time of day, gender, and age; measure and record stature (cm) and weight (kg).
7. Explain and briefly demonstrate the test:

a. Exercise protocol
   (1) Exercise mode—step, bicycle, or treadmill ergometer; dynamometer
   (2) Timing—cadence, rate, pace, stage, and duration
   (3) Intensity—submaximal (low, moderate, heavy, or percent maximal); maximal; supramaximal
b. Technique of exercising—proper stepping
c. Physiological measures
   (1) The variable and method: for example, heart rate by palpation
   (2) Timing of variable: onset and duration of measure
8. Ask performer if there are any questions.
9. Obtain performer's informed consent (agreement to be tested).
10. Provide a non-fatiguing practice period for the performer that includes stepping and palpating of pulse.

Testing

The testing procedures for various step tests are similar. The exercise protocol (Table 3) for the Forestry Step Test includes such factors as height of step, rate of stepping, duration of stepping, and time period of the pulse count. The procedures for the Forestry Step Test include such factors as paying attention to warning signs, timing of the test and heart rate, palpation of the heart rate, and the prevention of soreness in the performer.

Warning Signs

If the performer cannot complete the test due to fatigue or any stop-test characteristics listed in Table 4, then the

Table 3 Protocol for the Forestry Step Test[a]

Step Height	
Men:	40 cm (15.75 in.)
Women:	33 cm (13 in.)
Step Rate	22.5 steps per min; (metronome = 90 b·min⁻¹)
Stepping Duration	5 min
Pulse Count Time Period	15 s (5:15–5:30)

Note: [a]Same protocol as for Astrand-Ryhming Step Test.[13] YMCA test is 12 in., 24 steps per min, 3-min duration, and pulse period 3:05–4:05.

Procedures for the Forestry Step Test

The sequence of procedures may be summarized in thirteen steps as follows:

1. Performer stands facing 40-cm (men) or 33-cm (women) step bench.
2. Technician starts metronome, which is set for 90 beats per minute.
3. Technician requests performer to start stepping at any metronome beat.
4. Technician starts timer as soon as performer makes first movement.
5. Technician helps with cadence at beginning by counting aloud: "up-one, up-two, down-one, down-two."
6. Technician encourages the performer to straighten the back and the legs at top of step.
7. Technician encourages completion of the test while keeping aware of stop-test indicators (Table 4).
8. Technician stops test and metronome at 5th min.
9. Performer sits down immediately upon completion of test.
10. Technician and/or performer immediately palpate pulse and count silently for 15 s, starting the count at 5:15 (15 s after the test) and stopping at 5:30.
11. The technician records the 15-s pulse count on Form AS 1.
12. Performer cools down by walking and statically stretching the gastrocs and quads for the next 5–8 min.
13. The technician thanks the performer for such effort and cooperation.

Table 4 Stop-Test Indicators from Unmonitored Performer During Exercise Testing

Indicator	Performer Characteristics
1. [a]Request	Makes request to end the test
2. [a]Pallor	Skin becomes pale, cyanotic
3. [a]Ataxia	Lacks coordination; e.g., fails to keep proper cadence for *20 consecutive seconds*
4. [a]Confusion	Inability to focus attention; e.g., time disorientation
5. Syncope	Faintness, dizziness, or light-headedness
6. [a]Nausea	Sick to the stomach; vomiting symptoms
7. Dyspnea	Dysfunction in breathing
8. Angina	Chest pain
9. Muscular problem	Side stitch, cramp, strain, fatigue
10. Facial disorder	Panic look, blank stare, unresponsive

[a]From The American College of Sports Medicine, *Guidelines for Graded Exercise Testing and Prescription,* p. 72, 1991. Copyright © 1991 Lea & Febiger Publishers, Malvern, PA. Reprinted by permission.

technician should record the actual total time of the test in addition to the reason for terminating the test (e.g., fatigue, pallor, dyspnea). Stopping an exercise test for *specific* indications, such as a drop in blood pressure, are not applicable for the Forestry Step Test because the performer usually is not monitored for that variable. Therefore, the stop-test signs listed in Table 4 are general signs that are likely to indicate a deficiency in an unmonitored physiological system.

Timing

The laboratory clock should continue to run after the 5th min; the time for taking heart rate begins at 5:15 and ends at 5:30. The metronome is stopped, however, because it may be disconcerting while trying to count heartbeats.

Pulse Rate

The radial pulse is on the thumb side of the wrist; contrary to popular belief, it is acceptable to palpate your *own* pulse with your thumb; it is not acceptable to palpate someone else's pulse with your thumb.

The carotid pulse may be palpated on either side of the neck. There is some controversy over the bradycardiac (slowing) effect of carotid palpation. However, in a well-controlled study the investigators found no significant difference between carotid and radial palpation of heart rate.[14] They cautioned, however, against unnecessary pressure against the carotid artery.

The technician's and performer's 15-s pulse counts should not differ by more than three beats for laboratory purposes. (It is quite likely that only one person will take the pulse rate under field conditions.) If the difference is greater than three beats, then repeat the test after both palpators are confident that they are palpating correctly.

It is very important to get accurate heart rates. The heart rate will be used for estimating the individual's maximal oxygen consumption. In general, palpation errors are those of *underestimation* because people are more likely to miss pulses than add extra ones.[9]

Cool-Down

To alleviate possible delayed muscle stiffness, it is best to walk for about three minutes immediately following the test. After mild walking, the performer should stretch the calves (e.g., wall-lean exercise) and quadriceps (e.g., lean back while kneeling and sitting on heels) on three or four occasions for 3–60 s with 2-min relief intervals.

Table 5 Forestry Nonadjusted Aerobic Fitness ($\dot{V}O_2max$) for Men

Pulse Count (15 s)	Maximal Oxygen Consumption (ml·kg⁻¹·min⁻¹)												
45	33	33	33	33	33	32	32	32	32	32	32	32	32
44	34	34	34	34	33	33	33	33	33	33	33	33	33
43	35	35	35	34	34	34	34	34	34	34	34	34	34
42	36	35	35	35	35	35	35	35	35	35	35	34	34
41	36	36	36	36	36	36	36	36	36	36	36	35	35
40	37	37	37	37	37	37	37	37	35	35	35	35	35
39	38	38	38	38	38	38	38	38	38	38	38	37	37
38	39	39	39	39	39	39	39	39	39	39	39	38	38
37	41	40	40	40	40	40	40	40	40	40	40	39	39
36	42	42	41	41	41	41	41	41	41	41	41	40	40
35	43	43	42	42	42	42	42	42	42	42	42	42	41
34	44	44	43	43	43	43	43	43	43	43	43	43	43
33	46	45	45	45	45	45	44	44	44	44	44	44	44
32	47	47	46	46	46	46	46	46	46	46	46	46	46
31	48	48	48	47	47	47	47	47	47	47	47	47	47
30	50	49	49	49	48	48	48	48	48	48	48	48	48
29	52	51	51	51	50	50	59	50	50	50	50	50	50
28	53	53	53	53	52	52	52	52	51	51	51	51	51
27	55	55	55	54	54	54	54	54	54	53	53	53	52
26	57	57	56	56	56	56	56	56	56	55	55	54	54
25	59	59	58	58	58	58	58	58	58	56	56	55	55
24	60	60	60	60	60	60	60	59	59	58	58	57	
23	62	62	61	61	61	61	61	60	60	60	59		
22	64	64	63	63	63	63	62	62	61	61			
21	66	66	65	65	65	64	64	64	62				
20	68	68	67	67	67	67	66	66	65				
WT (lb)	120	130	140	150	160	170	180	190	200	210	220	230	240
WT (kg)	54.5	59.1	63.6	68.2	72.7	77.3	81.8	86.4	91	95.4	100	104.5	109

From B. J. Sharkey, *Physiology of Fitness*, Table B.1, p. 258, 1984. Copyright © 1984 Human Kinetics Publishers, Champaign, IL.

Derivation of Aerobic Fitness from the Forestry Step Test

The unit of measure derived from the heart rate response from the Forestry Step Test is a maximal oxygen consumption value (milliliters of oxygen per kilogram body weight per minute; ml·kg⁻¹·min⁻¹). Tables 5 (men), 6 (women), and 7 (age adjustment) minimize mathematical calculations.[17] The body weight and 15-s pulse count are needed to find the *nonadjusted* value of maximal oxygen consumption in the tables for men and women, respectively. Age and the nonadjusted value are needed to find the age-adjusted aerobic fitness for men and women 15–65 years of age.

Weight

The bottom two rows of Tables 5 and 6 are presented in 10-pound (lb) and 4.5-kilogram (kg) increments. The columns above each weight represent the predicted maximal oxygen consumption score for any given row of pulse counts that intersects the weight column. Because the efficiency of stepping (ml·kg⁻¹·min⁻¹) changes very little for any given change in weight (especially for men), there is no need to interpolate the weight columns for those weights that lie between the columns.

Pulse Count

The vertical column to the far left represents the post-step test heartbeats (15 s) from 20 to 45 (80 to 180 b·min⁻¹). The value at the intersection of the row for the pulse counts and the column for the weight lifted is the nonadjusted fitness score ($\dot{V}O_2max$ in ml·kg⁻¹·min⁻¹) for the Forestry Step Test. The Tables must be used because no regression equation has been derived from the original Sharkey data.

It is not essential to calculate heart rate in order to derive the aerobic fitness score. It should be recognized that the actual exercise heart rate during the last minute of the Forestry Step Test is really higher than that represented by the 15-s pulse count even after the 15-s count is converted to a minute rate. This is because heart rate would continue to decrease from the 15th to 30th s of postexercise.

As an example of using the nonadjusted fitness tables, suppose the number of pulse counts between the 15th and 30th s following the step test was 30 for a 110-lb (50.0-kg) woman. By reading horizontally along the 30 pulse-count row (or marking lightly with a pencil) to the point where it intersects the 110-pound vertical column (may also be marked with a pencil), the value 44 is found. This value represents a maximal oxygen consumption of

Table 6 Forestry Nonadjusted Aerobic Fitness Values (ml·kg^{-1}·min^{-1}) for Women

Pulse Count	HR (b·min^{-1})	Maximal Oxygen Consumption ($\dot{V}O_2$ max)											
45	180										29	29	29
44	176								30	30	30	30	30
43	172							31	31	31	31	31	31
42	168			32	32	32	32	32	32	32	32	32	32
41	164			33	33	33	33	33	33	33	33	33	33
40	160			34	34	34	34	34	34	34	34	34	34
39	156			35	35	35	35	35	35	35	35	35	35
38	152			36	36	36	36	36	36	36	36	36	36
37	148			37	37	37	37	37	37	37	37	37	37
36	144		37	38	38	38	38	38	38	38	38	38	38
35	140	38	38	39	39	39	39	39	39	39	39	39	39
34	136	39	39	40	40	40	40	40	40	40	40	40	40
33	132	40	40	41	41	41	41	41	41	41	41	41	41
32	128	41	41	42	42	42	42	42	42	42	42	42	42
31	124	42	42	43	43	43	43	43	43	43	43	43	43
30	120	43	43	44	**44**	44	44	44	44	44	44	44	44
29	116	44	44	45	45	45	45	45	45	45	45	45	45
28	112	45	45	46	46	46	47	47	47	47	47	47	47
27	108	46	46	47	48	48	49	49	49	49	49		
26	104	47	48	49	50	50	51	51	51	51			
25	100	49	50	51	52	52	53	53					
24	96	51	52	53	54	54	55						
23	92	53	54	55	56	56	57						
WT (lb)		80	90	100	**110**	120	130	140	150	160	170	180	190
WT (kg)		36.4	40.9	45.4	**50.0**	54.5	59.1	63.6	68.2	72.7	77.3	81.8	86.4

From B. J. Sharkey, *Physiology of Fitness*, Table B.2, p. 259, 1984. Copyright © 1984 Human Kinetics Publishers, Champaign, IL.

44 ml·kg^{-1}·min^{-1}. If a man weighing 150 lb (68.2 kg) had a pulse count response of 30 (120 b·min^{-1}), his nonadjusted maximal oxygen consumption is 49 ml·kg^{-1}·min^{-1}. However, both the woman's and the man's values need to be adjusted for age.

Age-Adjusted Aerobic Fitness

In order to derive a valid aerobic fitness score for persons 30 years of age or more, it is necessary to account for the natural decrease in maximal heart rate due to aging. This decrease was presented earlier as follows: maximal HR equals 220 minus age.

For example, if a 20-year-old man and 50-year-old man have the same pulse count after the step test, they do not have equal aerobic fitness levels. Theoretically, the 30 pulse counts (120 b · min^{-1}) for the 20-year-old only represent 120/200th (60%) of his maximal rate, whereas 30 counts represents 120/170th (70%) of the 50-year-old's maximal. Thus, the degree of stress for the older person was relatively greater during the step test because he was working closer to his maximal heart rate.

To find the age-adjusted fitness score, the first step is to round off the performer's age to the closest fifth year (y). For example, if the person is 33, then locate the 35-year row originating at the far left of Table 7;[17] if the subject is

32, then locate the 30-year row. Then read horizontally along the *age* row to where the age intersects with the nonadjusted fitness score. This is the age-adjusted fitness score, which should be used to categorize the aerobic fitness level found in Table 8.[17]

Results and Discussion

The interpretation of the predicted maximal oxygen consumption from the Forestry Step Test is made by consulting the aerobic fitness norms in Table 8. These fitness categories distinguish between gender and age groups.

If only one maximal oxygen consumption were chosen as the criterion for aerobic fitness, that value most likely would be the 45 ml·kg^{-1}·min^{-1} that Sharkey himself chose as the criterion for selecting wilderness firefighters.

References

1. American College of Sports Medicine. (1991). *Guidelines for graded exercise testing and prescription.* Philadelphia: Lea & Febiger.
2. American College of Sports Medicine. (1995). *ACSM's Guidelines for graded exercise testing and prescription.* Philadelphia: Williams & Wilkins.

Table 7 Age-Adjusted Fitness Scores for the Forestry Step Test

Age (y)	Nonadjusted Fitness Score																				
	30	31	32	33	34	35	36	37	38	39	40	41	42	43	44	45	46	47	48	49	50
	Age-Adjusted Score (ml·kg⁻¹·min⁻¹)																				
15	32	33	34	35	36	37	38	39	40	41	42	43	44	45	46	47	48	49	50	51	53
20	31	32	33	34	35	36	37	38	39	40	41	42	43	44	45	46	47	48	49	50	51
25	30	31	32	33	34	35	36	37	38	39	40	41	42	43	44	45	46	47	48	49	50
30	29	30	31	32	33	34	35	36	37	38	39	40	41	42	43	44	45	46	47	48	49
35	27	28	29	31	32	33	34	35	36	37	38	39	40	41	42	43	44	45	46	47	48
40	26	27	28	30	31	32	33	34	35	36	37	38	39	40	41	42	43	44	45	46	47
45	25	26	27	29	30	31	32	33	34	35	36	37	38	39	40	41	42	43	44	45	46
50	24	25	26	28	29	30	31	32	33	34	35	36	37	38	39	40	41	42	43	44	45
55	23	24	25	27	28	29	30	31	32	33	34	35	36	37	38	39	40	40	41	42	43
60	22	23	24	25	26	27	28	30	31	32	33	34	35	36	37	37	38	39	40	41	42
65	21	22	23	24	25	26	27	28	29	30	31	32	33	34	35	36	37	38	38	39	40

Example: If your age is 40 years and you score 50 on the step test, your age-adjusted score is 47.

(Continued)

Table 8 Aerobic Fitness Categories in Men (M) and Women (W) for the Forestry Step Test

Age (y)		Fitness Category[a]						
		Super	Excel	V Good	Good	Fair	Poor	V Poor
		Maximal Oxygen Consumption (ml·kg⁻¹·min⁻¹)						
15	M	57+	56–52	51–47	46–42	41–37	36–32	<32
	W	54+	53–49	48–44	43–39	38–34	33–29	<29
20	M	56+	55–51	50–46	45–41	40–36	35–31	<31
	W	53+	52–48	47–43	42–38	37–33	32–28	<28
25	M	55+	54–50	49–45	44–40	39–35	34–30	<30
	W	52+	51–47	46–42	41–37	36–32	31–27	<27
30	M	54+	53–49	48–44	43–39	38–34	33–29	<29
	W	51+	50–46	45–41	40–36	35–31	30–26	<26
35	M	53+	52–48	47–43	42–38	37–33	32–28	<28
	W	50+	49–45	44–40	39–35	34–30	29–25	<25
40	M	52+	51–47	46–42	41–37	36–32	31–27	<27
	W	49+	48–44	43–39	38–34	33–29	28–24	<24
45	M	51+	50–46	45–41	40–36	35–31	30–26	<26
	W	48+	47–43	42–38	37–33	32–28	27–23	<23
50	M	50+	49–45	44–40	39–35	34–30	29–25	<25
	W	47+	46–42	41–37	36–32	31–27	26–22	<22
55	M	49+	48–44	43–39	38–34	33–29	28–24	<24
	W	46+	45–41	40–36	35–31	30–26	25–21	<21
60	M	48+	47–43	42–38	37–33	32–28	27–23	<23
	W	45+	44–40	39–35	34–30	29–25	24–20	<20
65	M	47+	48–42	41–37	36–32	31–27	26–22	<22
	W	44+	43–39	38–34	33–29	28–24	23–20	<20

Note: [a]Super = superior; excel = excellent; v = very.
From B. J. Sharkey, *Physiology of Fitness*, Tables B.4 and B.5, p. 262, 1984. Copyright © 1984 Human Kinetics Publishers, Champaign, IL.

3. Andersen, K. L., Shephard, R. J., Denolin, H., Varnauskas, E., & Masironi, R. (1971). *Fundamentals of exercise testing*. Geneva: World Health Organization.
4. Brouha, L. (1943). The Step Test: A simple method of measuring physical fitness for muscular work in young men. *Research Quarterly, 14*, 30–35.
5. Cicutti, N., Jette, M., & Sidney, K. (1991). Effect of leg length on bench stepping efficiency in children. *Canadian Journal of Sport Science, 16*, 58–63.
6. deVries, H. A. (1971). *Lab experiments in exercise physiology*. Dubuque, IA: Wm. C. Brown.
7. Fox, E. L., Bowers, R. W., & Foss, M. L. (1993). The physiological basis for exercise and sport. Dubuque, IA: Brown & Benchmark.
8. Frohlich, E. D., Grim, C., Labarthe, D. R., Maxwell, M. H., Perloff, D., & Weidman, W. H. (1987).

Table 7 (continued)

Age (y)	51	52	53	54	55	56	57	58	Nonadjusted Fitness Score 59	60	61	62	63	64	65	66	67	68	69	70	71	72
									Age-Adjusted Score (ml·kg⁻¹·min⁻¹)													
15	54	55	56	57	58	59	60	61	62	63	64	65	66	67	68	69	70	71	72	74	75	76
20	52	53	54	55	56	57	58	59	60	61	62	63	64	65	66	67	68	69	70	71	72	73
25	51	52	53	54	55	56	57	58	59	60	61	62	63	64	65	66	67	68	69	70	71	72
30	50	51	52	53	54	55	56	57	58	59	60	61	62	63	64	65	66	67	68	69	70	71
35	49	50	51	52	53	54	55	56	57	58	59	60	60	61	62	63	64	65	66	67	68	69
40	48	49	50	51	52	53	54	55	55	56	57	58	59	60	61	62	63	64	65	66	67	68
45	47	48	49	50	51	52	52	53	54	55	56	57	58	59	60	61	62	63	64	65	65	66
50	45	46	47	48	49	50	51	52	53	53	54	55	56	57	58	58	59	61	61	62	63	64
55	44	45	46	46	47	48	49	50	51	52	53	53	54	55	56	57	58	59	59	60	61	62
60	42	43	44	45	46	46	47	48	49	50	51	51	52	53	54	55	56	57	57	58	59	60
65	41	42	42	43	44	45	46	46	47	48	49	50	50	51	52	53	54	54	55	56	57	58

From B. J. Sharkey, *Physiology of Fitness*, Table B.3, 260–1, 1984. Copyright © 1984 Human Kinetics Publishers, Champaign, IL.

Recommendations for human blood pressure determination by sphygmomanometers: Report of a special task force appointed by the steering committee, American Heart Association. Dallas: National Center, American Heart Association.

9. Greer, N. L., & Katch, F. I. (1982). Validity of palpation recovery pulse rate to estimate exercise heart rate following four intensities of bench step exercise. *Research Quarterly for Exercise and Sport, 53,* 340–343.

10. Howley, E. T., Colacino, D. L., & Swensen, T. C. (1992). Factors affecting the oxygen cost of stepping on an electronic stepping ergometer. *Medicine and Science in Sports and Exercise, 24,* 1055–1058.

11. Johnson, J., & Siegel, D. (1981). The use of selected submaximal step tests in predicting change in the maximal oxygen intake of college women. *Journal of Sports Medicine and Physical Fitness, 21,* 259–264.

12. McArdle, W. D., Katch, F. I., & Katch, V. L. (1996). *Exercise physiology: Energy, nutrition, and human performance.* Baltimore: Williams & Wilkins.

13. Ryhming (Astrand), I. (1953). A modified Harvard step test for the evaluation of physical fitness. *Arbeitsphysiologia, 15,* 235–250.

14. Sedlock, D. A., Knowlton, R. G., Fitzgerald, P. I., Tahamont, M. V., & Schneider, D. A. (1983, April).

Accuracy of subject-palpated carotid pulse after exercise. *The Physician and Sportsmedicine,* 106–108, 113–116.

15. Shahnawaz, H. (1978). Influence of limb length on a stepping exercise. *Journal of Applied Physiology, 44,* 346–349.

16. Sharkey, B. J. (1977). *Fitness and work capacity.* (Report FS-315.) Washington, D.C.: U.S. Department of Agriculture.

17. Sharkey, B. J. (1984). *Physiology of fitness.* Champaign, IL: Human Kinetics.

18. Shephard, R. J. (1969). Learning, habituation, and training. *Internationale Z. Angew. Physiologi, 28,* 38–48.

19. Shephard, R. J. (1971). Standard test of aerobic power. In R. J. Shephard (Ed.), *Frontiers in fitness,* (pp. 133–165). Springfield, IL: Charles C Thomas.

20. Thomas, S. G., Miller, I. M. R., & Cox, M. H. (1993). Sources of variation in oxygen consumption during a stepping task. *Medicine and Science in Sports and Exercise, 25,* 139–144.

21. Washburn, R. A., & Safrit, M. J. (1982). Physical performance tests in job selection—A model for empirical validation. *Research Quarterly for Exercise and Sport 53*(3): 267–270.

Form AS 1

Individual Data for Forestry Step Test

Basic Data

Name: TOYA HART

Date: 9-20-99 Time: 2 a.m. [ ] p.m. [✓]

Age: 22 y Gender (M or F): F Ht: 173 cm Wt: 64 kg

Meterological Data

Temperature (T): 21.8 °C Relative Humidity (RH): 60 %

Fan: Yes [ ] No [✓] Barometric Pressure (P_B): 749 torr

Test Data

Proper Cadence (check one): Always [✓] Usually [ ] Seldom [ ]

Proper Technique (check one): Always [✓] Usually [ ] Seldom [ ]

Comment, if applicable, on cadence and technique: _____

15-s Pulse Count (5:15–5:30): 38 ; × 4 = HR 152 b/min

AMANDA = 40
HR = 160

Aerobic Fitness ($ml \cdot kg^{-1} \cdot min^{-1}$):

Nonadjusted: 36 Age Adjusted: 37

Aerobic Fitness Category (check one):

Superior [ ] Excellent [ ] Very Good [ ] Good [ ]

Fair [✓] Poor [ ] Very Poor [ ]

Qualification as Wilderness Firefighter (45^+ $ml \cdot kg^{-1} \cdot min^{-1}$): Yes [ ] No [✓]

Form AS 2

Group Data for Forestry Step Test

MEN

Initials/I.D.	$\dot{V}O_2max$ $(ml \cdot kg^{-1} \cdot min^{-1})$
1.	
2.	
3.	
4.	
5.	
6.	
7.	
8.	
9.	
10.	
11.	
12.	
13.	
14.	
15.	
16.	
17.	
18.	
19.	
20.	
21.	
22.	
M	

WOMEN

Initials/I.D.	$\dot{V}O_2max$ $(ml \cdot kg^{-1} \cdot min^{-1})$
1.	
2.	
3.	
4.	
5.	
6.	
7.	
8.	
9.	
10.	
11.	
12.	
13.	
14.	
15.	
16.	
17.	
18.	
19.	
20.	
21.	
22.	
M	

Chapter 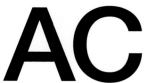AC   Aerobic Cycling

The Astrand Cycle Test is one of the most popular submaximal exercise tests in exercise physiology laboratories and fitness clinics. It is a more sophisticated field/lab test than the step test, partially due to its more complicated procedures and its more expensive and less portable ergometer. Group testing is severely restricted due to the need for numerous cycle ergometers. It nearly qualifies as a laboratory test because heart rate can be measured *during* exercise by a more sophisticated method (e.g., ECG or auscultation) than palpation. However, it probably does not qualify as a laboratory test because it is not a direct measure of maximal oxygen consumption.

Purpose of the Astrand Cycle Test

The purpose of this submaximal exercise test is similar to the run tests and the step tests, that is, to estimate a person's aerobic fitness. Additionally, the designers'[2,3] original purposes are expanded to include educational objectives such as familiarization with cycle ergometry, achievement of the skill in auscultation of heartbeats, and the understanding of the rationale for the test.

Physiological Rationale

All submaximal cycle ergometer tests rely predominantly upon the oxidative metabolic pathway (aerobic) in order to supply the majority of the energy substrate, ATP, to the muscles. As is typical of exercise meant to promote aerobic fitness, the muscles used in cycling are relatively large. For example, the extension of the hip and knee joints for the downstroke in cycling is accomplished mainly by the gluteus maximus, rectus femoris, and the vastus lateralis. Knee flexion, on the other hand, is accomplished by the biceps femoris and the gastrocnemius during the upstroke, while hip flexion is accomplished by the rectus femoris during the latter part of the upstroke.[11]

The Astrand Test *predicts* maximal oxygen consumption based upon the steady-state heart rate of a person exercising at a submaximal power level for 6 min. Thus, the rationale is similar to that of step tests in that the test is dependent upon the direct relationships between power level, oxygen consumption, and heart rate. The relationship between power and oxygen consumption was described in Chapter UN. The positive relationship between heart rate and oxygen consumption is most linear between 50% and

---

Accuracy of the Astrand Cycle Test

Reliability

The test-retest reliability coefficients were acceptable for older men (r = .835)[6] and college women (r = .87)[32] who twice performed the Astrand Cycle Test. When heart rates are taken daily on a person exercising at the same exercise power level, they vary by about ±5 b·min^{-1}.[22]

Validity

All *predictive* tests should be interpreted with caution, especially if the original data from the test were from a different type of population. For example, both age and fitness are characteristics that may influence the interpretation of a test. With respect to age, low validity coefficients (approximately .60) were reported between the Astrand Cycle Test and the directly measured maximal oxygen consumption of middle-aged men.[15] With respect to fitness, untrained persons are more likely to be underestimated by the Astrand Cycle Test, whereas the highly trained are more likely to be overestimated in their maximal oxygen consumptions.[4]

The ability of the Astrand Test to predict or estimate the actual measured maximal oxygen consumption varies considerably. The standard error of the estimate (*SEE*) has ranged from as low as 6% to 10%[30] to as high as 15% to 20%.[15,21,23]

One investigator reported a validity coefficient of .74 between the Astrand predicted values and the directly measured maximal oxygen consumption values.[7] In a review of thirteen studies, validity coefficients ranged from as low as .34 to as high as .94, with the average being .64.[15]

90% of maximal heart rate.[10] Expressed in terms of the respective units of measure, the physiological rationale for the Astrand Test can be stated as: A prediction of maximal oxygen consumption (L·min^{-1}) based upon the performer's heart-rate response at a given power (W) level or submaximal oxygen consumption.

Method

As with all field or laboratory tests, the methodology of the Astrand Cycle Test includes such factors as (a) equipment, (b) technician and participant preparations, (c) test procedures, and (d) calculations. Many of these methods apply to other cycle ergometer tests that predict aerobic fitness, such as the YMCA Test.[13]

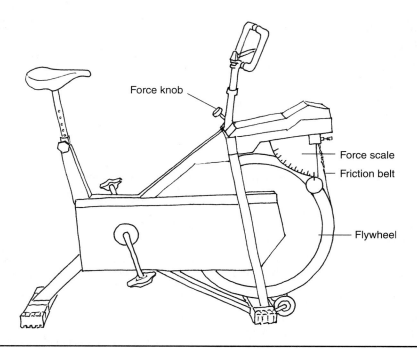

Labels on figure: Force knob, Force scale, Friction belt, Flywheel

Figure 1 A mechanically braked bicycle ergometer; the force (load) remains constant at its setting regardless of pedal revolutions.

Equipment

The equipment used to administer the Astrand Cycle Test varies according to the purposes of the investigator, technician, teacher, or student. For example, no equipment is necessary to palpate the pulse; but if the goal of students is to develop auscultatory (listening to heart sounds) skills, then stethoscopes will be needed. Additionally, if assured accuracy is required, then an investigator would need an electrocardiogram to measure heart rate. Also, heart-rate telemetry may be used, whereby chest electrodes send electrocardiographic signals to an FM radio transmitter that relays the heart rate to an external display or receiver "wristwatch."

The equipment needed for the purposes presented in this manual are (a) cycle ergometer, (b) seconds stopwatch, (c) laboratory timers, (d) metronome, (e) stethoscope, and (f) calculator.

Cycle Ergometer

There are various types of bicycle ergometers. Most ergometers may be classified in two ways, either according to their braking method or according to the constancy of the power level. There are usually two types of braking methods—mechanical or electrical; similarly, there are two types of power controls—one that is constant regardless of pedal speed and one that changes power according to pedal speed.

Mechanically braked cycles (e.g., Monark™ and Bodyguard™) used in laboratories are usually of a superior quality compared to most of those sold in department stores. The resistance to the wheel of a mechanically braked bike is based upon the tightening (friction) of the belt that surrounds the flywheel (Fig. 1). The typical force settings range from 5 N (0.5 kg) to a high of 70 N (7.0 kg).

Mechanically braked ergometers provide a constant force, but a nonconstant power at varying pedal revolutions. Thus, any increase in the rate of pedal revolutions ($r \cdot min^{-1}$; rpm) causes an increase in work (w) and power (P). This is because any change in pedal revolutions (r) changes the distance (D) factor of the work and power equations. The Monark™ ergometer's flywheel has a circumference of 1.62 m (often stated in rounded figures as 2 m) and travels 6 m in 3.7 circuits (often stated as 3 circuits) with each pedal revolution (r).[12] Thus, in mechanically braked ergometers any change in pedal revolutions per minute ($r \cdot min^{-1}$; rpm) will alter the work (w) and power (P) as presented in Equation 1.

*Constant **Force** Ergometer:*

$$\text{Change in } r \cdot min^{-1}; \text{ rpm} = \text{change in D}$$
$$= \text{change in w and P} \qquad \text{Eq. 1}$$

When combining the force (F) component with the distance (D) per minute component, the product becomes a power unit, that is, work rate. Although watts (W) is the preferred expression of the power unit, kilogram meters per minute ($kg \cdot m \cdot min^{-1}$) is still popular; newton meters per minute $N \cdot m \cdot min^{-1}$ may be used also. Thus, the power for any force or distance can be calculated from Equation 2.

$$P = F \times D/t \qquad \text{Eq. 2}$$

For example, if the force setting is 20 N (or 2 kg) and the distance traveled in 1 min is 300 m, then the power is

$$20 \text{ N} \times 300 \text{ m·min}^{-1} = 6000 \text{ N·m·min}^{-1} \text{ or}$$
$$2 \text{ kg} \times 300 \text{ m·min}^{-1} = 600 \text{ kg·m·min}^{-1}$$

Because 1 watt is equal to approximately 60 N·m·min^{-1} and 6 kg·m·min^{-1}, the watt value is 100 W.

On the other hand, **electromagnetically braked** cycle ergometers (e.g., Tectrix™ and Collins Pedal-Mode™) do not require strict attention to pedal frequency. If the distance (D) changes because the pedal revolutions increase or decrease on a constant-power ergometer, the force (F) factor compensates electronically to maintain a constant power level (Eq. 3).

*Constant **Power** Ergometer:*

Change in rpm = change in D but compensating change in F;
$\qquad$ = no change in w and P $\qquad$ Eq. 3

Obviously, these constant power ergometers simplify matters. However, the relationships among force, distance, work, time, and power are more easily conceptualized by students of exercise physiology when using the constant force ergometer. It should be noted for the pure measure of work, these calculations do not consider the internal work from the rotation of the lower limbs themselves during cycling.[31]

Timing Mechanisms

Three types of timers can be used to administer the Astrand Cycle Test. Stopwatches (or wristwatches capable of measuring tenths of a second) are mandatory for measuring heart rate, while either a laboratory set-clock or wall clock is acceptable for elapsed time, that is, the continuous running time.

Metronome or Tachometer

Metronomes are probably more accurate than most bicycle tachometers. The purpose of the metronome for the cycle test is the same as that for the step tests—to provide the prescribed cadence for the exerciser.

The Astrand Test often prescribes a pedal frequency of 50 r·min^{-1} when using mechanically braked, nonconstant-power ergometers (e.g., Monark™). This 50-rpm speed is equivalent to a metronome setting of 100 based on either foot of the cyclist being at the bottom of the stroke at each beat of the metronome. The tachometer on the ergometer should display a speed of 18 km·h^{-1} (11.2 mph) at a 50-rpm setting.

The Monark ergometer's flywheel has a circumference of 1.62 m and travels 6 m in 3.7 circuits with each pedal revolution (r).[12,a] Equation 4 states that the cycling distance is a function of pedal rpm and flywheel circumference and wheel circuits per pedal rpm.

$$D \text{ (m·min}^{-1}) = \text{r·min}^{-1} \times \text{wheel circumference (m)}$$
$$\times \text{ wheel circuits per pedal r} \qquad \text{Eq. 4}$$

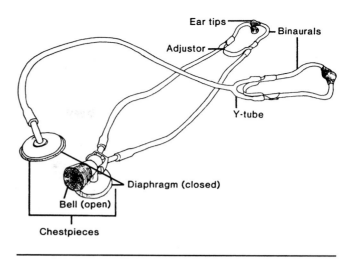

Figure 2 Stethoscopes for auscultation of heart rate.

The calculation of total distance (D) in 1 min for the Astrand Test uses Equation 5.

$$D \text{ (m·min}^{-1}) = 50 \text{ rpm} \times 6 \text{ m} = 300 \text{ m·min}^{-1} \qquad \text{Eq. 5}$$

where:

$\qquad$ 50 rpm = commonly prescribed rpm for Astrand Test
$\qquad$ 6 m = 1.62 m × 3.7 circuits

Constant power ergometers should approximate the prescribed 50 rpm because of the known change in metabolic efficiency ($\dot{V}O_2$) at varying pedal frequencies.[31]

Stethoscope

Auscultatory (by ear) heart rates are preferred over palpatory ones (by pulse or apical beat) for some tests when performed by experienced technicians.[13] In fact, the standard error between auscultation by stethoscope and recording by electrocardiograph for measuring heart rate is less than 2 b·min^{-1}.[b] The chestpiece of a stethoscope (Fig. 2) may be an open (bell-shaped) or closed diaphragm. The flatter and larger closed diaphragm is preferred for auscultating heart rates.

The basic purpose of the stethoscope—to bring the ear of the listener closer to the source of the sound—has not changed since a one-piece hollow tube first was used in 1819.[18] Typical stethoscopes do not amplify sounds, although some battery-powered ones may amplify by 100 times. The length of the tubing makes little, if any, practical difference in the sound intensity unless it exceeds three feet.[25]

Technician Preparations

To adequately prepare for the administration of the Astrand Cycle Test certain preparations must be made, such as (1) development of auscultatory and timing skills by the

---

[a]The bodyguard™ 990 ergometer's flywheel is only 0.73 m. Therefore, one pedal revolution equals 8.2 circuits of the flywheel to achieve an effective distance of 300 m (0.73 × 8.2 × 50) in one min.[12]

[b]H. A. deVries, personal communication, December 6, 1965.

technician, (2) recording of basic and meteorological data, (3) orientation of the participant, and (4) establishment of the power level for the exercise protocol. Additionally, periodic calibrations of equipment may be necessary. Some preparations were discussed in more detail in other chapters.

Technician's Preparatory Steps for the Astrand Cycle Test

1. Calibrate the cycle ergometer and metronome. (Instructor may have done this.)
2. Measure and record basic and meteorological data.
3. Practice auscultating the subject's heart rate while he or she is seated comfortably in a chair; record quality and rate onto Form AC 1.
4. Orient the performer by:
   a. Stating the purpose of the test to the subject, i.e., ". . . to record heart rate during cycling exercise so that aerobic power ($\dot{V}O_2$max) may be estimated."
   b. Explaining the protocol of the test (e.g., duration, intensity, mode, and technique).
5. Adjust the seat height so that the cyclist's leg is nearly straight with the ball of the foot on the down pedal (Fig. 5).
6. Record the seat-post number onto form AC 2.
7. Establish the cadence (100 b·min⁻¹; or 18 km·h⁻¹) of cycling:
   a. Show how one foot is at the bottom of the stroke with each metronome beat.
   b. Show where the tachometer indicates 18 "km/h" or 50 rpm.
8. Establish the diaphragm site for auscultation (see Fig. 3).
9. Measure heart rate while performer is seated at rest on the cycle; record onto Form AC 2.
10. Establish the power (kg·m·min⁻¹; N·m·min⁻¹; W) level for the exercise protocol.

Auscultation of Heartbeats

The vibrations of the heart valves and blood are responsible for the heart sounds. Their sounds are of low frequency and low decibel, making them difficult to hear for inexperienced technicians. The two distinct sounds of the heart heard under resting conditions are often referred to as *lub-dup*. The first sound, *lub,* is a systolic (ventricles contract) sound, and the second sound, *dup,* is the diastolic (ventricles relax) sound. The sound of systole is due primarily to the closing of the atrioventricular valves (mitral and tricuspid) and secondarily to the opening of the semilunar valves (aortic and pulmonic); *lub* is heard best at the 4th to 5th intercostal space near the midclavicular line.[17,18] The *dup* sound of diastole is due mainly to the closing of the semilunar valves[19] and is heard best at the pulmonic area near the base of the heart, which is externally marked between the 2nd and 3rd intercostal space at a point about 2–3 cm left of the sternum.[5,17,18] Under exercise conditions the duration between the *lub* and *dup* is usually too short to distinguish as two separate sounds. Thus, at exercise each sound is equivalent to one heartbeat.

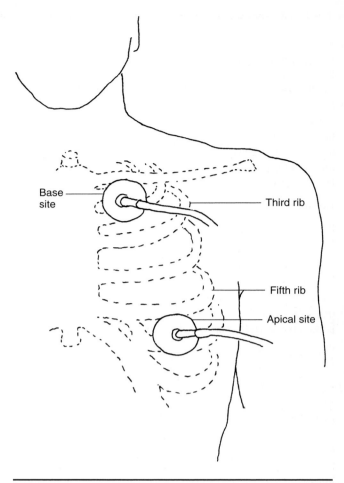

Figure 3 Two practical stethoscopic sites (base and apical) for auscultating heartbeats.

In general, the heartbeat is heard best at the apical region just below the pectoralis major muscle and the left nipple. Occasionally, it is more convenient to auscultate heartbeat at its base area just below and to the left of the sternum's manubrium.

Stethoscopes have binaurals, which sometimes curve near the ear tips; the direction of the binaurals should point toward the nose because the ear canals normally are oriented in that direction. By tapping gently on the diaphragm, the listener can assure that the sound is being transmitted adequately. The diaphragm of a stethoscope should not be used over cloth and should be flush with the skin (i.e., no air spaces between it and the skin surface).

Technicians should learn to feel comfortable testing members of the opposite sex. For example, the subject should not be asked to hold the diaphragm of the stethoscope in position while the technician listens. The technician should not be shy about placing the diaphragm of the stethoscope against skin at the appropriate site even if that site is near the breasts. Because heart sounds cannot be heard well through breast tissue, there is no need to place the diaphragm on the breasts. Participants should

Calibration of the Cycle Ergometer

Mechanically braked ergometers

The mechanically braked (friction belt) ergometer (Fig. 1) can be statically (no pedalling) calibrated based upon the movement of the pendulum to a given reading on the force scale which corresponds to the amount of weight suspended from the friction belt.

Zero

1. Remove the belt from the spring-belt junction at the front of the ergometer (see Fig. 1).
2. Adjust the "winged-bolt" screw at the front rim of the Force scale "quadrant" so that the zero point of the scale coincides with the index mark on the pendulum weight.
3. Tighten the lock nut of the thumb screw.

Range

1. Hang a known weight from the spring or suspension hook where the friction belt attaches; possibly incline the ergometer slightly forward to assure that the weight hangs freely.
2. The pendulum weight should move to the corresponding marker on the Force scale (e.g., a 4-kg weight moves the pendulum to the 40-N or 4-kp [kilopond] marker). *Note:* kp is essentially the same as kg.
3. If not in agreement, adjust the weight pin inside the pendulum weight with the lock screw in the center of the backside of the pendulum weight.
4. A less sophisticated adjustment can be made by taping over the present numbers and writing in the correct values.[c]

Electronically Braked Constant-Power Cycle Ergometer

Although these cycle ergometers are calibrated by the manufacturer, they can lose their calibration with constant use. Advertisers of electronic calibrators claim that the typical accuracy of the power setting is 5–20%. These cycles require either a technician's expertise in interfacing the cycle's electronic output to a volt/watt meter, or purchasing an expensive special calibrating dynamometer (e.g., Quinton, model 805; Vacu · Med). The calibrators can measure the accuracy of powers up to 600 W from 40–120 rpm (Vacu · Med®). Some dynamometric calibrators are capable of detecting power variations of about 1 watt. Manufacturers may perform the calibration periodically; however, this can be expensive. Rough checks of the accuracy can be made with a conventional torque wrench, following instructions from the manufacturer.

---

[c]The friction in the transmission (mainly the chain) of the Monark cycle increases the stated power level by 9%. All of the tables relating power to oxygen consumption have been corrected to conform to this increase. Thus, the stated and calculated (F × D) power level of 600 kg·m·min^{-1} is really 650 kg·m·min^{-1}, a power of 1200 kg·m·min^{-1} is 1300 kg·m·min^{-1}. Consequently, 1.5 L·min^{-1} of oxygen consumption is actually atatined at 109 W and 650 kg·m·min^{-1}, not at 100 W or 600 kg·m·min^{-1} as listed.[3]

avoid talking while the technician is listening to their heart beats.

Timing of Heartbeats

Heart rates are timed differently for the Astrand Cycle Test than for the Run Tests and the Step Tests. The following procedures are used for timing the heart beats and converting the number of beats to heart rate:

1. Start the watch on a heart beat while silently saying "zero."
2. Count 30 heart beats (30-b).
3. Stop the watch on the 30th beat.
4. Record the time (t) to closest 0.1 s for the 30 beats (30-b t)
5. Calculate the heart rate (HR) by using Equation 6.

$$HR \ (b\cdot min^{-1}) = 60 \ s \times (30 \ b/30\text{-}b \ t) \qquad Eq. \ 6a$$
$$= 1800/30\text{-}b \ t \qquad Eq. \ 6b$$

Because 30 b and 60 s are constants for one form of the equation (6a), the equation may be simplified by using the value 1800 found in the second form (6b). As an example, suppose that the time for 30 b under resting conditions was 26.0 s. The heart rate then is 69 b·min^{-1}, found by dividing 1800 by 26.0.

This 30-b method of obtaining heart rate is considered more exact than the 15-s method that was prescribed for the field tests.[3] This is due to the partial intervals between beats at the start and finish of a timing period; there are only whole intervals in the 30-b method because the stopwatch is started and stopped on the respective beats, not on a go and stop signal.

By auscultating heart rate while the performer sits at rest on the ergometer prior to the test, the technician may be alerted to any difficulties associated with hearing the heartbeat. It may also reveal any anxiety in the participant. The resting heart rate, however, is not used to estimate the maximal oxygen consumption, but it can serve as a starting point if graphing the relationship between time and exercise.

In cases where auscultation is difficult, it is helpful to get second opinions from more experienced technicians or to use double-headed and amplifying stethoscopes (Fig. 4). Also, telemetered heart rate monitors have been perfected to provide accurate and practical measures.[16]

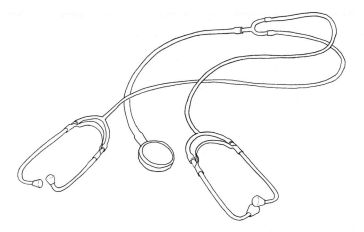

Figure 4 A "double-headed" stethoscope.

Orientation of the Participant

The orientation of the performer by the technician includes such factors as (1) the establishment of the standard condition, (2) the explanation of the purpose and basic features of the test, and (3) a brief demonstration of the cadence for the test.

The performer should be in a condition that is standard for field or laboratory testing. This means that he or she is relaxed, drug free, euhydrated, appropriately dressed, and neither hungry nor full.

Power Prescription for Exercise Protocol

The technician must understand the relationship between force (F), work (w), and power (P) in order to make the proper exercise prescription on mechanically braked cycle ergometers. The force component of work is often displayed on the ergometer as kg, kp, or N. For practical purposes, the kg and kp are identical. The power units are often expressed as $kg \cdot m \cdot min^{-1}$ or watts (W). Table 1 shows the relationship between these units when the mechanically braked ergometer's rpm range is from 40 to 80; special attention should be given to the 50-rpm column because it is the prescribed rpm for the Astrand Cycle Test.

An estimation of the appropriate power dosage for the participant can be made by following the guidelines in Table 2. It prescribes the power based on (1) age and/or (2) the best guess or estimate ("guesstimate") of the participant's fitness level.

Ideally, for persons under 30 years of age, the power level of the protocol should elicit a heart rate between 150 and 160 beats per minute ($b \cdot min^{-1}$). This target heart rate may be reduced by about one-half beat per minute for each year over 30 years of age. Table 2 also shows that the prescribed power level for *sedentary* persons may be based upon a general rule of $10 \ kg \cdot m \cdot min^{-1}$ (~1.65 W) per kilogram of body weight. For example, if a sedentary person weighs 75 kg, then the prescribed power level is $750 \ kg \cdot m \cdot min^{-1}$; if expressing it in watts, then 1.65×75 is equal to 123.75 W, or approximately 125 W.

Seat Adjustment

The position of the cycle seat affects the efficiency of the rider.[27] Mechanical efficiency may vary by plus or minus 6% on the cycle ergometer even when appropriate seat adjustments are made.[4] For example, at a power level of $600 \ kg \cdot m \cdot min^{-1}$, two-thirds of the population will consume between 1.41 and 1.59 liters of oxygen per minute [1.5 + or $- (6\% \times 1.5)$]. In order to assure that the efficiency remains within this narrow range, or is optimal for the performer, the seat adjustment should be based upon various accepted criteria.[1,8,24]

With the ball of the cyclist's foot on the pedal, as it should be during the test, the leg should have a bend of only 5% to 10% at the bottom of the stroke[1] (Fig. 5a). The leg should be straight when the heel of the foot is on the pedal at the bottom of the stroke (Fig. 5b). A quick guideline for preventing seat heights from being too high is for the performer to try backpedalling while the technician observes the hips. If the hips are rocking or if the heels slip off the pedals, then the seat is too high. Most seat posts have numbers at about 2- to 3-cm intervals. Once the proper seat height has been established the seat setting should be recorded on Form AC 2.

Test Procedures

The normal duration of the Astrand Cycle Test is six minutes. During this time, the technicians are mainly responsible for auscultating heart beats, calculating and recording heart rates, adjusting the power level, and observing the performer. The procedures during the test are summarized as follows:

1. Start the metronome if using a nonconstant-power ergometer.
2. Ask the participant to begin cycling at the proper cadence using the metronome or tachometer as an aid.

Table 1 Force (F) and Power (P) on a Mechanically Braked Ergometer

							Speed					
rpm		40		50		60		70		80	
km·h⁻¹		14.4		18		21.6		25.2		28.8	

Force kg (kp)	N	kg·m/min	W	kg·m/min	W	Power kg·m/min	W	kg·m/min	W	kg·m/min	W
0.5	5	120	20	150	25	180	30	210	35	240	40
1.0	10	240	40	300	50	360	60	420	70	480	80
1.5	15	360	60	450	75	540	90	630	105	720	120
2.0	20	480	80	600	100	720	120	840	140	960	160
2.5	25	600	100	750	125	900	150	1050	175	1200	200
3.0	30	720	120	900	150	1080	180	1260	210	1440	240
3.5	35	840	140	1050	175	1260	210	1470	245	1680	280
4.0	40	960	160	1200	200	1440	240	1680	280	1920	320
4.5	45	1080	180	1350	225	1620	270	1890	315	2160	360
5.0	50	1200	200	1500	250	1800	300	2100	350	2400	400
5.5	55	1320	220	1650	275	1980	330	2310	385	2640	440
6.0	60	1440	240	1800	300	2160	360	2520	420	2880	480
6.5	65	1560	260	1950	325	2340	390	2730	455	3120	520
7.0	70	1680	280	2100	350	2520	420	2940	490	3360	560

Table 2 Prescription of the Initial Power Level for the Astrand Cycle Test

Age (y)	Target HR (b·min⁻¹)		Trained (Power)		Sedentary (Power)	
			Men	Women	Men	Women
<30	150–160	kg·m·min⁻¹:	>900	>600	900	600
30–39	145–155	W:	>150	>100	150	100
40–49	140–150				or:	
50–59	135–145				10 kg·m·min⁻¹·kg wt⁻¹	
60–69	130–140				or: 1.65 W·kg wt⁻¹	
70–79	125–135					

3. Once the performer has achieved the proper cadence, increase the power level to the prescribed setting.
4. Start the timer.
5. Auscultate and time 30 heartbeats starting between 1:30–1:45 of the test; repeat this at 1-min intervals through the last minute (sixth) of the test.
6. Record the 30-beat time on the data form; while waiting for the next auscultation period, calculate the heart rate using Equation 6.
7. Readjust the power level after the 3-min heart rate if heart rate target zone is unlikely to be achieved. Use Table 3 as a guide.
8. After the 6th min, if no power adjustments were made, set the force level to 0.5 kg (5 N) and ask the performer to continue cycling for recovery/cool-down purposes until the heart rate is less than 100 b·min⁻¹.
9. As usual, at the end of the test thank the participant for such effort and cooperation, in addition to asking how he or she feels.

Power Adjustments

The power levels of most mechanically braked ergometers cannot be adjusted precisely to the prescribed level unless the performer is cycling. Additionally, the flywheel tension may slip or drift upward occasionally during the test,[26] requiring readjustment and periodic monitoring.

Table 3 and Figure 6 provide guides for changing the original power level after the third minute of the cycle test. For example, if a 30-year-old's heart rate (HR) is less than 110 b·min⁻¹ at the end of the third minute (2:30–3:00), then the power level should be raised by 50–75 W (300–450 kg·m·min⁻¹). If a change is made immediately after the third minute, a steady state will likely be achieved by the end of the 6-min test. Each change in power level after this change requires an extension of one minute to the typical 6-min test. In general, if the heart rate is between 140 and 149 b·min⁻¹ at the end of the third minute, the power level does not need to be changed.

Time Adjustments

If the difference between the heart rates during minutes 5 and 6 exceeds 10 beats, then the performer should continue to exercise until the difference between the final two heart rates is 10 or less. If the difference between the final two heart rates is between 6 and 10 beats, then ignore the earlier minute's rate and use only the final minute's heart

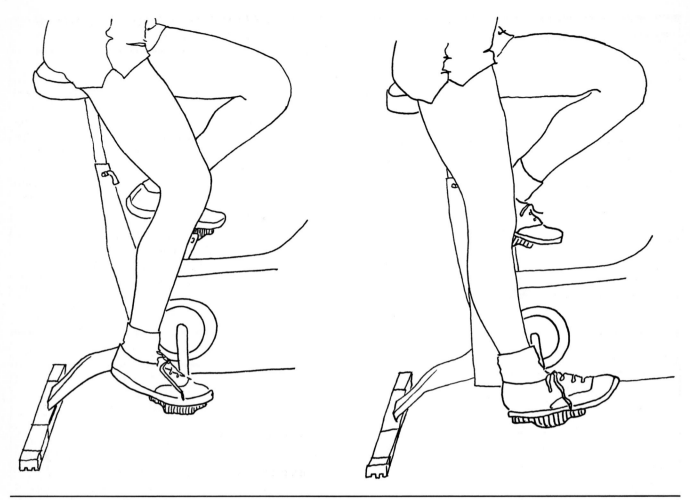

Figure 5 Adjusting the seat for the Astrand Cycle Test: (a) Slight bend in knee when the ball of the foot is on the pedal at the bottom of the pedal stroke; (b) Straight leg when the heel is on the pedal.

Table 3 Possible Power Adjustments After the Third Minute (2:30–3:00) of the Astrand Cycle Test[a]

A. Raise Power Level by:		Heart Rate	Force	
kg·m·min^{-1}	W	b·min^{-1}	kg	N
300–450	50–75	if HR is <110	1.0–1.5	10–15
150–300	25–50	if HR is 110–129	0.5–1.0	5–10
≤150	≤25	if HR is 130–139	≤0.5	≤5
B. Lower Power Level by:				
150–300	25–50	if HR is 160	0.5–1.0	10
≤150	≤25	if HR is 150–159	≤0.5	≤5

Note: [a]Subtract (>30 y) or add (<30 y) one-half beat per minute for each year above or below 30 years of age, respectively.

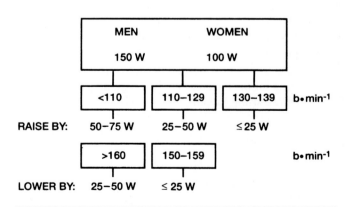

Figure 6 Schematic of power adjustments after the third minute (2:30–3:00) of the Astrand Cycle Test. Also adjust for age by subtracting or adding one-half b·min^{-1} for each year above or below 30 years of age, respectively.

rate to make the calculation for predicting maximal oxygen consumption.[9]

Cool-Down

It is important that the cyclist be given a low intensity exercise level after the regular test protocol. This will prevent the pooling of blood in the legs, which could lead to fainting if the performer were to stand still immediately after finishing the test. In general, the recovery exercise may end when the heart rate is 100 beats per minute or less (18.0 s for 30 beats). It is very unlikely that muscle soreness will occur as a result of this aerobic submaximal test.

Estimation of $\dot{V}O_2max$ from Steady-State Heart Rate

The prediction of the maximal oxygen consumption ($\dot{V}O_2max$) can be made by equation, table, or nomogram, all of which are based on the heart rate at the steady state of exercise during the Astrand Test.

Equation Method of Calculating $\dot{V}O_2max$

Usually, the final two heart rates of the exercise test are averaged in order to determine the steady state heart rate that is used in the calculations. The averaged rate is then used with either the Astrand-Ryhming nomogram[2,3] or derived equations; both are based on the ratio between submaximal oxygen consumption ($\dot{V}O_2SM$) and maximal oxygen consumption. This ratio is expressed in terms of maximal (HRmax) and submaximal (HRsm) heart rates and put in equation form;[28,29] the generalized form of that equation is presented in Equation 7. The prediction of maximal oxygen consumption is more accurate if the popular formula for predicting maximal heart rate (220 − age) is substituted[20] for the original HR Range values. Thus, Equations 8 and 9 are suggested for calculating maximal oxygen consumption for men and women, respectively. Presumably, it would be best to use the individual's known maximal heart rate if such data are available from previous maximal exercise testing.

$$\dot{V}O_2max \ (L \cdot min^{-1}) = \dot{V}O_2 \times \frac{HR\ Range}{HRsm\ Range} \qquad \text{Eq. 7}$$

$$\text{Men:} = \dot{V}O_2 \times \frac{(220 - age) - 61}{HRsm - 61} \qquad \text{Eq. 8}$$

$$\text{Women:} = \dot{V}O_2 \times \frac{(220 - age) - 72}{HRsm - 72} \qquad \text{Eq. 9}$$

where:

$\dot{V}O_2$ = L of oxygen required for the Astrand power level (Eq. A, B, or C) used during the Astrand Test.

$\dot{V}O_2 \ (l \cdot min^{-1}) =$

$$[P \text{ (in N·m·min}^{-1}) \times 0.0002] + 0.3 \qquad \text{Eq. A}$$
$$[P \text{ (in kgm·min}^{-1}) \times 0.002] + 0.3 \qquad \text{Eq. B}$$
$$[P \text{ (in W)} \times 0.012] + 0.3 \qquad \text{Eq. C}$$

HR Range = HRmax (known value or 220 − age) minus resting HR (men = 61; women = 72).

HRsm = the steady state heart rate (b·min^{-1}) during the Astrand Test

Thus, to calculate maximal oxygen consumption, one needs only to insert three values into Equation 8 or 9: (1) maximal heart rate, (2) the submaximal heart rate (HRsm) elicited during the Astrand Bike Test, and (3) the submaximal oxygen consumption ($\dot{V}O_2$) value for the power level that elicited that submaximal heart rate.

For example, if a 25-year-old man's heart rate (HRsm) was 155 b·min^{-1} at 150 W (900 kg·m·min^{-1}), then the maximal oxygen consumption may be calculated as follows:

$$\dot{V}O_2 \ (L \cdot min^{-1}) = (0.002 \times 900 \text{ kg·m·min}^{-1}) + 0.3$$
$$= 2.1 \text{ L·min}^{-1}$$
$$or = (0.012 \times 150 \text{ W}) + 0.3$$
$$= 2.1 \text{ L·min}^{-1}$$

$$\dot{V}O_2max \ (L \cdot min^{-1}) = 2.1 \times \frac{(220 - 25) - 61}{155 - 61}$$

$$= 2.1 \times \frac{134}{94}$$

$$= 2.1 \times 1.43$$

$$= 3.0 \text{ L} \cdot min^{-1}$$

Table Method for Predicting $\dot{V}O_2max$

The same $\dot{V}O_2max$ value as in the example of the 25-year-old man could have been found by using Table 4 (men). Accordingly, Table 5 (women) may be used to predict maximal oxygen consumption (L·min^{-1}) from the steady-state heart rates of women at given power levels (kg·m·min^{-1}) of the Astrand Cycle Test.[3] For example, if a 20-year-old woman has a heart rate of 168 b·min^{-1} at 750 kg·m·min^{-1}, then Table 5 shows that the maximal oxygen consumption is 2.4 L·min^{-1}.

Calculations for the Age-Adjusted $\dot{V}O_2Max$

When the maximal oxygen consumption value of persons over 25 years of age is derived from the tables, but not Equations 8 or 9, an adjustment is needed to account for the decrease in maximal heart rate with increased age. The maximal oxygen consumption value, which was derived from the tables, is based upon a constant maximal heart rate of 195 for men and 192 for women, regardless of age. Because maximal heart rate decreases with age, a proper correction must be used (unless the man and woman are 25 and 28 years of age, respectively). The correction factor (HRmax CF) for various ages may be found by combining the HR Range component (220 − age) of Equations 8 and 9 with the constants 195 and 192, respectively (Eqs. 10 and 11).

Table 4 Prediction of Maximal Oxygen Consumption from Heart Rate (HR) and Cycling Power (Men)

Maximal Oxygen Consumption (L·min⁻¹)						Maximal Oxygen Consumption (L·min⁻¹)				
HR bpm	Power (kg·m·min⁻¹; W)					HR	Power (kg·m·min⁻¹; W)			
	300; 50	600; 100	900; 150	1200; 200	1500; 250		600; 100	900; 150	1200; 200	1500; 250
120	2.2	3.5	4.8			146	2.4	3.3	4.4	5.5
121	2.2	3.4	4.7			147	2.4	3.3	4.4	5.5
122	2.2	3.4	4.6			148	2.4	3.2	4.3	5.4
123	2.1	3.4	4.6			149	2.3	3.2	4.3	5.4
124	2.1	3.3	4.5	6.0		150	2.3	3.2	4.2	5.3
125	2.0	3.2	4.4	5.9		151	2.3	3.1	4.2	5.2
126	2.0	3.2	4.4	5.8		152	2.3	3.1	4.1	5.2
127	2.0	3.1	4.3	5.7		153	2.2	3.0	4.1	5.1
128	2.0	3.1	4.2	5.6		154	2.2	3.0	4.0	5.1
129	1.9	3.0	4.2	5.6		155	2.2	3.0	4.0	5.0
130	1.9	3.0	4.1	5.5		156	2.2	2.9	4.0	5.0
131	1.9	2.9	4.0	5.4		157	2.1	2.9	3.9	4.9
132	1.8	2.9	4.0	5.3		158	2.1	2.9	3.9	4.9
133	1.8	2.8	3.9	5.3		159	2.1	2.8	3.8	4.8
134	1.8	2.8	3.9	5.2		160	2.1	2.8	3.8	4.8
135	1.7	2.8	3.8	5.1		161	2.0	2.8	3.7	4.7
136	1.7	2.7	3.8	5.0		162	2.0	2.8	3.7	4.6
137	1.7	2.7	3.7	5.0		163	2.0	2.8	3.7	4.6
138	1.6	2.7	3.7	4.9		164	2.0	2.7	3.6	4.5
139	1.6	2.6	3.6	4.8		165	2.0	2.7	3.6	4.5
140	1.6	2.6	3.6	4.8	6.0	166	1.9	2.7	3.6	4.4
141		2.6	3.5	4.7	5.9	167	1.9	2.6	3.5	4.4
142		2.5	3.5	4.6	5.8	168	1.9	2.6	3.5	4.3
143		2.5	3.4	4.6	5.7	169	1.9	2.6	3.5	4.3
144		2.5	3.4	4.5	5.7	170	1.8	2.6	3.4	4.3
145		2.4	3.4	4.5	5.6					

Modified from nomogram in I. Astrand, *Acta Physiologica Scandinavica, 49,* suppl. 169, 1960, by P. O. Astrand in *Work Test with Bicycle Ergometer,* Varberg, Sweden, Monark, 1988.

$$\text{Men:} \quad \text{HRmax CF} = \frac{220 - \text{age} - 61}{195 - 61} \qquad \text{Eq. 10}$$

$$\text{Women:} \quad \text{HRmax CF} = \frac{220 - \text{age} - 72}{195 - 72} \qquad \text{Eq. 11}$$

For example, a man who is 40 years of age would have a correction factor of 0.89 based upon the following calculation:

$$\text{CF} = \frac{220 - 40 - 61}{195 - 61}$$
$$= \frac{119}{134}$$
$$= 0.89$$

Thus, if this man has a table-derived maximal oxygen consumption value of 3.0 L·min⁻¹, then 3.0 multiplied by the HRmax CF 0.89 provides an adjusted value of 2.7 L·min⁻¹.

Calculations for the Weight-Adjusted $\dot{V}O_2max$

The equations and the nomogram value may also be adjusted to account for differences in body weight. The nomogram is not presented here but can be found in various texts of exercise physiology.[3] Maximal oxygen consumption, expressed as liters per minute, is closely related to

body size; it is sometimes referred to as the raw or absolute value. However, maximal oxygen consumption is usually expressed relative to body weight when predicting performance in activities that require the performer to lift his/her own weight. The unit of measure denoting relative oxygen consumption is milliliters per kilogram per minute (ml·kg⁻¹·min⁻¹). To convert the raw score to the relative score, Equation 12 is used, whereby the absolute value is multiplied by 1000 (1 L = 1000 ml) and the product is divided by the body weight (kg).

For example, if a subject who weighs 68.0 kg has an age-adjusted $\dot{V}O_2max$ of 2.35 L·min⁻¹, then the relative $\dot{V}O_2max$ is 2350 ml·min⁻¹ divided by body weight; thus, the relative $\dot{V}O_2max$ is 35 ml·kg⁻¹·min⁻¹.

$$\text{Relative } \dot{V}O_2max \left(\text{ml} \cdot \text{kg}^{-1} \cdot \text{min}^{-1}\right) = \frac{\dot{V}O_2max \left(\text{L} \cdot \text{min}^{-1}\right) \times 1000}{\text{kg}} \qquad \text{Eq. 12}$$

Results and Discussion

The original norms of Astrand were derived from the Swedish population, most of whom were physical education students. The original norms had higher standards than the ones presented in Table 6, which are based on 450

Table 5 Prediction of Maximal Oxygen Consumption from Heart Rate (HR) and Cycling Power (Women)

Maximal Oxygen Consumption (L·min⁻¹)

HR bpm	Power (kg·m·min⁻¹; W) 300; 50	450; 75	600; 100	750; 125	900; 150
120	2.6	3.4	4.1	4.8	
121	2.5	3.3	4.0	4.8	
122	2.5	3.2	3.9	4.7	
123	2.4	3.1	3.9	4.6	
124	2.4	3.1	3.8	4.5	
125	2.3	3.0	3.7	4.4	
126	2.3	3.0	3.7	4.4	
127	2.2	2.9	3.5	4.2	
128	2.2	2.8	3.5	4.2	
129	2.2	2.8	3.4	4.1	
130	2.1	2.7	3.4	4.0	4.7
131	2.1	2.7	3.4	4.0	4.6
132	2.0	2.7	3.3	4.0	4.5
133	2.0	2.6	3.2	3.8	4.4
134	2.0	2.6	3.2	3.8	4.4
135	2.0	2.6	3.1	3.7	4.3
136	1.9	2.5	3.1	3.6	4.2
137	1.9	2.5	3.0	3.6	4.2
138	1.8	2.4	3.0	3.5	4.1
139	1.8	2.4	2.9	3.5	4.0
140	1.8	2.4	2.8	3.4	4.0
141	1.8	2.3	2.8	3.4	3.9
142	1.7	2.3	2.8	3.3	3.9
143	1.7	2.2	2.7	3.3	3.8
144	1.7	2.2	2.7	3.2	3.8
145	1.6	2.2	2.7	3.2	3.7

Maximal Oxygen Consumption (L·min⁻¹)

HR bpm	Power (kg·m·min⁻¹; W) 300; 50	450; 75	600; 100	750; 125	900; 150
146	1.6	2.2	2.6	3.2	3.7
147	1.6	2.1	2.6	3.1	3.6
148	1.6	2.1	2.6	3.1	3.6
149		2.1	2.6	3.0	3.5
150		2.0	2.5	3.0	3.5
151		2.0	2.5	3.0	3.4
152		2.0	2.5	2.9	3.4
153		2.0	2.4	2.9	3.3
154		2.0	2.4	2.8	3.3
155		1.9	2.4	2.8	3.2
156		1.9	2.3	2.8	3.2
157		1.9	2.3	2.7	3.2
158		1.8	2.3	2.7	3.1
159		1.8	2.2	2.7	3.1
160		1.8	2.2	2.6	3.0
161		1.8	2.2	2.6	3.0
162		1.8	2.2	2.6	3.0
163		1.7	2.2	2.6	2.9
164		1.7	2.1	2.5	2.9
165		1.7	2.1	2.5	2.9
166		1.7	2.1	2.5	2.8
167		1.6	2.1	2.4	2.8
168		1.6	2.0	2.4	2.8
169		1.6	2.0	2.4	2.8
170		1.6	2.0	2.4	2.7

Modified from nomogram in I. Astrand, *Acta Physiologica Scandinavica, 49,* suppl. 169, 1960, by P. O. Astrand in *Work Test with Bicycle Ergometer,* Varberg, Sweden, Monark, 1988.

Table 6 Norms for Evaluating Astrand Cycle Test Performance

Age	Very High (VH)	High (H)	Aerobic Fitness Categories Good (G)	Average (Ave)	Fair (F)	Low (L)
			Maximal Oxygen Consumption (mL·kg⁻¹·min⁻¹)			
Men						
20–29	>61	53–61	43–52	34–42	25–33	<25
30–39	>57	49–57	39–48	31–38	23–30	<23
40–49	>53	45–53	36–44	27–35	20–26	<20
50–59	>49	43–49	34–42	25–33	18–24	<18
60–69	>45	41–45	31–40	23–30	16–22	<16
Women						
20–29	>57	49–57	38–48	31–37	24–30	<24
30–39	>53	45–53	34–44	28–33	20–27	<20
40–49	>50	42–50	31–41	24–30	17–23	<17
50–59	>42	38–42	28–37	21–27	15–20	<15
60–69	>39	35–39	24–34	18–23	13–17	<13

Source: Preventive Medicine Center, Palo Alto, CA; National Athletic Health Institute, Inglewood, CA.

healthy Americans, who mainly were tested on cycle ergometers (Preventive Medicine Center, Palo Alto, CA, and NAHI, Inglewood, CA).

It is also important to consider the mode of exercise for establishing the norms. For example, maximal (peak) oxygen consumptions elicited from treadmill tests are typically 5% to 10% greater than those elicited by cycle ergometry.[7,14]

References

1. American College of Sports Medicine. (1991). *Guidelines for exercise testing and prescription.* Philadelphia: Lea & Febiger.
2. Astrand, I. (1960). Aerobic work capacity in men and women with special reference to age. *Acta Physiologica Scandinavica, 49* (Suppl. 169).
3. Astrand, P. O. (1988). *Work tests with the bicycle ergometer.* Varberg, Sweden: Monark Crescent AB.
4. Astrand, P. O., & Rodahl, K. (1977). *Textbook of work physiology.* San Francisco: McGraw-Hill.
5. DePasquale, N. P., Burch, G. E., & Philips, J. H. (1968). The second heart sound. *American Heart Journal, 76,* 419–431.
6. deVries, H. A. (1971). Prescription of exercise for older men from telemetered exercise heart rate data. *Geriatrics, 26,* 102–111.
7. deVries, H. A. (1986). *Physiology of exercise.* Dubuque, IA: Wm. C. Brown.
8. Dickson, T. B. (1985, October). Preventing overuse cycling injuries. *Physician and Sportsmedicine,* 118–123.
9. Edgren, B., Marklund, G., Nordesjo, L., & Borg, G. (1976). The validity of four bicycle ergometer tests. *Medicine and Science in Sports, 8,* 179–185.
10. Edington, D. W., & Cunningham, L. (1975). *Biological awareness.* Englewood Cliffs, NJ: Prentice-Hall.
11. Faria, I. E., & Cavanagh, P. R. (1978). *The physiology and biomechanics of cycling.* New York: John Wiley & Sons.
12. Gledhill, N., & Jamnik, R. (1995). Determining power outputs for cycle ergometers with different sized flywheels. *Medicine and Science in Sports and Exercise, 27,* 134–135.
13. Golding, L. A., Myers, C. R., & Sinning, W. E. (1989). *Y's way to fitness: The complete guide to fitness testing and instruction.* Champaign, IL: Human Kinetics.
14. Hermansen, L., & Saltin, B. (1969). Oxygen uptake during maximal treadmill and bicycle exercise. *Journal of Applied Physiology, 26,* 31–37.
15. Kasch, F. W. (1984, August). The validity of the Astrand and Sjostrand submaximal tests. *The Physician and Sportsmedicine,* 47–51, 54.
16. Leger, L., & Thivierge, M. (1988). Heart rate monitors: Validity, stability, and functionality. *The Physician and Sportsmedicine, 16*(5): 143–151.
17. Lehmann, J. (1972). Auscultation of heart sounds. *American Journal of Nursing, 72,* 1242–1246.
18. Littmann, D. (1972). Stethoscope and auscultation. *American Journal of Nursing, 72,* 1238–1241.
19. Luisada, A. A., & Zalter, R. (1960). Phonocardiography. In American College of Chest Physicians (Eds.), *Clinical Cardiopulmonary Physiology*, pp. 75–83, New York: Grune and Stratton.
20. Mahar, M., Jackson, A. S., Ross, R. L., Pivarnik, J. M., & Pollock, M. L. (1985). Predictive accuracy of single and double stage submax treadmill work for estimating aerobic capacity. *Medicine and Science in Sports and Exercise, 17,* 206–207, Abstract #4.
21. Mathews, D. K., & Fox, E. L. (1976). *The physiological basis of physical education and athletics.* Philadelphia: W. B. Saunders.
22. McArdle, W. D., Katch, F. I., & Katch, V. L. (1991). *Exercise physiology: Energy, nutrition, and human performance.* Philadelphia: Lea & Febiger.
23. Noble, B. J. (1986). *Physiology of exercise and sport.* St. Louis: Times Mirror/Mosby College Publishing.
24. Powell, B. (1982, October). Correction and prevention of bicycle saddle problems. *The Physician and Sportsmedicine,* 60–64, 67.
25. Rappaport, M. B., & Sprague, H. B. (1941). Physiologic and physical laws that govern auscultation, and their clinical application. *American Heart Journal, 21,* 257–318.
26. Seifert, J. G. (1991). The comparison of physiological responses from cycling on friction-braked and electromagnetic ergometers. *Research Quarterly for Exercise and Sport, 62,* 115–117.
27. Shennum, P. L., & deVries, H. A. (1976). The effect of saddle height on oxygen consumption during bicycle ergometer work. *Medicine and Science in Sports, 8,* 119–121.
28. Shephard, R. J. (1970). Computer programs for solution of the Astrand nomogram and the calculation of body surface area. *Journal of Sports Medicine and Physical Fitness, 10,* 206–210.
29. Shephard, R. J. (1972). *Alive man: The physiology of physical activity.* Springfield, IL: Charles C Thomas.
30. Terry, J. W., Tolson, H., Johnson, D. J., & Jessup, G. T. (1977). A workload selection procedure for the Astrand-Ryhming test. *Journal of Sports Medicine and Physical Fitness, 17,* 361.
31. Widrick, J. J., Freedson, P. S., & Hamill, J. (1992). Effect of internal work on the calculation of optimal pedaling rates. *Medicine and Science in Sports and Exercise, 24,* 376–382.
32. Williams, L. (1975). Reliability of predicting maximal oxygen intake using the Astrand-Ryhming nomogram. *Research Quarterly, 46,* 12–16.

Form AC 1

Practice of Heart Rate (HR) Auscultation, Timing, and Calculation

Auscultation Quality

Initials | Apical | (check one at each site) | Base

Men | Excellent | Good | Fair | Poor | Excellent | Good | Fair | Poor

1. ☐ ☐ ☐ ☐ ☐ | ☐ ☐ ☐ ☐

2. ☐ ☐ ☐ ☐ ☐ | ☐ ☐ ☐ ☐

Women | Apical | Base

1. ☐ ☐ ☐ ☐ ☐ | ☐ ☐ ☐ ☐

2. ☐ ☐ ☐ ☐ ☐ | ☐ ☐ ☐ ☐

Initials $1800/(30\text{-}b\ t)$ in s = HR (b·min^{-1}; closest 0.1 s) Site (check one)

Men | | Apical | Base

1. ☐ 1800/☐ · ☐ s = ☐ b·min^{-1} ☐ ☐

2. ☐ 1800/☐ · ☐ s = ☐ b·min^{-1} ☐ ☐

Women

1. ☐ 1800/[23] · [6] s = [76.3] b·min^{-1} ☐ ☐

2. ☐ 1800/[21] · [5] s = [83.7] b·min^{-1} ☐ ☐

Maximal Heart Rate Correction Factor (HRmax CF):

Men: HRmax CF = (220 – age – 61)/(195 – 61)

$= (220 - \boxed{}\ y - 61)/134$

$= \boxed{}\ /134 = \boxed{}$

Women: HRmax CF = (220 – age – 72)/(192 – 72)

$= (220 - \boxed{22}\ y - 72)/120$

$= \boxed{126}\ /120 = \boxed{1.05}$

Form AC 2

Handwritten annotations at top:
IF HR IS NOT WHAT IS SUPPOSED TO BE AT 2-3 MIN MARK - DECREASE/INCREASE WORK LOAD
CHANGE PER MIN SHOULDN'T BE MORE THAN 10 BEATS
WOMEN - START AT 600 KGM
MEN - START AT 900 KGM
RPM - 50

Individual Data for Astrand Cycle Test

Name: TOYA HART   Date: 9-27-99   Time: [ ] a.m. [ ] p.m.

Age: 22 y   Gender (M or F): F   Ht: 173 cm   Wt: 63.6 kg

T: 21.3 °C   RH: 60 % P_B: 755 torr   Fan: Yes [ ] No [ ]

Bike Model: Combi   Seat-post ht: N/A   Bike-Seated HR = 1800/ 22.5 s = 79.8 b·min⁻¹

Target HR Range: < 30 y = 150–160 b·min⁻¹   30 + y (see Table 2) = b·min⁻¹

Initial Power: [ ] kgm·min⁻¹; × 2 (+ 300) = $\dot{V}O_2SM$ [ ] mL·min⁻¹; = [ ] L·min⁻¹

100 W; × 12 (+ 300) = $\dot{V}O_2SM$ 1500 mL·min⁻¹ = 1.5 L·min⁻¹

Time min:s	1800/	Exercise HR 30-b time (s) = b·min⁻¹	
1:30–2:00	1800/	_____	136
2:30–3:00	1800/	_____	143
3:30–4:00	1800/	_____	155
4:30–5:00	1800/	_____	159
5:30–6:00	1800/	_____	164
6:30–7:00	1800/	_____	166
7:30–8:00	1800/	_____	

Adjusted Power if Warranted: [ ] W [ ] kgm·min⁻¹
Average of 5th & 6th min HR (if differ by < 6 b/min) 165
6th min HR (if 5th & 6th min differ between 6–10 b/min)
HR if 5th & 6th min HR differ by > 10 b/min or if power adjustment was made.

$\dot{V}O_2max$ (L·min⁻¹; mL·kg⁻¹·min⁻¹) for MEN (M) and WOMEN (W) using equations 8 and 9:

$\dot{V}O_2SM$ 1.8 L·min⁻¹ × {[(220 − Age 22 y) − 61 M]/(HRsm 165 − 61)} [− 72 W above both]

= $\dot{V}O_2SM$ 1.8 L·min⁻¹ × (126 / 93)

= $\dot{V}O_2SM$ 1.8 L·min⁻¹ × 1.4 = 2.52 ; × 1000 = 2520 mL·min⁻¹;

divided by body wt 63.6 kg = Relative $\dot{V}O_2max$ 39.6 mL·kg⁻¹·min⁻¹

$\dot{V}O_2max$ using Table Method for Men (table 4) and Women (5):

$\dot{V}O_2max$ 2.5 L·min⁻¹ (from Table) × HRmax CF (from Form AC 1) 1.05

= 2.625 L·min⁻¹ = 2625 mL·min⁻¹; divided by body wt 63.6 kg = 41.3 mL·kg⁻¹·min⁻¹

Fitness Category (circle one): Very High   High   (Good)   Ave   Fair   Low

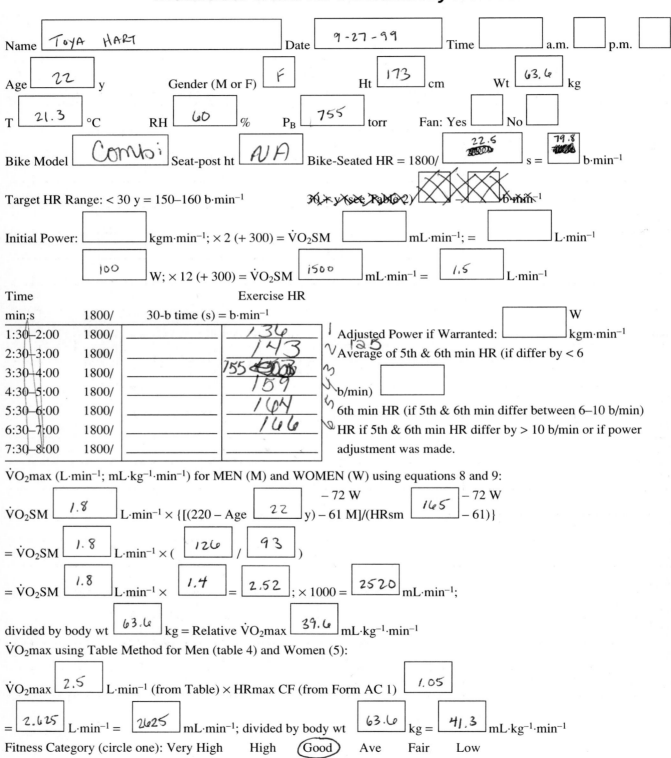

152 Aerobic Cycling   AC-14

Form AC 3

Group Data for Astrand Cycle Test

MEN

Initials or I.D.	$\dot{V}O_2max$ (ml·kg⁻¹·min⁻¹)	Fitness Category
1.		
2.		
3.		
4.		
5.		
6.		
7.		
8.		
9.		
10.		
11.		
12.		
13.		
14.		
15.		
16.		
17.		
18.		
19.		
20.		
21.		
22.		
M		

WOMEN

Initials or I.D.	$\dot{V}O_2max$ (ml·kg⁻¹·min⁻¹)	Fitness Category
1.		
2.		
3.		
4.		
5.		
6.		
7.		
8.		
9.		
10.		
11.		
12.		
13.		
14.		
15.		
16.		
17.		
18.		
19.		
20.		
21.		
22.		
M		

Chapter OC Maximal Oxygen Consumption

A test of aerobic fitness that truly qualifies as a lab test is the Maximal Oxygen Consumption ($\dot{V}O_2$max) Test. Although this test may involve a substantial anaerobic contribution to metabolism at the terminal portion of the test, it is primarily an aerobic test.

Whereas the running and cycling tests attempt to *predict* aerobic power as accurately as possible, the $\dot{V}O_2$max Test actually *measures* aerobic power. The run/walk tests, for example, predict maximal oxygen consumption based on the relationship between maximal oxygen consumption and time or distance of running or walking; the step tests and cycle tests *estimate* the maximal oxygen consumption based on the relationship between heart rate, oxygen consumption, and power level. Because the $\dot{V}O_2$max Test directly measures oxygen consumption, it requires more expensive and sophisticated equipment than that required by field or field/lab tests.

In this chapter, the direct measurement of oxygen consumption is described for submaximal and maximal exercise. Special importance is given to the latter stages of exercise, because that is when the *maximal* oxygen consumption typically occurs.

Purpose of the Maximal Oxygen Consumption Test

The purpose of the Maximal Oxygen Consumption Test is to measure aerobic fitness. Aerobic fitness is synonymous with several other terms such as aerobic power, aerobic capacity, cardiovascular endurance, circulorespiratory endurance, and cardiorespiratory endurance.

The Maximal Oxygen Consumption Test has received more recognition than any other exercise physiology lab test. Testimony to this is the fact that the purpose of many field and field/lab tests is to predict maximal oxygen consumption–the variable that often has been used synonymously with aerobic fitness.[48,59,65] Traditionally, no other single lab test has been used as frequently to indicate a person's aptitude for success in events calling upon maximal efforts longer than 3 min. In addition, combined with some anaerobic tests, it helps indicate success for events lasting 1.5 to 3 min. In conjunction with tests of efficiency (economy), ventilatory threshold/breakpoint, glycogen storage, acclimatization, and fractional utilization of maximal oxygen consumption, this test is also an important indicator of success for all-out events lasting between 20 min and 4 h.[58]

Also, the Maximal Oxygen Consumption Test provides insight into the cardiorespiratory system. For example, the clinical severity of disease has been shown to decrease with an increase in functional aerobic capacity.[13] Thus, the Maximal Oxygen Consumption Test has been used to assess not only aerobic power but also to assess the role of the cardiovascular and respiratory systems in the transport and diffusion of oxygen.

Physiological Rationale

The ability to consume oxygen is important for the metabolic function of body cells. Cell activity is dependent upon oxygen because the cell derives its energy from adenosine triphosphate (ATP), which is produced mainly by aerobic metabolism. Aerobic metabolism produces large volumes of ATP via the oxidative pathway. This pathway reflects the ability of the muscles' mitochondria to synthesize the phosphagen ATP. The maximal consumption of oxygen is not only dependent upon the cells' ability to extract and use oxygen, but upon the ability of the cardiovascular and respiratory systems to transport this oxygen to the cells. Cardiovascularly, the transport of oxygen is represented by the cardiac output, the amount of blood pumped by a heart ventricle per minute. Thus, a greater cardiac output leads to a greater maximal oxygen consumption under normal conditions. The respiratory system's transport of oxygen is represented by ventilation, which is measured as liters of air per minute. Although a greater ventilation capacity usually is associated with a greater maximal oxygen consumption, it is not a limiting factor in the average person.

The highest oxygen value achieved during the $\dot{V}O_2$max Test represents the maximal oxygen consumption. This peak is most likely to occur at the final minute of the progressive exercise test. Because the peak oxygen consumption value may vary with the mode of exercise and limiting symptoms, the term **peak oxygen consumption** denotes the highest oxygen consumption for a specific type of exercise, and the term **maximal oxygen consumption** denotes the single highest possible oxygen consumption elicited among the different modes of exercise.[9] For example, peak oxygen consumption values are similar for treadmill and step tests for most people, but they are about 5%–10% higher on a treadmill than on a bicycle ergometer.[35] For trained cyclists, however, similar results may be achieved on bicycle and treadmill ergometry. Another example is the $\dot{V}O_2$ peak

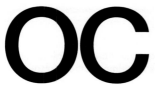

Accuracy of the $\dot{V}O_2$max Test

The accuracy of the Maximal Oxygen Consumption Test is maximized by achieving the traditional criteria of the max test, such as (1) the plateau of the oxygen consumption despite an increase of power level, (2) the attainment of respiratory exchange ratios of 1.0 or higher, (3) the plateau of heart rate, (4) high blood lactates, and (5) the exhaustion of the performer.

Validity

The validity of any exercise test, as noted previously, is partly dependent on the exercise modality and the specific fitness of the performer. Although not supported by all physiologists,[24,51] most investigators and reviewers[48,59,65] have supported the maximal oxygen consumption value as probably the best single physiological indicator of a person's capacity for maintaining endurance-type activity. High maximal oxygen consumption values, when expressed relative to body weight (ml·kg^{-1}·min^{-1}), are associated with successful running performance in events lasting more than 5 min. For example, correlations of .90 and .91 have been reported between $\dot{V}O_2$max and 12-min distance.[22,31] However, a lower correlation of –.74 was reported between $\dot{V}O_2$max and 1.5-mile time.[44]

Reliability

The test-retest reliability of maximal oxygen consumption tests is high—about .95[52,65] to .99.[13] The standard error (*SE*) of the $\dot{V}O_2$max Test may range from a low of about 2.5%[65] to a high of about 5%–6%[40] of the mean score for an average person; it may extend up to about 8% in aerobically trained males.[18] Thus, an individual would be expected to vary by about 2–4 ml·kg^{-1}·min^{-1}, even when tested weeks apart.[13,46,65] For example, if a person's maximal oxygen consumption is truly 40 ml·kg^{-1}·min^{-1}, then repeated tests with an *SE* of 5% would be expected to vary between 38.0 and 42.0 ml·kg^{-1}·min^{-1} [calculated as: 40 ml·kg^{-1}·min^{-1} ± (5% × 40)]. The $\dot{V}O_2$max is highly consistent even over a 4-month period, having an average coefficient of variation [(*SD/M*) × 100] of about 4.3%.[73]

elicited by arm ergometry, which is 63% of that elicited by the treadmill.[7] Thus the term *peak* should be used to denote the highest oxygen consumption value achieved for a particular mode of exercise, and the term *maximal* should be used for the highest value achieved among all the modes, which is usually treadmill ergometry. Symptom-limited peak $\dot{V}O_2$ is the highest value achieved before disease symptoms dictated the halt of the test rather than physiological limits. In general, the peak oxygen consumption is directly related to the muscle mass involved in the ergometric task.

Method

The methods and procedures for the administration of oxygen consumption (metabolic) testing may seem complicated, especially for first-year exercise physiology students. However, it is certainly possible for novices to gain an appreciation and understanding of maximal oxygen consumption testing simply by observing the performer and by monitoring the instruments during the exercise test. The methods include a description of the equipment, the exercise protocol, procedures, and calculations.

Equipment

Until the 1970s, the equipment used for measuring oxygen consumption consisted of several instruments purchased from separate manufacturers. The investigator then would either interface the individual instruments so that on-line testing could be accomplished, or the investigator would collect the exhaled air in special bags for posttest analysis of oxygen and carbon dioxide concentrations and ventila-

tion volumes. Today there are a variety of manufacturers who combine the individual components into a single package. These interfaced consoles often include a computer to make all the calculations for deriving the metabolic and respiratory values. Improved and consolidated instrumentation has led to portable and breath-by-breath capabilities in measuring oxygen consumption.

The equipment for Maximal Oxygen Consumption Tests may be categorized into four areas: (1) ergometers, (2) respiratory equipment, (3) metabolic equipment, and (4) auxiliaries.

Ergometers

It is best to use the type of ergometer that simulates the type of movement for which the subject has been training. For example, runners should be tested on treadmills, cyclists on bicycle ergometers, rowers on rowing ergometers, wheelchair athletes on wheelchair or arm ergometers, cross-country skiers on ski ergometers, and swimmers in swim flumes, on swim benches, or in a pool while tethered to weighted pulleys. Another consideration is the norms by which the subject will be evaluated. The Maximal Oxygen Consumption Test should be performed on the same ergometer as that which was used by the subjects who generated the norms. A practical consideration is the cost and ancillary objectives of the test. For example, a step bench is inexpensive, while a cycle ergometer facilitates the measurement of blood pressure.

The treadmill (TM) has two basic units of measure: (1) speed and (2) slope or grade (Fig. 1; Table 1). Maximal speeds (mph or m·h^{-1}; kph or km·h^{-1}) may vary with different treadmills from 12 mph (19.3 kph) to 15 mph (24 kph) to 25 mph (40.2 kph). The maximal slopes or

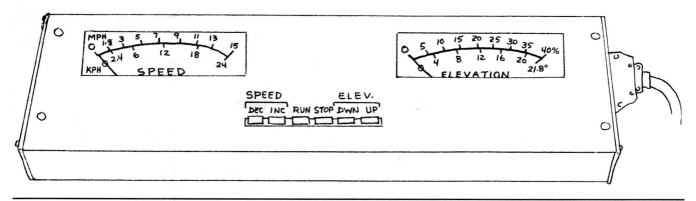

Figure 1 A treadmill's control panel displaying the speed (mph or m·h^{-1}; kph or km·h^{-1}) and elevation (%; degrees).

Table 1 Conversions for Speed and Slope for Treadmill Ergometry

Speed (based upon 1 mph = 1.609 kph = 26.8 m·min^{-1})					
mph	kph	m·min^{-1}	mph	kph	m·min^{-1}
1.7	2.74	45.6	8.5	13.68	228.0
2.0	3.22	53.6	9.0	14.48	241.4
2.5	4.02	66.7	9.5	15.29	254.8
3.0	4.83	80.4	10.0	16.09	268.2
3.5	5.63	94.0	10.5	16.89	281.6
4.0	6.44	107.2	11.0	17.70	295.0
4.5	7.24	121.0	11.5	18.50	308.5
5.0	8.04	134.1	12.0	19.31	322.0
5.5	8.85	148.0	12.5	20.11	335.3
6.0	9.65	161.0	13.0	20.92	348.7
6.5	10.46	174.3	13.5	21.72	362.1
7.0	11.26	188.8	14.0	22.53	375.5
7.5	12.07	201.2	14.5	23.33	389.0
8.0	12.87	215.0	15.0	24.13	402.3

Slope			
Degree (°)	Grade (%)	Degree (°)	Grade (%)
1	1.75	6	10.51
2	3.49	7	12.28
3	5.24	8	14.05
4	6.99	9	15.84
5	8.75	10	17.63

grades of laboratory treadmills are about 25%, but some can reach 40% (21.8°). Table 1 provides the equivalent speeds in the American and metric systems, along with the slopes in degrees and percent grade. The calibration of treadmills is described in the "Calibration of the Treadmill" box.

Respiratory and Metabolic/Gas Equipment (Fig. 2)

The pieces of equipment that aid in the measurement of the volume of air breathed by the subject are (1) a noseclip, (2) a mouthpiece, (3) an air meter, (4) a respiratory valve, and (5) ventilatory hoses. The pieces of equipment that promote the measurement of the metabolic gases are (1) an oxygen analyzer, (2) a carbon dioxide analyzer, (3) a mixing chamber, and (4) a drying tube.

Respiratory Equipment. A **noseclip** prevents the inhalation and exhalation of air through the nose. Otherwise, if air is breathed through the nose, it is unaccounted for at the air meter.

A **rubber mouthpiece** attaches to the respiratory valve and is similar to a scuba mouthpiece. The flanges of the mouthpiece prevent the leakage of air around the subject's mouth, while the protruding tabs allow the subject to grip the piece with the teeth.

An **air meter** of some sort (electronic pneumotachometer, turbine flow, tissot spirometer, or mechanical bellows) is used to measure the volume of air inspired or expired (V_I or V_E). The recorded unit of measure is liters per minute (L·min^{-1}). Either the inspiratory or expiratory volumes, or both, are measured by the air meter. When measuring inspired air, the inspiratory air flows from the inlet of the air meter to its outlet and on toward the subject's respiratory valve.

A **respiratory valve** (Fig. 3) is a one-way valve that allows the inspiration of normal air via the air meter. The inspired air comes into the inlet side of the respiratory valve but cannot return out the same inlet during expiration. The expired air is directed to the outlet of the respiratory valve. Contrarily, when measuring expired air volume, the expiratory air flows from the respiratory valve outlet to the inlet of the air meter.

Ventilatory hoses are internally smooth (noncorrugated) flexible tubes that conduct air to and from the air meter.

Metabolic/Gas Equipment. The metabolic/gas equipment directs, dries, and analyzes the subject's expired air as it passes from the ventilatory tube at the outlet of the respiratory valve and through the mixing chamber to the respective gas analyzers.

Many electronic **oxygen analyzers** use paramagnetic or galvanic fuel cell principles to determine the fractional (or percentage) concentration of oxygen in the expired air (F_EO_2). Most metabolic analyzers are designed to be most accurate between oxygen concentrations of 15% to 21%. Many electronic **carbon dioxide analyzers** use an infrared

Calibration of the Treadmill (TM)

Both the speed and slope of a treadmill (TM) should be calibrated annually. Instructions for TM calibration are usually found in the manufacturer's instruction manual and can be found in other sources.[19,33]

Speed Calibration
1. If the length of the TM belt is not given in the manufacturer's instruction manual, then measure the belt length as follows:
   a. Mark (#1) the exposed belt with a piece of easily visible tape at the front of the TM (but not on the curved surface).
   b. Place a chalk or pen mark at a second point (mark #2) at the rear flat portion of the TM belt.
   c. Using a meter-stick or metric tape, measure the distance between marks #1 and #2 to the nearest 0.1 cm; record the value (e.g., 153.2 cm; 1.532 m).
   d. Expose another belt portion by pushing it clockwise with your foot, but stop it when the tape mark is at back of TM.
   e. Make mark #3 at the front flat portion of the TM belt.
   f. Measure the distance from the tape mark now at the back of the belt to the mark #3; record the value (e.g., 144.3 cm).
   g. Again move the belt, then stop it when the original rear chalk or pen mark (#2) is visible at a flat portion at the front of the TM belt.
   h. Measure the distance between mark #3 and mark #2; record the value (e.g., 141.0 cm; 1.410).
   i. Add the three values; the total is the length of the belt (e.g., 438.5 cm, or 4.385 m, for Quinton™ (18–60).
2. Measure the number of revolutions as follows if the TM has no automatic counter:
   a. Start the treadmill and set the speed control to a slow speed (e.g., 4.0 kph).
   b. Mark a fixed point outside the TM belt (e.g., the inside edge at the rear of the TM where the belt descends or disappears).
   c. Start a stopwatch the instant that the tape mark (#1) passes the fixed mark.
   d. Count the number of belt revolutions by counting the number of times the belt mark passes the fixed point.
   e. Stop the watch at a complete (whole) revolution that is closest to 60 s; record the number of revolutions.
   f. Record the time to closest tenth of a second (e.g., 59.6).
3. Convert the revolutions to revolutions per minute (rpm) by using Equation 1:

$$rpm = \text{revolutions (\#)} \div (t \text{ in s/60 s}) \qquad \text{Eq. 1}$$

   Sample calculation: If revolutions = <u>17</u> and time = <u>59.6</u> s
   then rpm = 17 ÷ 59.6 / 60;
   $\qquad$ = 17 ÷ 0.99;
   $\qquad$ = 17.17

4. The distance (D) covered in 1 min is calculated according to Equation 2:

$$D \cdot min^{-1} = rpm \times \text{belt length in m}$$

   Using the prior example, then $D \cdot min^{-1} = 17.17 \times 4.385$ m = 75.30 m·min^{-1}, which is faster than the expected 66.7 m·min^{-1} (Table 1).
5. The distance in m·h^{-1} is calculated by multiplying the m·min^{-1} by 60:

$$75.30 \times 60 = 4518 \text{ m·h}^{-1}$$

6. The distance in kph (km·h^{-1}) = 4.518, which is faster than the expected 4.0 km·h^{-1} (Table 1).
7. The distance in mph = 4.518 km·h^{-1} ÷ 1.609 = 2.80 mph, which is faster than the expected 2.50 mph (Table 1).
8. The treadmill controller's zero set screw must be adjusted until the speed reads the same as the controller's gauge.

Slope Calibration
Zero:
1. Run the treadmill at a slow speed while the elevation setting is at 0% or 0°.
2. Stop the treadmill.
3. Place a carpenter's level on the TM belt.
4. Check the bubble on the level to make sure it is centered.
5. If it is not centered, then run and stop the TM repeatedly while changing the slope setting until the carpenter's level indicates zero slope.
6. Once the TM is level, change the slope indicator to zero by making an adjustment at a small screw usually found on the meter's face.

Range:
1. Place the treadmill to a given percent slope (e.g., 20%).
2. Measure a fixed distance on the floor parallel and at the edge of the treadmill (e.g., 20 in.).
3. Measure the perpendicular height of the treadmill at the low part of the parallel distance (e.g., 15 in.).
4. Measure the perpendicular height of the treadmill at the high part of the parallel distance (e.g., 19 in.).
5. Calculate the percent slope according to the following formula:

$$\% \text{ slope} = [(\text{Highest ht} - \text{lowest ht}) \div \text{parallel distance}] \times 100$$

   E.g., 20% = [(19 – 15) ÷ 20] × 100 = (4 ÷ 20) × 100
6. Adjust, if necessary, the potentiometer on the control-meter to the appropriate percent slope (e.g., 20%).

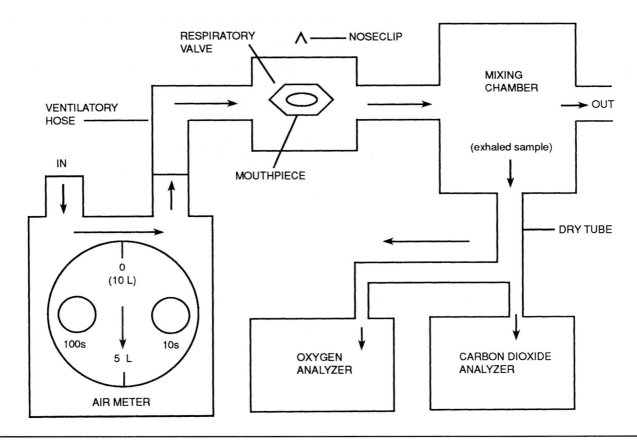

Figure 2 Schematic depiction of the air flow circuit for measuring the inspiratory volume of air (V_I) and the expired fractional concentrations of oxygen (F_EO_2) and carbon dioxide (F_ECO_2). The air meter has three dials—the big circle representing 0–10 L, the two smaller circles representing 10–100 L and 100–1000 L, respectively.

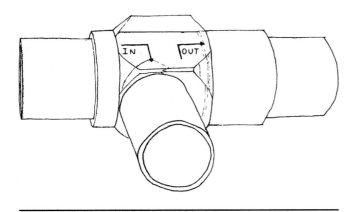

Figure 3 A one-way respiratory valve.

principle to determine the fractional (F) concentration (or %) of carbon dioxide in the expired air (F_ECO_2). Mass spectrometers can measure both carbon dioxide and oxygen concentrations. Nitrogen analyzers are not necessary for measuring oxygen consumption because nitrogen concentration can be calculated as the balance from the other two gas measures.

The samples of gas can be directed to and from a mixing chamber, or be sampled after being collected in small rubber bags (aliquots), or large collection bags (meteoro-logical; Douglas). The **mixing chamber,** usually a 4- to 10-L box or cylinder made of clear plexiglass, allows the expired air to be uniformly distributed before passing into the gas analyzers for on-line sampling.

A **drying tube** consists of a small (3–4 in. × 0.5 in.) container holding a suitable drying agent or desiccant (e.g., calcium sulfate) and filter that prevents damp (saturated) and dusty air from entering the analyzers. Although not universally used, it may prolong the life of the analyzers, and it eliminates the need to correct mathematically for the percentage of water vapor in the gas samples. Because the airflow through the drying tube is slower than normal, a delay in the circuit of about 15,[66] or up to 30 s, should be accounted for when analyzing the data.

Auxiliaries

The need for auxiliary equipment is dependent upon the type of basic equipment available to the investigator. For example, some computerized metabolic consoles also contain gauges for monitoring temperature and pressure. To measure oxygen consumption, a laboratory needs auxiliary equipment for such purposes as (1) monitoring the environment; (2) measuring the performer's height and weight; (3) providing comfort to the subject, (4) calibrating instruments and gases, (5) timing, (6) recording, and (7) protecting the instruments.

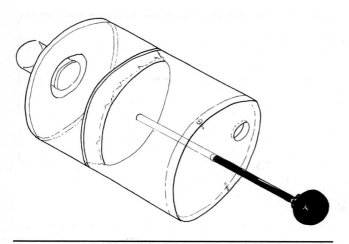

Figure 4 A one-liter syringe for calibrating air meters.

Various **meteorological gauges** for measuring environmental air temperature, barometric pressure, and relative humidity are necessary to correct for temperature, pressure, and saturation of the observed inspiratory and/or expiratory air volumes.

Either a **platform** or **electronic scale** may be used to measure the subject's height and weight just prior to the test. These techniques are described in Chapter UN.

A **respiratory valve support** may consist of a support from an overhead rail or ceiling, or from a commercially available waist-harness. Without such a support the performer has trouble keeping the valve in the mouth, especially during treadmill exercise.

Calibrative auxiliaries include such items as gas cylinders and air volume syringes. The cylinders should contain certified precise CO_2, O_2, and N_2 gases; substantiation of such gases can be made with a Scholander apparatus. The 1- to 5-L air volume syringes (Fig. 4) insert a precise volume of air into the air meter, pneumotach, or metabolic instrument.

A **laboratory timer**, easily visible to all technicians, is used for timing various events such as exercise protocol and air/gas recordings. Timers are described in the chapter for the Wingate Anaerobic Test.

A **ventilation recorder** is an optional auxiliary instrument. Some are capable of graphing inspirations and expirations, thus enabling the calculation of such respiratory parameters as ventilatory volume, frequency, and tidal volume. Of these three parameters, only ventilatory volume is essential for the calculation of oxygen consumption. If the airflow meter has no electrical output by which to record the volume electronically, then the technician must simply record the values indicated by the pointers on the airflow meter.

Exercise Protocol

The Maximal Oxygen Consumption Test usually requires the performer to exercise to exhaustion, although it need not be totally exhaustive as long as the other traditional criteria are met. Usually the test duration is a minimum of 5–9 min to a maximum of 15–20 min. The longer tests are usually associated with other objectives, such as the monitoring of the electrocardiogram. The exercise may be performed on various modalities, such as (a) step bench, (b) cycle ergometer, (c) treadmill, (d) swim flume, (e) wheelchair ergometer, (f) rowing ergometer, (g) skiing ergometer, and others. The test protocol, which consists of the prescription for time spent at each power level, is often a continuous and progressive type that eventually exceeds the aerobic power of the exerciser. Thus, the test includes submaximal, maximal, and supramaximal exercise relative to $\dot{V}O_2max$. The supramaximal portion leads to the performer's exhaustion.

Several protocols may be used to elicit peak or maximal oxygen consumption.[3] Some of these are described in the chapter on the ECG Test of this manual, while two protocols are presented for the cycle ergometer, and one for the treadmill, in this chapter.

Although it is possible to reach nearly the maximal oxygen consumption level in 1 min when performing an all-out 90-s cycling task,[62] the test (excluding warmup) is seldom less than 5 min and often no longer than 9 min. Occasionally, it may be as long as 20 min for exceptional individuals, or if a longer time for monitoring the electrocardiogram is desired, or if mechanical efficiency is being measured simultaneously. Some investigators recommend a continuous protocol that brings performers to their limit of tolerance in about 10 min ± 2 min.[15]

Cycling Protocols

Prior to the test, the estimated $\dot{V}O_2max$ of the performer should be made from previous field or field/lab predictive tests. It can also be estimated by questioning the performer about training habits.

$\%\dot{V}O_2max$ *Protocol.* If technicians are reasonably confident in predicting the subject's $\dot{V}O_2max$, one recommended protocol is to start at 25 to 40% of the predicted $\dot{V}O_2max$ and then progress through the 1–3 min stages by 10–15% $\dot{V}O_2max$.[66]

If no predictive $\dot{V}O_2max$ is available, but the subject knows the highest power level that he or she can sustain for three or more minutes on a cycle ergometer, then Table 2 can be used to approximate the maximal oxygen consumption. Table 2 gives MET values, multiples of resting metabolism, at various power levels during cycle ergometry for persons weighing between 50 and 100 kg.[3] The approximate oxygen cost (not maximal) may be found by multiplying the MET value by 3.5 ml·kg^{-1}·min^{-1}. The predicted $\dot{V}O_2max$ likely would be greater than the oxygen cost derived from the power level in which the performer sustains longer than 3 min. Once the $\dot{V}O_2max$ value has been estimated, either the $\%\dot{V}O_2max$ protocol or a protocol from Table 3 may be used.

Table 2 Conversion of Power to Energy Cost (MET) of Cycle Ergometry

Weight (kg)	50	75	100	Power (W) 125	150	175	200
50	5.1	6.9	8.6	10.3	12.0	13.7	15.4
60	4.3	5.7	7.1	8.6	10.0	11.4	12.9
70	3.7	4.9	6.1	7.3	8.6	9.8	11.0
80	3.2	4.3	5.4	6.4	7.5	8.6	9.6
90	2.9	3.8	4.8	5.7	6.7	7.6	8.6
100	2.6	3.4	4.3	5.1	6.0	6.9	7.7

"Zero load" (0 N or 0 kg) on load or force indicator is equivalent to about 550 ml·min^{-1}·$\dot{V}O_2$ for 70–80 kg performers.
From The American College of Sports Medicine, *Guidelines for Exercise Testing and Prescription,* Table D-4, p. 299, 1991. Copyright © 1991 Lea & Febiger Publishers, Malvern, PA. Reprinted by permission.

Table 3 Cycle Ergometer Protocols for $\dot{V}O_2$max Test

Time (min:s)	Power (W; N·m·min^{-1}; kg·m·min^{-1})					
	"Guesstimated" Maximal Oxygen Consumption (L·min^{-1})					
	< 3.0 L·min^{-1}			> 3.0 L·min^{-1}		
Warmup	W	N·m·min^{-1}	kg·m·min^{-1}	W	N·m·min^{-1}	kg·m·min^{-1}
0:00–5:00	75	4500	450	150	1500	900
"Rest"	0–25	0–1500	0–150	25–50	1500–3000	150–300
Max Test						
0:00–2:00	100	6000	600	175	10 500	1050
2:00–4:00	125	7500	750	200	12 000	1200
4:00–6:00	150	9000	900	225	13 500	1350
6:00–8:00	175	10 500	1050	250	15 000	1500
8:00–10:00	200	12 000	1200	275	16 500	1650
10:00–12:00	225	13 500	1350	300	18 000	1800
12:00–14:00	250	15 000	1500	325	19 500	1950
Recovery						
0:00–3:00	50–75	3000–4500	300–450	125–150	7500–9000	750–900

Table-3 Protocols. The two cycle protocols presented in Table 3 are modifications of a former continuous protocol,[43] and are based on the aerobic fitness status of the performer. They are for persons who are "guesstimated" to have maximal oxygen consumptions above and below 3.0 L·min^{-1}. For persons with an estimated $\dot{V}O_2$max less than 3.0 L·min^{-1}, the initial power level is 100 W (600 kg·m·min^{-1}) and increases by 25 W for subsequent 2-min power intervals. A similar protocol is followed for persons with estimated $\dot{V}O_2$max levels greater than 3.0 L·min^{-1}, except that the initial power level is 175 W. For persons with suspected $\dot{V}O_2$max levels that are exceptionally high, the starting power level can be higher than 175 W in order to keep the time for the test close to a 9-min maximum. Often, the final power level of a performer cannot be sustained for the entire 2 min due to the performer's fatigue.

$\dot{V}O_2$max Criteria. The performer is encouraged to exercise to exhaustion in order to assure that peak oxygen consumption has been achieved. A primary criterion for attainment of peak, or maximal, is an increase in oxygen consumption no greater than 150 ml·min^{-1} at a succeeding power level.[65] This means, for example, that for a change in power level equivalent to 25 W (or 150 kg·m·min^{-1}), or a treadmill power level of 2.5% grade and 7 mph, the change

in oxygen consumption should not exceed 150 ml·min^{-1}. An expected increase for 25 W is 300 ml·min^{-1}, thus the lower value of 150 indicates that the performer cannot meet the oxygen requirement. In MET terms, an expected increase of 2.5 MET is achieved with only a 0.6 MET increase.[36] Thus it is likely that performers truly reach peak oxygen consumptions when this criterion is met. If oxygen consumptions at the last power level increase by more than 150 ml · min^{-1}, then it is more likely that they might reach a higher oxygen consumption if proceeding to a higher power level.[17] However, reviewers note that a significant percentage of persons, especially children, elderly, and low-fit persons, fail to reach an oxygen plateau as defined by this criterion.[37]

If this primary criterion is not met, peak oxygen consumption may still have occurred if secondary criteria have been met. For example, the respiratory exchange ratio serves as an excellent indicator of $\dot{V}O_2$max achievement. Investigators would expect a ratio greater than 1.0;[10,45,49,71] some exercise physiologists recommend minimum ratios from 1.05[27] to 1.1[36] or 1.15[5,60] or 1.2.

Other secondary criteria (1) high blood lactates (e.g., >7.9 mM); (2) rate of perceived exertion (RPE) greater than 17 and 8 for the original category scale and the category-ratio scale, respectively; (3) reaching previously *measured* maximal heart rate; and (4) exhaustion of the performer.

Table 4 Bruce Treadmill Protocol for the $\dot{V}O_2$max Test

Time min:s	Bruce Stage	Speed mph	kph	Slope %	MET
Walk/Warmup					
0:00–3:00	1	1.7	2.7	10	5
3:00–6:00	2	2.5	4.0	12	7
Walk/Run					
6:00–9:00	3	3.4	5.5	14	10
9:00–12:00	4	4.2	6.8	16	13
Run					
12:00–15:00	5	5.0	8.0	18	16
15:00–18:00	6	5.5	8.0	20	18
18:00–21:00	7	6.0	9.7	22	22
Recovery (Walk/Run)					
0:00–2:00	2	2.5	4.0	12	7

Because of the large standard deviation in maximal heart rate between persons (± 10–12 b·min^{-1}), the *predicted* maximal heart rate should not be used as a criterion. In summary, if the attainment of $\dot{V}O_2$max criteria is questionable, then the more apt term may be peak $\dot{V}O_2$ rather than maximal $\dot{V}O_2$.

Pedal Revolutions Per Minute (RPM). Although economy or efficiency of cycling may vary with pedal rpm,[20,29,34,54,55,61,64] it does not mean that rpm will necessarily alter the peak oxygen consumption value.[57] Also, although some suggest that cyclists stand on the pedals during the last moments of cycling in order to cause the cycling peak $\dot{V}O_2$ value to approximate more closely the treadmill value, this has not been confirmed.[2,32]

Treadmill (TM) Protocol

It appears that similar results are obtained with a variety of treadmill protocols, although some take less time than others.[30] One of the most popular treadmill tests is the Bruce test, the earliest standard treadmill test.[46] Although it is often used for cardiovascular screening purposes,[14] it also is a common protocol for predicting[1,8,42] and directly measuring maximal oxygen consumption.[52]

The Bruce protocol (Table 4) consists of seven 3-min stages. Most performers should walk during the initial three stages in the first nine minutes.[10] Although the initial stages are important for cardiovascular screening (e.g., ECG monitoring), they are sometimes deleted when the primary purpose is to measure maximal oxygen consumption; in these cases the initial stage for $\dot{V}O_2$max testing is dependent upon the fitness level of the performer. Table 4 also lists the approximate MET for each completed stage of the Bruce protocol.[3]

Treadmill Technique. A person should never be standing on a stationary treadmill belt when it is placed in the On position. To enter and exit a moving belt of a treadmill, both sides of the hand-rails should be used. There are two acceptable ways of stepping onto the moving belt of a

Instrument Calibration

Calibration can be performed by the instructor or lab assistants prior to the test. The gold-standards of gas calibration are based on the measurement of oxygen and carbon dioxide from one of three methods: (1) Scholander technique; (2) Haldane technique; and (3) mass spectrometry. The former two methods require inexpensive apparatuses that measure volumes of oxygen and carbon dioxide after each has been absorbed by respective chemical reagents.[21] These two methods are gradually giving way to the more rapid mass spectrometry method.

Some commercial metabolic instruments (e.g., Sensor Medics MMC4400) have autocalibration devices using gas tanks with 24% and 12% oxygen, and 8% and 0% carbon dioxide.[50]

It is not unusual to calibrate the analyzers against standardized gas tanks of known concentrations before each test. Ideally, a three-point calibration is recommended,[37] whereby certified calibrated gases at the zero are at 0%, with the high span for carbon dioxide and oxygen at 6% and 18%, respectively, and the mid-ranges at 3% and 15%.

treadmill. One way is to stand alongside the moving belt and then to lean over the belt while grasping both rails for support. Then one foot is placed onto the belt and allowed to coast briefly; that foot is then returned to its original position. This is repeated until the performer establishes a rhythm or pace. Once the performer feels secure about the pace, the other foot is placed on the belt while the upper body is still substantially supported by the handrails; finally, the performer releases the handrails. The other method is to straddle the moving belt and then proceed as in the previous method. In order to reduce testing variability, the performer should not rely on the handrails for upper-body support.[12] While on the treadmill, the performer should look straight ahead to prevent possible nausea from viewing the moving belt.

Procedures for the Maximal Oxygen Consumption Test

The initial steps for the $\dot{V}O_2$max Test consist of calibrating the instruments (see "Instrument Calibration" box) and preparing the performer for exercise.

Preparations

The **performer** should arrive for testing under similar conditions as those presented for performers of the Step Test (see Chapter AS). Thus, the performer should be refreshed, euhydrated, dressed in lightweight exercise clothes, and not under the influence of drugs, hunger, or fullness.

The technician assigned as the performer's **caretaker** should oversee the gathering of the basic data such as height, weight, and age. The caretaker should also prepare the performer for the ergometer (e.g., adjust the seat post of cycle ergometer) and the respiratory valve, in addition to explaining the exercise protocol and objectives of the Maximal Oxygen Consumption Test.

The technician assigned as the **meteorologist** is responsible for observing and recording the environmental temperature, barometric pressure, and relative humidity (see Chapter UN).

Procedures During the Exercise Test

After these initial steps, the exercise begins, and various technicians perform their specific duties at significant times in the exercise protocol (Form OC 1).

The warmup and initial stages of the exercise protocol are not critical for measuring maximal oxygen consumption, but they are important for submaximal measures. They also allow the technicians to become familiar with their roles and possibly alert them to any technical or performer problems. The step-by-step procedures are as follows:

1. Start laboratory timer when performer is at the chosen power level.
2. Record the fraction of expired oxygen (F_EO_2) every 15 s.
3. Record the fraction of expired carbon dioxide (F_ECO_2) every 15 s.
4. Record ventilation (V_E or V_I) from the air meter every 60 s early in the test, but every 30 s as the performer nears the expected maximal level.
5. Change the power level at the appropriate time in the exercise protocol.
6. If using a treadmill, record the first complete minute of running; usually between the 6th and 12th min.
7. Because the valve restricts the speech of performers, periodically have them indicate their condition by a thumb-up, thumb-sideways, or thumb-down signal, or use a Rate-of-Perceived-Exertion chart.
8. As the performer begins to lose coordination due to fatigue (e.g., lots of extraneous movements), encourage continuation to exhaustion.
9. Place a spotter near the performer.
10. When the performer reaches exhaustion, record the exact time of stopping the test.
11. After stopping the treadmill, restart it in order to provide a recovery period on the treadmill; ask the performer to walk-in-place on the platform alongside the treadmill belt, until the proper recovery speed of the treadmill is obtained; if there is no space alongside the treadmill, ask the subject to grasp the siderails for support while continuing to jog/walk as the technician decreases the slope and speed of the treadmill. If using a cycle ergometer, quickly adjust to the proper recovery level and ask the performer to resume pedaling.
12. Remove the noseclip and respiratory valve from the performer.
13. Thank the performer for such cooperation and effort.
14. Calculate the maximal oxygen consumption.

Calculation of Maximal Oxygen Consumption

The equations used to calculate $\dot{V}O_2$max can look rather intimidating. Some of this might be lessened by first trying to grasp the concepts surrounding the calculation.

Concepts

Several concepts can help us to understand the calculation of maximal oxygen consumption. One concept (Eq. 1) presents oxygen consumption as the product of **true oxygen** (true O_2) and ventilation (V_I or V_E) as the oxygen consumption ($\dot{V}O_2$). The true O_2 represents the oxygen percentage extracted from the ventilation, or stated differently, the amount of oxygen (ml) consumed for every 100 ml of air inspired or expired; it also reflects the respiratory exchange ratio (R) (i.e., the ratio of carbon dioxide produced to oxygen consumed). Ventilation is the volume of air expired (V_E) or inspired (V_I) during each minute (L · min^{-1}) of the test.

$$\dot{V}O_2 \ (L{\cdot}min^{-1}) = true \ O_2\% \times V_E \qquad \text{Eq. 1}$$

where:

$$true \ O_2 \ \% = \frac{1 - F_EO_2 - F_ECO_2}{0.7904} \times (0.2093 - 0.162)$$

The **subtraction** concept leads to the calculation of oxygen consumption by subtracting the amount of oxygen in the expired air from that in the inspired air (Eq. 2). The fraction of oxygen in inspired air (F_IO_2) and expired air (F_EO_2) is usually expressed as a percentage or a decimal (e.g., 20.93% or 0.2093), rather than a fraction (20.93/100). The direct application of this concept requires the measurement of both the inspired and expired volumes, but eliminates the need to measure carbon dioxide.

$$\dot{V}O_2 \ (L{\cdot}min^{-1}) = (V_I \times F_IO_2) - (V_E \times F_EO_2) \quad \text{Eq. 2}$$

The **carbon dioxide** concept is a more complex concept than those that led to Equations 1 and 2. As with the true O_2 concept, it considers the fraction of carbon dioxide in the expired air (F_ECO_2) as a result of its metabolic production. This may be presented in Equation 3 as[68]

$$\dot{V}O_2 \left(L \cdot min^{-1}\right) = V_I \times \left[\frac{\left[0.2093 \times \left(1 - F_ECO_2\right) - F_EO_2\right]}{1 - F_EO_2 - F_ECO_2} \right]$$

$$\text{Eq. 3}$$

Application of the Calculation Concepts

In order to make the necessary calculations, of course, the values of the components in each equation must be known. Two components required for all of the conceptual equations are ventilatory volume and fractional concentration of oxygen. Two of the equations require the value for the fractional concentration of carbon dioxide in the expired air.

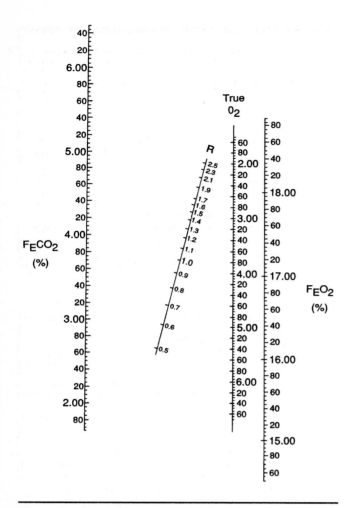

Figure 5 Nomogram for determination of R and true O_2 from the fractional concentrations of expired oxygen (F_EO_2) and carbon dioxide (F_ECO_2). Both the true O_2 and R may be found simultaneously by placing a straightedge at the F_ECO_2 and F_EO_2 points of the outside vertical lines, and then reading the R and true O_2 values on the inside lines.
From figure 1 on p. 134 of Dill, D. B., & Folling, A. (1928). Studies in muscular activity. II. A nomographic description as published in *Journal of Physiology, 66* and in Consolazio et al., 1963, p. 10. Copyright © 1963 The Physiological Society, Oxford.

Calculation of the Ventilatory Volume (V_E or V_I)

A nomogram (Fig. 5) facilitates the calculation of oxygen consumption via the true O_2 concept. However, after inserting the nomogram's true O_2 value into Equation 1, the second part of the equation—ventilatory volume—must be corrected for the effects of temperature (T), barometric pressure (torr), saturation (S), and dryness (D). By convention, it is universally accepted that all ventilatory volumes used to express a *metabolic* amount (such as oxygen consumption) should be presented in *standard* terms.[21] The term *standard* (*S*) is used to refer to a dry (D) gas (e.g., oxygen) that is of a universally designated temperature (0 °C; 273 °K) and pressure (760 torr; sea level). The volume of air the technician observes at the air meter is ex-

pressed in terms of ambient (A) or environmental conditions. Thus the ambient air volume (ATPS) is the volume of air under its measured conditions. The specific letters in the abbreviation *ATPS* represent the following:

A = ambient (environmental; laboratory; air meter)
T = temperature of the expired or inspired air (°C); it is based on the thermometer reading at a specific site within the airflow circuit near or at the air meter.
P = barometric pressure (P_B; torr) in the laboratory
S = saturation; wet expiratory air; air in a wet spirometer is always 100% saturated; the vapor pressure (P-H_2O; torr) of inspiratory air is dependent upon relative humidity (RH) and temperature.

When the air is saturated, which is always the case with expired air from living organisms, it has a greater volume than when it is dry. Because scientific convention requires that all metabolic volumes be expressed in standard (thus, dry and freezing—0 °C) conditions, the volume must be converted to the smaller STPD volume. This universal volume then can be compared with other STPD volumes derived from tests under different meteorological conditions.

Correction Factors (CF). The ATPS volume may be converted to STPD by finding the correction factor (cf) in Table 5[16,47,56] or by calculating STPDcf by multiplying the correction factors for standard (S) air temperature (STcf) and air pressure dry (SPDcf) as in Equation 4.

$$STPDcf = STcf \times SPDcf \qquad \text{Eq. 4}$$

When the appropriate constant values for temperature (273 °K) and barometric pressure (760 torr) are inserted into Equation 4 along with the measured values, the former equation now appears as Equation 5:

$$STPDcf = \frac{273\ °K}{273\ °K + T_A} \times \frac{P_B - P\text{-}H_2O}{760} \qquad \text{Eq. 5}$$

The kelvin scale is used for the **temperature** correction because of its absolute zero property, that is, no minus values. The STPD correction factor will never be a number greater than 1.0 because both the temperature and pressure parts of Equation 4 produce a fraction which, in turn, results in a ratio (correction factor) less than 1.0. Thus the standard volume will always be less than the ambient volume under normal laboratory conditions. For example, under normal laboratory conditions, the temperature and humidity (P-H_2O) will be greater than 0 °C and 0 torr (dry), respectively. When the STPDcf is known, the standard air volume can be found by multiplying the ATPS volume by the STPD correction factor according to Equation 6.

$$V_E \text{ or } V_I \text{ (STPD)} = STPDcf \times V_E \text{ or } V_I \text{ (ATPS)} \quad \text{Eq. 6}$$

where: V_E or V_I (ATPS) = the measured volume of air (L·min^{-1})

Air becomes saturated and warmed (or cooled if the ambient air temperature is >37 °C) by being exposed to the

Table 5 Correction Factors for Reducing ATPS Expiratory Volume (100% Saturated) to STPD Volume

P_B (torr)	Temperature (°C)										
	16	17	18	19	20	21	22	23	24	25	26
740	0.900	.896	.892	.887	.883	.878	.874	.869	.864	.860	.855
742	.903	.898	.894	.890	.885	.881	.876	.871	.867	.862	.857
744	.906	.901	.897	.892	.888	.883	.878	.874	.869	.864	.859
746	.908	.903	.899	.895	.890	.886	.881	.876	.872	.867	.862
748	.910	.906	.901	.897	.892	.888	.883	.879	.874	.869	.864
750	.913	.908	.904	.900	.895	.890	.886	.881	.876	.872	.867
752	.915	.911	.906	.902	.897	.893	.888	.883	.879	.874	.869
754	.918	.913	.909	.904	.900	.895	.891	.886	.881	.876	.872
756	.920	.916	.911	.907	.902	.898	.893	.888	.883	.879	.874
758	.923	.918	.914	.909	.905	.900	.896	.891	.886	.881	.876
760	.925	.921	.916	.912	.907	.902	.898	.893	.888	.883	.879
762	.928	.923	.919	.914	.910	.905	.900	.896	.891	.886	.881
764	.930	.926	.921	.916	.912	.907	.903	.898	.893	.889	.884

lungs. The air in the lungs is about 37 °C and 100% saturated. This corresponds to a **water vapor pressure** of 47 torr (P-H$_2$O). As the air is expelled into the gas meter under normal laboratory conditions, however, the air is condensed and cooled from a typical mouth temperature of about 33 °C to approximately 31 °C and 28 °C at the respiratory valve and unheated pneumotach or air meter, respectively.[41] This lower temperature decreases the amount of water vapor pressure in the expired air. The farther the thermometer is from the subject's mouth, the lower the exhaled air temperature, and consequently the P-H$_2$O, under normal laboratory conditions. Table 6 provides estimates of P-H$_2$O at various ambient temperatures; as the temperature increases at 100% RH, the P-H$_2$O increases.

Inspired volumes usually are not 100% saturated and thus do not exert water vapor pressures quite as high as those presented in Table 6.[17,53,69,70] By measuring the relative humidity (RH) with a hygrometer or sling psychrometer, the pressure of water vapor (P-H$_2$O) for any given temperature may be found by using Equation 7 in conjunction with Table 6.

$$\text{P-H}_2\text{O (torr)} = \text{RH\%} \times \text{P-H}_2\text{O value at 100\% RH} \qquad \text{Eq. 7}$$

For example, Table 6 shows that an ambient temperature of 25 °C is equivalent to a water vapor pressure of 24 torr. Because this table value represents 100% saturation (RH), it must be corrected to the observed ambient relative humidity (e.g., 60% RH) by using Equation 7. Thus, the water vapor pressure becomes 0.60×24 torr $= 14.4$ torr.

Minute (min) Volumes. If the performer stops exercising before 30 s of air has been measured during the last starting minute of exercise, then only the preceding minute's volume should be used to calculate $\dot{V}O_2$max. If the performer stops between 30 and 60 s, then the appropriate arithmetical adjustment should be made to account for a minute's worth of ventilation (e.g., double the volume based on 30-s value).

Table 6 Water Vapor Pressure (P-H$_2$O) at 100% Saturation at Given Temperatures (T)

°C	T °K	P-H$_2$O torr	°C	T °K	P-H$_2$O torr
20	293	18	31	304	34
21	294	19	32	305	36
22	295	20	33	306	38
23	296	21	34	307	40
24	297	22	35	308	42
25	298	24	36	309	45
26	299	25	37	310	47
27	300	27	38	311	50
28	301	28	39	312	52
29	302	30	40	313	55
30	303	32			

Fractions of Inspired and Expired Gases

One must know the fractional concentration of three gases in order to calculate oxygen consumption. The major gases are oxygen, carbon dioxide, and nitrogen (Table 7). All other gases (e.g., helium and argon) are either inert or insignificant for calculating oxygen consumption. An inert gas does not enter into biological metabolism. One of the three major components of the environmental air, nitrogen, is an inert gas.

The fractional concentrations of the expired gases (F_EO_2 or F_ECO_2) are expressed as percentages or decimals. Expired nitrogen concentration (dry) may be calculated from Equation 8.[26]

$$F_EN_2 = 1.0 - F_EO_2 - F_ECO_2 \qquad \text{Eq. 8}$$

Expired concentrations of oxygen and carbon dioxide are dependent upon the intensity of exercise. Expected fractional concentrations of expired gases in exercising persons usually will range according to those listed in Table 7. For

Table 7 Fractions (%) of Inspired (F_I) and Expired (F_E) Gases

Gas	Fractional Concentrations	
	Inspired	Expired at Exercise
Oxygen (O_2)	20.93	14.5–18.5
Carbon Dioxide (CO_2)	0.03–0.04	2.5–5.5
Nitrogen (N_2)	79.03–79.04	78.5–82.5

example, if the F_EO_2 is 16% (0.16) and the F_ECO_2 is 5.0% (0.05), then by substitution, Equation 8 becomes:

$$F_EN_2 = 1.0 - 0.16 - 0.05 = 0.79$$

The exact amount of oxygen extracted from the volume of air (V_E or V_I) cannot be calculated directly by multiplying this minute volume (L·min^{-1}) by the fractional concentration of oxygen unless the respiratory exchange ratio is equal to 1.0. This is because the volume of oxygen consumed is dependent not only upon the fractional concentration of the expired oxygen but also upon the fractional concentration of expired carbon dioxide. Consequently, when F_ECO_2 is included in the calculation of oxygen consumption the term used to represent the true amount of oxygen extracted is called the true O_2. This can be calculated from Equation 1 or from the nomogram in Figure 5.

Respiratory Exchange Ratio

True O_2 is dependent upon the ratio of carbon dioxide produced to oxygen consumed. This ratio is called the respiratory exchange ratio (R), although it has sometimes been referred to as the respiratory quotient (RQ). However, *R* should be reserved for respiratory purposes while *RQ* should be used for nutritional or dietary considerations. As exercise intensifies, the R value increases due to the release of greater quantities of carbon dioxide from the buffering of lactic acid. The R may change from typical resting values between 0.85 to typical maximal exercise values between 1.0 and 1.25; values at supramaximal exercise may reach as high as 1.3 and during recovery, lower than 0.7.[38] As mentioned previously, the R is often used as a criterion to indicate the achievement of true maximal oxygen consumption. When the R is 1.0 it means that the production of carbon dioxide ($\dot{V}CO_2$) is equivalent to the consumption of oxygen ($\dot{V}O_2$). The respiratory exchange ratio is calculated either from a nomogram using the F_EO_2 and F_ECO_2 values, or from the STPD volumes of carbon dioxide and oxygen (Eq. 9).

$$R = \dot{V}CO_2/\dot{V}O_2 \qquad \text{Eq. 9}$$

For example, if the volume of carbon dioxide produced is 3.5 L·min^{-1} and the consumption of oxygen is 3.5 L·min^{-1}, then the respiratory exchange ratio is calculated as follows:

$$R = 3.5/3.5 = 3.5 \div 3.5 = 1.0$$

Although the *percent* of carbon dioxide is necessary to calculate oxygen consumption, it is not necessary to know the *volume* of carbon dioxide. Its volume may be calculated easily from Equation 10.

$$\dot{V}CO_2 \text{ (L·min}^{-1})STPD = \dot{V}_E \times (F_ECO_2 - F_ICO_2) \qquad \text{Eq. 10}$$

For example, if expired ventilation STPD is 100 L·min^{-1} and F_ECO_2 is 5.0% and F_ICO_2 is .03%, then

$$\dot{V}CO_2 = 100 \times (5.0 - 0.03) = 100 \times 4.97\% = 4.97 \text{ L·min}^{-1}$$

After calculating the volume of carbon dioxide produced by using Equation 10, the respiratory exchange ratio may be calculated from Equation 11 as soon as the volume of oxygen consumed is known, or simply from the nomogram (Figure 5) when the F_ECO_2 and F_EO_2 are known.

For example, if the $\dot{V}CO_2$ is 4.97 and the $\dot{V}O_2$ is 4.93, then solving for Equation 9 is as follows:

$$R = \dot{V}CO_2/\dot{V}O_2 = 4.97 \div 4.93 = 1.01$$

Interaction of Ventilatory Volume and Gas Concentrations

The volume of inspired and expired air differs at rest and throughout most stages of exercise intensity. Because maximal oxygen consumption can be measured using either the inspired and expired volumes alone or together, all three methods are explained here. The inspired or expired[26,72] air volumes may be calculated from the known value of the other by using Haldane Equations 11 and 12, respectively.

$$\dot{V}_I = \dot{V}_E \times (F_EN_2 \div F_IN_2) \qquad \text{Eq. 11}$$
$$= \dot{V}_E \times [(1.0 - F_EO_2 - F_ECO_2) \div 0.7904]$$

where: $F_IN_2 = 79.04\%$

$$\dot{V}_E = \dot{V}_I \times (F_IN_2/F_EN_2) \qquad \text{Eq. 12}$$
$$= \dot{V}_I \times (0.79/F_EN_2)$$

Expired Air Volume. The concentrations of the inspired gases are essentially constant. Thus, when using expired ventilation to calculate oxygen consumption, Equation 13 may be used.

$$\dot{V}O_2 = \dot{V}_E \times \left[\left(F_EN_2 / F_IN_2 \right) \times \left(F_IO_2 - F_EO_2 \right) \right]$$
$$= \dot{V}_E \times \left[\frac{(1.0 - F_EO_2 - F_ECO_2)}{0.79)} \times (0.209 - F_EO_2) \right]$$
$$\text{Eq. 13}$$

Both Expired and Inspired Air Volumes. If both the volume of inspired and expired air are measured, then carbon dioxide need not be measured and the Haldane transformation equations are not necessary;[67] thus oxygen consumption is calculated according to the conceptual Equation 2[45] presented earlier as

$$\dot{V}O_2 = (\dot{V}_I \times F_IO_2) - (\dot{V}_E \times F_EO_2)$$

where $F_IO_2 = 20.93\%$ (0.2093)

Inspired Air Volume. If only the inspired volume is measured, oxygen consumption can be calculated from Equation 14[45] or simply by converting the V_I to V_E by the Haldane Equation (Eq. 12) and then using the nomogram to find true O_2% or using Equation 13.

$$\dot{V}O_2 = \dot{V}_I \times \{F_IO_2 - [(F_IN_2 / F_EN_2) \times F_IO_2]\} \quad \text{Eq. 14}$$

Calculating Relative Maximal Oxygen Consumption

When other factors are equal, larger persons (especially those with larger muscle mass) will have higher maximal oxygen consumptions. It is often appropriate to convert the absolute value of liters per minute to milliliters per minute (Eq. 15); this is then divided by body weight in order to derive the *relative* value, which is expressed in units of $ml \cdot kg^{-1} \cdot min^{-1}$ (Eq. 16). Sometimes the absolute value is divided by the fat-free mass if the latter is known.

$$\dot{V}O_2max \ (ml \cdot min^{-1}) = 1000 \times L \cdot min^{-1} \quad \text{Eq. 15}$$

$$\text{relative } \dot{V}O_2max \ (ml \cdot kg^{-1} \cdot min^{-1}) = (ml \cdot min^{-1}) \div kg \ wt \quad \text{Eq. 16}$$

For example, if a person weighing 65 kg is found to have a maximal oxygen consumption of 4.0 liters per minute, then the following calculations would be made in order to find the relative maximal oxygen consumption:

$$ml \cdot min^{-1} = 1000 \times 4.0 \ L \cdot min^{-1} = 4000$$
$$ml \cdot kg^{-1} \cdot min^{-1} = 4000 \ ml \cdot kg^{-1} \cdot min^{-1} \div 65 \ kg = 61.5$$

Calculating MET Values

MET is the term used to denote the multiple of the resting oxygen consumption. The maximal MET value is calculated from Equation 17 by simply dividing the relative maximal oxygen consumption by the assumed resting value of $3.5 \ ml \cdot kg^{-1} \cdot min^{-1}$.[3]

$$\text{MET} = \text{relative } \dot{V}O_2 \div 3.5 \quad \text{Eq. 17}$$

Thus, using the previous example, the calculation appears as

$$\text{MET} = 61.5 \ ml \cdot kg^{-1} \cdot min^{-1} \div 3.5 = 17.6$$

Ventilatory Threshold/Breakpoint ("Anaerobic Threshold")

The ventilatory breakpoint occurs at the lowest point of a line, just before it rises, on a graph describing the relationship between ventilation and oxygen consumption (V_E vs. $\dot{V}O_2$). It is sometimes referred to as the "anaerobic threshold,"[69] but not without controversy. Although computer programs can select the ventilatory breakpoint by plotting the change in linearity between $\dot{V}O_2$ and V_E, it can be estimated by plotting the points on a graph and noting the point where the line changes slope.

Summary of the Calculation of Maximal Oxygen Consumption

Although the numerous equations presented appear to be quite formidable, the tables and nomogram simplify the calculation of oxygen consumption. The summarized steps and examples for calculating $\dot{V}O_2max$ with and without the nomogram and using inspired or expired ventilatory volumes are presented.

Nomogram Method If Expired Air Volume

1. Convert the volume of air (V_E) from ATPS to STPD by consulting Table 5 or completing Equations 5 and 6.
2. Determine the R and true O_2 values by placing a straight edge on the two vertical lines denoting fractions of expired gases and reading the answers on the diagonal R line and vertical true O_2 line of the nomogram (Fig. 5).
3. Insert the values found in Steps #1 (V_E STPD) and #2 (true O_2) into Equation 1.
   For example, if V_E is 100 $L \cdot min^{-1}$ and true O_2 is 4.0%, then

$$\dot{V}O_2 = V_E \ STPD \times true \ O_2$$
$$= 100 \ L \cdot min^{-1} \ (STPD) \times 4.0\% \ (or \ 0.04)$$
$$= 4.0 \ L \cdot min^{-1}$$

4. Convert $L \cdot min^{-1}$ to $ml \cdot min^{-1}$ by using Equation 15.
5. Convert $ml \cdot min^{-1}$ to relative $\dot{V}O_2max$ ($ml \cdot kg^{-1} \cdot min^{-1}$) by using Equation 16.
6. Calculate MET value by using Equation 17.

Example of Nomogram Method If Expired Air Volume

> **Given Conditions:**
> Performer's weight: 70 kg
> $\dot{V}_E$ ATPS = 100 $L \cdot min^{-1}$
> Saturation = 100%
> T = 25.0 °C
> P_B = 751 torr
> F_EO_2 = 16.2%; F_ECO_2 = 5.0%

1. Convert the volume of expired air from ATPS to STPD:

$$\dot{V}_E \ STPD = 100 \ L \cdot min^{-1} \ ATPS \times STPDcf$$
$$= 100 \times [273/(273 + 25)] \times [(751 - 24)/760]$$
$$= 100 \times (273/298) \times (727/760)$$
$$= 100 \times (0.916 \times 0.956)$$
$$= 100 \times 0.876^a \ (slightly >0.873 \ from \ Table \ 5)$$
$$= 87.6 \ L \cdot min^{-1} \ STPD$$

---

[a]Agrees with table in Wasserman et al., 1994, p. 469.

2. The R and true O_2 values from the nomogram (Fig. 5) are

R = 1.08 (but not needed for the $\dot{V}O_2$ max calculation)
True O_2 = 4.65% (0.0465)

3. The volume of oxygen consumed (STPD) found from Equation 1 is:

$$\dot{V}O_2 \text{ STPD} = 87.6 \text{ L·min}^{-1} \times 0.0465$$
$$= 4.073 \text{ L·min}^{-1}$$

4. The value of 4.073 L·min⁻¹ converted to ml·min⁻¹ is

$$4.073 \text{ L·min}^{-1} \times 1000 = 4073 \text{ ml·min}^{-1}$$

5. The relative value is

$$4073 \div 70 \text{ kg} = 58.2 \text{ ml·kg}^{-1}\text{·min}^{-1}$$

6. The MET value is

$$58.2 \div 3.5 \text{ ml·kg}^{-1}\text{·min}^{-1} = 16.6$$

Nomogram Method If Inspired Air Volume

1. Convert the volume of inspired air from ATPS to STPD by using Table 6 (P-H_2O vs T) and Equation 7 (RH%), along with Equations 5 (V_I) and 6 (STPD).
2. Convert the STPD inspired volume to an expired volume by using Equation 12 (Haldane).
3. Then follow the same steps #2 through #5 as used for expired air.

Example of Nomogram Method If Inspired Air Volume

Given Conditions:
Performer's weight: 70 kg
$\dot{V}_I$ ATPS = 100 L·min⁻¹
Saturation (RH) = 40%
T = 25.0 °C
P_B = 751 torr
F_EO_2 = 16.5%; F_ECO_2 = 4.5%

1. The volume of inspired air is converted from ATPS to STPD:

$$\dot{V}_I \text{ STPD} = 100 \text{ L·min}^{-1} \times \text{STPDcf}$$

a. Find P-H_2O at 100% RH (Table 6) and convert to 40% RH:

P-H_2O (torr at 40% RH) = 40% RH x 24 (Table 6 value)
= 9.6 torr or rounded-off to 10 torr

b. Now the torr and temperature are inserted into Equation 5:

$$\dot{V}_I \text{ STPDcf} = \frac{273 \text{ °K}}{273 \text{ °K} + 25 \text{ °C}} \times \frac{751 - 10}{760}$$

$$= (273 / 298) \times (741 / 760)$$
$$= 0.916 \times 0.975$$
$$= 0.893$$

c. Thus,

$$V_I \text{ STPD} = 100 \text{ L·min}^{-1} \times 0.893$$
$$= 89.3 \text{ L·min}^{-1}$$

2. Convert the V_I STPD value to V_E STPD by using Haldane Equation 12

$$V_E \text{ STPD} = 89.3 \times [0.79 \div (1.0 - 0.165 - 0.045)]$$
$$= 89.3 \times (0.79 \div 0.79)$$
$$= 89.3 \times 1.0$$
$$= 89.3 \text{ L·min}^{-1}$$

3. Now follow same steps #2 through #6 as for expired volume.
4. The R and true O_2 values from the nomogram (Fig. 5):

R = 1.0 (but not needed for the $\dot{V}O_2$max calculation)
True O_2 = 4.50% (when R = 1.0, the F_EO_2% = true O_2%, and $\dot{V}_I = \dot{V}_E$)

5. The volume of oxygen consumed (STPD) found from Equation 1 is:

$$\dot{V}O_2 \text{ STPD} = 89.3 \text{ L·min}^{-1} \times 0.045$$
$$= 4.019 \text{ L·min}^{-1}$$

6. The value of 4.019 L·min⁻¹ converted to ml·min⁻¹ is

$$4.019 \text{ L·min}^{-1} \times 1000 = 4019 \text{ ml·min}^{-1}$$

7. The relative value is

$$4019 \div 70 \text{ kg} = 57.4 \text{ ml·kg}^{-1}\text{·min}^{-1}$$

8. The MET value is

$$57.4 \div 3.5 \text{ ml·kg}^{-1}\text{·min}^{-1} = 16.4$$

Non-Nomogram Method If Expired Air Volume

1. Same as step #1 for nomogram method using expired air: Correct the volume of expired air to STPD from Table 5 or Equations 5 and 6 with Table 6.
2. Find oxygen consumption (L·min⁻¹) using Equation 13.
3. Follow same steps #4 through #6 as nomogram method if expired air:

Convert the L·min⁻¹ value to ml·min⁻¹ by multiplying the L·min⁻¹ by 1000 (Equation 15).

4. Find the relative $\dot{V}O_2$max by dividing the ml·min⁻¹ value by the body weight (kg) of the performer.
5. Find the MET value by dividing ml·kg⁻¹·min⁻¹ by 3.5.

Example of Non-Nomogram Method If Expired Air Volume

> **Given Conditions:**
> Same as for nomogram method for expired air volume:
> 70 kg; 100 L·min⁻¹; 25 °C; 100% saturation; 751 torr;
> $F_EO_2 = 16.2\%$; $F_ECO_2 = 5.0\%$

1. Same as step #1 for nomogram method if expired air: The volume of expired air is converted from ATPS to STPD:

$$\dot{V}_E \, STPD = 100 \, L·min^{-1} \, ATPS \times STPDcf$$
$$= 100 \, L·min^{-1} \, ATPS \times 0.876 \, (or \, 0.873)$$
$$= 87.6 \, L·min^{-1}$$

2. Find $\dot{V}O_2max$ by inserting the appropriate conditions into Eq. 13:

$$\dot{V}O_2 = 87.6 \times \frac{1 - 0.162 - 0.05}{0.79} \times (0.2093 - 0.162)$$

$$= 87.6 \times [(0.788/0.790) \times (0.0473)]$$
$$= 87.6 \times (0.997 \times 0.0473)$$
$$= 87.6 \times 0.0472$$
$$= 4.134 \, L·min^{-1} \, (slight \, difference \, from \, nomogram$$
method due to imprecise reading of nomogram and rounding-off)

3. The value of 4.134 L·min⁻¹ converted to ml·kg⁻¹·min⁻¹ is

$$4.134 \, L·min^{-1} \times 1000 = 4134 \, ml·min^{-1}$$

4. The relative value is

$$4134 \div 70 \, kg = 59.1 \, ml·kg^{-1}·min^{-1}$$

5. The MET value is

$$59.1 \, ml·kg^{-1}·min^{-1} \div 3.5 = 16.9$$

Non-Nomogram Method If Inspired Volume

1. Same as nomogram method for inspired air: Convert the volume of inspired air from ATPS to STPD by using Table 6 (P-H₂O vs T) and Equation 7 (RH%), along with Equations 5 (V_I) and 6 (STPD).
2. Insert the inspired STPD volume into Equation 3.
3. Follow same last three steps as for the other methods:
   a. Convert L·min⁻¹ to ml·min⁻¹ by multiplying L·min⁻¹ by 1000.
   b. Find the relative $\dot{V}O_2max$ by dividing ml·min⁻¹ by body weight.
   c. Find Met value by dividing ml·kg⁻¹·min⁻¹ by 3.5.

Example of Non-Nomogram Method If Inspired Air Volume

> **Given Conditions:**
> Same as for nomogram inspired air volume: 70 kg; V_IATPS =
> 100 L·min⁻¹; RH = 40%; T = 25.0 °C; P_B = 751 torr; F_EO_2 =
> 16.5%; F_ECO_2 = 4.5%

1. See step #1 for nomogram method using inspired air to convert 100 L·min⁻¹ ATPS to 89.3 STPD.
2. Insert appropriate values into Equation 3:

$$\dot{V}O_2 \left(L·min^{-1}\right) = 89.3 \times \left[\frac{[0.2093 \times (1 - 0.045) - 0.165]}{1 - 0.165 - 0.045} \right]$$

$$= 89.3 \times \{[(0.2093 \times 0.955) - 0.165] / 0.79\}$$
$$= 89.3 \times [(0.1999 - 0.165)/0.79]$$
$$= 89.3 \times 0.0349/0.79$$
$$= 89.3 \times 0.044$$
$$= 3.929 \, L·min^{-1} \, (slight \, difference \, from \, nomogram$$
method)

or (a) change V_I to V_E and (b) solve for $\dot{V}O_2$ with V_E

(a) $$V_E = 89.3 \, L·min^{-1} \times \frac{0.79}{1 - 0.165 - 0.045}$$

$$= 89.3 \, L·min^{-1} \times (0.79/0.79)$$
$$= 89.3 \, L·min^{-1} \, (when \, R = 1.0, \, then \, V_I = V_E)$$

(b) Follow step #2 of *expired* non-nomogram method:

$$\dot{V}O_2 = 89.3 \times \left[\left(\frac{1 - 0.165 - 0.045}{0.790} \right) \times (0.2093 - 0.165) \right]$$

$$= 89.3 \times [(0.79/0.790) \times (0.2093 - 0.165)]$$
$$= 89.3 \times (1.0 \times 0.0443)$$
$$= 89.3 \times 0.0443$$
$$= 3.956 \, L·min^{-1} \, (slight \, difference \, due \, to \, rounding$$
off)

3. Convert L·min⁻¹ by

$$1000 \times 3.956 = 3956 \, ml·min^{-1}$$

4. Find relative $\dot{V}O_2max$ by

$$\dot{V}O_2max \, (ml·kg^{-1}·min^{-1}) = 3956 \div 70 \, kg = 56.5$$

5. Find the MET value by

$$MET = 56.5 \, ml·kg^{-1}·min^{-1} \div 3.5 = 16.1$$

Results and Discussion

Earlier investigators and reviewers[48,59,65] supported the maximal oxygen consumption value as probably the best single physiological indicator of a person's capacity for

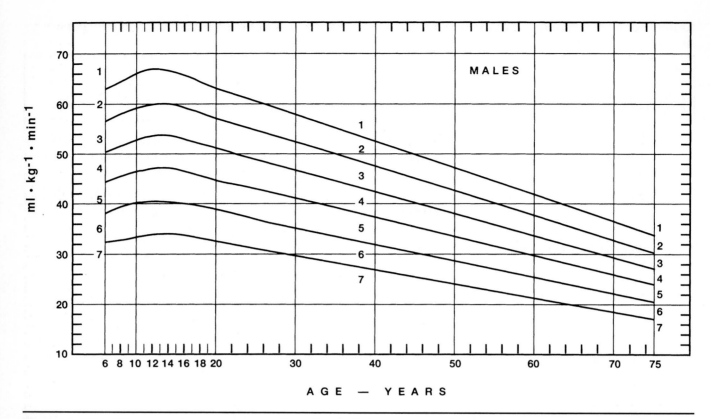

Figure 6 The relative maximal oxygen consumption (ml·kg⁻¹·min⁻¹) in **males** aged 6–75 y. 1 = excellent; 2 = very good; 3 = good; 4 = average; 5 = fair; 6 = poor; 7 = very poor.
From E. Shvartz and R. C. Reibold, "Aerobic Fitness Norms for Males and Females. . . ," in *Aviation Space, and Environmental Medicine,* 61, 3–11, 1990. Copyright © Aerospace Medical Association, Alexandria, VA.

maintaining endurance-type activity. This contrasts with one authority who questions the interpretation of maximal oxygen consumption[24] and with those who caution that other factors such as running economy[25] and the ability to use a high percent of the maximal oxygen consumption (fractional utilization)[23] and ventilatory threshold[68] also are important indicators of success in aerobic performance. For example, two investigators[44] found a higher correlation ($r = -0.86$) between fractional utilization and 1.5-mile time than between $\dot{V}O_2max$ and 1.5-mile time ($r = -0.74$). In fact, $\dot{V}O_2max$ has been shown to be an ineffective discriminator of aerobic endurance time among persons with fairly similar maximal oxygen consumptions.[23]

In general, maximal oxygen consumption is higher in men than in women, in younger adults than in older adults, and in aerobically conditioned persons than in untrained persons.

$\dot{V}O_2Max$ Values on Treadmill Versus Cycling and Stepping

Typically, treadmill protocols elicit maximal oxygen consumption values that are from 5%–8%,[27] or up to 10%[35] higher than cycle protocols. Due to the "law of the specificity of training," however, trained cyclists may achieve similar values on treadmill and bicycle protocols. Maximal oxygen consumption values during certain step-test protocols appear to compare favorably ($r = .95$) with those during treadmill protocols.[39]

Norms for $\dot{V}O_2Max$

Cycling Norms

Some popular norm tables were derived mainly by performers using cycle ergometers.[4,6,11] Therefore, in order to make valid comparisons, the values from treadmill testing should be adjusted downward by 5%–10%.

Generic Norms

Adjustments for treadmill testing are not necessary if using the norms (Figs. 6–9) compiled from 62 studies of apparently healthy but untrained men and women aged six to seventy-five years from the United States, Canada, and seven European countries.[63] These norms are based on directly measured maximal oxygen consumption tests from treadmill, cycle, and stepping ergometry.

In summary of these norms, the **absolute $\dot{V}O_2max$ (L·min⁻¹)** increases in male youths from about 1.0 L·min⁻¹ at age six to over 3.0 at age eighteen. The males then decline to about 1.5 L·min⁻¹ by age seventy-five. The females

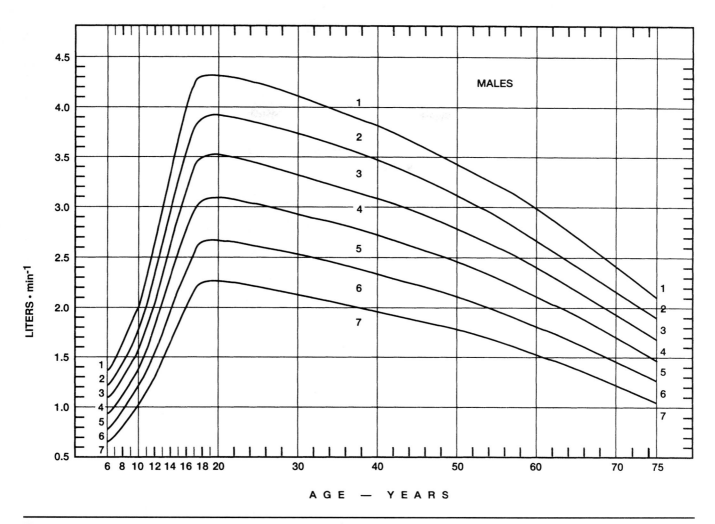

Figure 7 The absolute maximal oxygen consumption (l·min⁻¹) in **males** aged 6–75 y. 1 = excellent; 2 = very good; 3 = good; 4 = average; 5 = fair; 6 = poor; 7 = very poor.
From E. Shvartz and R. C. Reibold, "Aerobic Fitness Norms for Males and Females. . . ," in *Aviation Space, and Environmental Medicine,* 61, 3–11, 1990. Copyright © Aerospace Medical Association, Alexandria, VA.

follow a similar trend by increasing initially from about 0.8 L·min⁻¹ at age six to about 2.2 at age eighteen, then by decreasing to about 1.0 L·min⁻¹ by age seventy-five.

Relative $\dot{V}O_2$max shows smaller differences between the sexes and not nearly as great an increase during youth than that of absolute maximal oxygen consumption. The relative $\dot{V}O_2$max decreases in males from about 50 ml·kg⁻¹·min⁻¹ during late adolescence to about 25 in seventy-five year-old persons; females decrease from about 40 ml·kg⁻¹·min⁻¹ in early adolescence to about 17 "ml's" at age seventy-five.

The seven **fitness categories** depicted in Figures 6–9 represent the following percentages of the population based on the means and standard deviations:

Very poor and Excellent = 3% each
Poor and Very Good = 8% each

Fair and Good = 22% each
Average = 34%

For example, Figure 6 shows that an excellent rating is warranted for all adult males age twenty-six if their relative maximal oxygen consumption is 60 ml·kg⁻¹. Figure 8 shows that women at age twenty-six obtain an excellent rating if reaching 50 ml·kg⁻¹.

Comparison of Predicted and Direct $\dot{V}O_2Max$. The results of the Maximal Oxygen Consumption Test can be compared to those from previous predictive tests (Form OC 6). It would be interesting to see which predictive test came the closest to predicting the actual $\dot{V}O_2$max value for those students who performed the direct test. Conclusions would be tentative if only a few students performed the direct test.

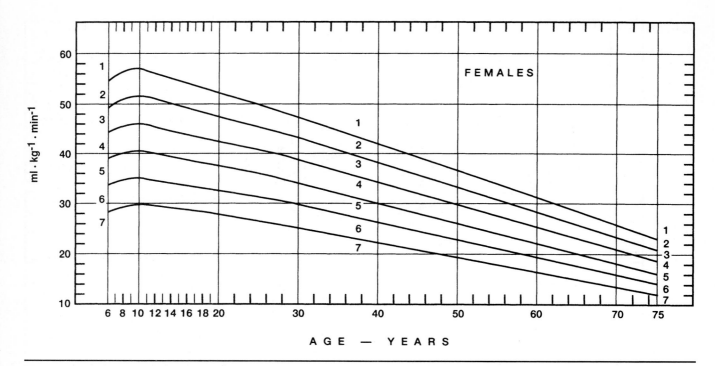

AGE — YEARS

Figure 8 The relative maximal oxygen consumption (ml·kg^{-1}·min^{-1}) in **females** aged 6–75 y. 1 = excellent; 2 = very good; 3 = good; 4 = average; 5 = fair; 6 = poor; 7 = very poor.
From E. Shvartz and R. C. Reibold, "Aerobic Fitness Norms for Males and Females. . . ," in *Aviation Space, and Environmental Medicine,* 61, 3–11, 1990. Copyright © Aerospace Medical Association, Alexandria, VA.

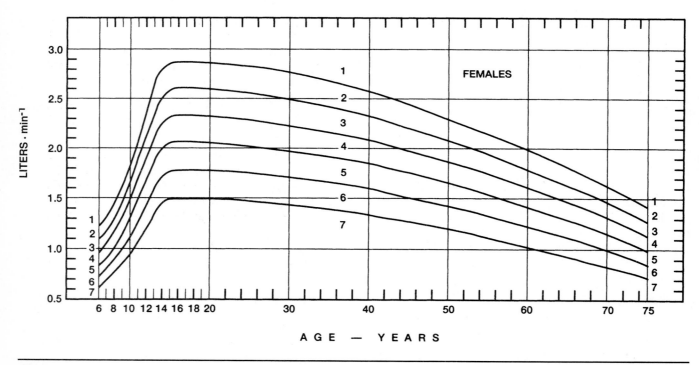

AGE — YEARS

Figure 9 The absolute maximal oxygen consumption (l·min^{-1}) in **females** aged 6–75 y. 1 = excellent; 2 = very good; 3 = good; 4 = average; 5 = fair; 6 = poor; 7 = very poor.
From E. Shvartz and R. C. Reibold, "Aerobic Fitness Norms for Males and Females. . . ," in *Aviation Space, and Environmental Medicine,* 61, 3–11, 1990. Copyright © Aerospace Medical Association, Alexandria, VA.

References

1. Alexander, J. F., Liang, M. T. C., Stull, G. A., Serfass, R. C., Wolfe, D. R., & Ewing, J. L. (1984). A comparison of the Bruce and Liang equations for predicting $\dot{V}O_2$max in young adult males. *Research Quarterly for Exercise and Sport, 55,* 383–387.

2. Allen, T. E., Hatcher, P. G., Lewis, J. B., Adams, F. S., & Brown, P. M. (1988). Standing and seated bicycle ergometry for elicitation of maximum oxygen uptake in women. *Medicine and Science in Sports and Exercise, 20* (Suppl.), Abstract #100, S17.

3. American College of Sports Medicine. (1986; 1991). *Guidelines for graded exercise testing and exercise prescription.* Philadelphia: Lea & Febiger.

4. American Heart Association Committee on Exercise. (1972). *Exercise testing and training in apparently healthy individuals: A handbook for physicians.* New York: Author.

5. Andersen, K. L., Shephard, R. J., Denolin, H., Varnauskas, E., & Masironi, R. (Eds.). (1971). *Fundamentals of exercise testing.* Geneva, Switzerland: World Health Organization.

6. Astrand, P. O., & Ryhming, I. (1954). A nomogram for calculation of aerobic capacity (physical fitness) from pulse rate during submaximal work. *Journal of Applied Physiology, 7,* 218–221.

7. Bar-Or, O., & Zwiren, L. D. (1975). Maximal oxygen consumption test during exercise—Reliability and validity. *Journal of Applied Physiology, 38,* 424–426.

8. Baumgartner, T. A., & Jackson, A. S. (1987). *Measurement for evaluation in physical education and exercise science.* Dubuque, IA: Wm. C. Brown.

9. Brooks, G. A., & Fahey, T. D. (1984). *Exercise physiology: Human bioenergetics and its application.* New York: John Wiley & Sons.

10. Brooks, G. A., & Fahey, T. D. (1987). *Fundamentals of human performance.* New York: Macmillan.

11. Bruce, R. A. (1972). Multi-stage treadmill test of submaximal and maximal exercise. In *Exercise testing and training of apparently healthy individuals: A handbook for physicians* (Ed.), American Heart Association's Committee on Exercise, 32–34. New York: American Heart Association.

12. Bruce, R. A. (1974). Methods of exercise testing. *The American Journal of Cardiology, 33,* 715–720.

13. Bruce, R. A., Kusumi, F., & Hosmer, D. (1973). Maximal oxygen intake and nomographic assessment of functional impairment in cardiovascular disease. *American Heart Journal, 85,* 546–562.

14. Bruce, R. A., & McDonough, J. R. (1969). Stress testing in screening for cardiovascular disease. *Bulletin of New York Academy of Medicine, 45,* 1288.

15. Buchfuhrer, M. J., Hansen, J. E., Robinson, T. E., Sue, D. Y., Wasserman, K., & Whipp, B. J. (1983). Optimizing the exercise protocol for cardiopulmonary assessment. *Journal of Applied Physiology, 55,* 1558–1564.

16. Carpenter, T. M. (1948). *Tables, factors, and formulas for computing respiratory exchange and biological transformations of energy.* 4th ed., Publication 303C. Washington, D.C.: Carnegie Institute of Washington.

17. Clarke, D. H. (1975). *Exercise physiology.* Englewood Cliffs, NJ: Prentice-Hall.

18. Clear, M. S., & Frisch, F. (1984). Intra-individual biological variability in maximum aerobic power of trained and untrained individuals [Abstract]. *International Journal of Sportsmedicine, 5,* 162.

19. Coast, J. R., Crouse, S. F., & Jessup, G. (1995). *Exercise physiology videolabs.* Dubuque, IA: Brown & Benchmark.

20. Coast, J. R., & Welch, H. G. (1985). Linear increase in optimal pedal rate with increased power output in ergometry. *European Journal of Applied Physiology, 53,* 339–342.

21. Consolazio, C. F., Johnson, R. E., & Pecora, L. J. (1963). *Physiological measurements of metabolic functions in man.* New York: McGraw-Hill.

22. Cooper, K. H. (1968c). Testing and developing cardiovascular fitness within the United States Air Force. *Journal of Occupational Medicine, 10,* 636–639.

23. Costill, D. L., Thomason, H., & Roberts, E. (1973). Fractional utilization of the aerobic capacity during distance running. *Medicine and Science in Sports and Exercise, 5,* 248–252.

24. Cureton, T. K. (1973). Interpretation of the oxygen intake test—What is it? *American Corrective Therapy Journal, 27,* 17–23.

25. Daniels, J. T. (1985). A physiologist's view of running economy. *Medicine and Science in Sports and Exercise, 17,* 332–338.

26. Davis, J. A., Caiozzo, V. J., Lamarra, N., Ellis, J. F., Vandagriff, R., Prietto, C. A., & McMaster, W. C. (1983). Does the gas exchange anaerobic threshold occur at a fixed blood lactate concentration of 2 or 4 mM? *International Journal of Sports Medicine, 4,* 89–93.

27. deVries, H. A. (1986). *Physiology of exercise for physical education and athletics.* Dubuque, IA: Wm. C. Brown.

28. Dill, D. B., & Folling, A. (1928). Studies in muscular activity. II. A nomographic description of expired air. *Journal of Physiology, 66,* 133.

29. Eckermann, P., & Millahn, H. P. (1967). Der einfluss der drehzahl auf die herzfrequenz und die sauerstoffaufnahme bei konstanter leistung am fahrradergometer. *Int. Z. Angew. Physiol. Arbeitsphysiol, 23,* 340–344.

30. Falls, H. B., & Humphrey, D. H. (1973). A comparison of methods for eliciting maximum oxygen uptake from

college women during treadmill walking. *Medicine and Science in Sports, 5,* 239–241.

31. Getchell, L. H., Kirkendall, D., & Robbins, G. (1977). Prediction of maximal oxygen uptake in young adult women joggers. *Research Quarterly, 48,* 61–67.

32. Goffredo, M. A., Rich, G. Y., & Holland, G. J. (1983). The influence of treadmill, sitting, and standing bicycle ergometry upon maximal oxygen uptake and anaerobic threshold [Abstract]. *International Journal of Sports Medicine, 4,* 136.

33. Grantham, W. C., & Howley, E. T. (1993). Facility design, equipment selection, and calibration. In American College of Sports Medicine (Eds.), *ACSM's resource manual for guidelines for exercise testing and prescription* (pp. 539–550). Philadelphia: Lea & Febiger.

34. Hagberg, J. M., Mullin, J. P., Giese, M. D., & Spitznagel, E. (1981). Effect of pedaling rate on submaximal exercise responses of competitive cyclists. *Journal of Applied Physiology, 51,* 447–451.

35. Hermansen, L., & Saltin, B. (1969). Oxygen uptake during maximal treadmill and bicycle exercise. *Journal of Applied Physiology, 26,* 31–37.

36. Holly, R. G. (1988). Measurement of the maximal rate of oxygen uptake. In *Resource manual for guidelines for exercise testing and prescription* (Ed.), ACSM. Philadelphia: Lea & Febiger.

37. Howley, E. T., Bassett, D. R., & Welch, H. G. (1995). Criteria for maximal oxygen uptake: Review and commentary. *Medicine and Science in Sports and Exercise, 27,* 1292–1301.

38. Issekutz, B., & Rodahl, K. (1961). Respiratory quotient during exercise. *Journal of Applied Physiology, 16,* 606–610.

39. Kasch, F. W., Phillips, W. H., Ross, W. D., Carter, J. E. L., & Boyer, J. L. (1966). A comparison of maximal oxygen uptake by treadmill and step test procedures. *Journal of Applied Physiology, 21,* 1387–1388.

40. Katch, V. L., Sady, S. S., Freedson, P. (1982). Biological variability in maximum aerobic power. *Medicine and Science in Sports and Exercise, 14,* 21–25.

41. Kolkhorst, F. W., Toepfer, T. D., & Dolgener, F. A. (1995). Expired air temperature during steady-state running. *Medicine and Science in Sports and Exercise, 27,* 1621–1625.

42. Liang, M. T. C., Alexander, J. F., Stull, G. A., & Serfass, R. C. (1982). The use of the Bruce equation for predicting $\dot{V}O_2$max in healthy young men. *Medicine and Science in Sports and Exercise, 14,* Abstract #129.

43. Luft, V. C., Cardus, D., Lim, T. P. K., Anderson, E. C., & Howarth, J. L. (1963). Physical performance in relation to body size and composition. *Annals of N.Y. Academy of Science, 110,* 795–808.

44. Mayhew, J. L., & Andrew, J. (1975). Assessment of running performance in college males from aerobic capacity percentage utilization coefficients. *Journal of Sports Medicine and Physical Fitness, 15,* 342–346.

45. McArdle, W. D., Katch, F. I., & Katch, V. L. (1991). *Exercise physiology.* Philadelphia: Lea & Febiger.

46. McDonough, J. R., & Bruce, R. A. (1969). Maximal exercise testing in assessing cardiovascular function. *Journal of South Carolina Medical Association, 65,* (Suppl.) 26–33.

47. Michael, E. D., Burke, E. J., & Avakian, E. V. (1979). *Laboratory experiments in exercise physiology.* Ithaca, New York: Mouvement Publications.

48. Mitchell, J. H., Sproule, B. J., & Chapman, C. B. (1958). The physiological meaning of the maximal oxygen intake test. *Journal of Clinical Investigation, 37,* 538.

49. Myerson, M., Gutin, B., Warren, M. D., May, M. T., Contento, I., Lee, M., Pi-Sunyer, F. Y., Pierson, R. N., & Brooks-Gunn, J. (1988). Resting metabolic rate and energy balance in amenorrheic and eumenorrheic runners. *Medicine and Science in Sports and Exercise, 23,* 15–22.

50. Nieman, D. C., Berk, L. S., Simpson-Westerberg, M., Arabatzis, K., Youngberg, S., Tan, S. A., Lee, J. W., & Eby, W. C. (1989). Effects of long-endurance running on immune system parameters and lymphocyte function in experienced marathoners. *International Journal of Sports Medicine, 10,* 317–323.

51. Noakes, T. D. (1988). Implications of exercise testing for prediction of performance: A contemporary perspective. *Medicine and Science in Sports and Exercise, 20,* 319–330.

52. Noble, B. J. (1986). *Physiology of exercise and sport.* Santa Clara, CA: Times Mirror/Mosby College.

53. Norton, A. C. (1976). *Technical memorandum. Methodologies for metabolic measurements.* Schiller Park, IL: Beckman.

54. Patterson, R. P., & Moreno, M. I. (1990). Bicycle pedalling forces as a function of pedalling rate and power output. *Medicine and Science in Sports and Exercise, 22,* 512–516.

55. Patterson, R. P., & Pearson, J. L. (1983). The influence of flywheel weight and pedalling frequency on the biomechanics and psychological responses to bicycle exercise. *Ergonomics, 26,* 659–668.

56. Peters, J. P., & Van Slyke, D. D. (1932). *Quantitative clinical chemistry. Vol. II (Methods).* Baltimore: Williams & Wilkins.

57. Pivarnik, J. M., Montain, S. J., Graves, J. E., & Pollock, L. (1988). Effects of pedal speed during incremental cycle ergometer exercise. *Research Quarterly for Exercise and Sport, 59,* 73–77.

58. Powers, S. K., & Howley, E. T. (1990). *Exercise physiology.* Dubuque, IA: Wm. C. Brown.

59. Robinson, S. (1938). Experimental studies of physical fitness in relation to age. *Arbetsphysiologia, 10,* 251–323.
60. Rogers, M. A., Yamamoto, C., Hagberg, J. M., Martin, W. H., Ehsani, A. A., & Holloszy, J. O. (1988). Effect of six days of exercise training on responses to maximal and submaximal exercise in middle-aged men. *Medicine and Science in Sports and Exercise, 20,* 260–264.
61. Seabury, J. J., Adams, W. C., & Ramey, M. R. (1977). Influence of pedalling rate and power output on energy expenditure during bicycle ergometry. *Ergonomics, 20,* 491–498.
62. Serresse, O., Lortie, G., Bouchard, C., & Boulay, M. R. (1988). Estimation of the contribution of the various energy systems during maximal work of short duration. *International Journal of Sports Medicine, 9,* 456–460.
63. Shvartz, E., & Reibold, R. C. (1990). Aerobic fitness norms for males and females aged 6 to 75 years: A review. *Aviation, Space, and Environmental Medicine, 61,* 3–11.
64. Tanaka, H., Bassett, D. R., Swensen, T. C., & Sampredo, R. M. (1993). Aerobic and anaerobic power characteristics of competitive cyclists in the United States Cycling Federation. *International Journal of Sports Medicine, 14,* 334–338.
65. Taylor, H. L., Buskirk, E., & Henschel, A. (1955). Maximal oxygen intake as an objective measure of cardiorespiratory performance. *Journal of Applied Physiology, 8,* 73–80.

66. Thoden, J. S. (1991). Testing aerobic power. In J. D. MacDougall, H. A. Wenger, & H. J. Green (Eds.), *Physiological testing of the high performance athlete* (pp. 107–173). Champaign, IL: Human Kinetics.
67. Thomson, J. M., & Garvie, K. J. (1981). A laboratory method for determination of anaerobic energy expenditure during sprinting. *Canadian Journal of Applied Sport Science, 6,* 21–26.
68. Vago, P., Mercier, J., Ramonatxo, M., & Prefant, C. (1987). Is ventilatory anaerobic threshold a good index of endurance capacity? *International Journal of Sports Medicine, 8,* 190–195.
69. Wasserman, K., Hansen, J. E., Sue, D. Y., Whipp, B. J., & Casaburi, R. (1994). *Principles of exercise testing and interpretation.* Philadelphia: Lea & Febiger.
70. Weast, R. C. (Ed.). (1967). *Handbook of chemistry and physics,* 54th ed., Cleveland, OH: The Chemical Rubber Co.
71. Wilmore, J. H., & Costill, D. L. (1974). Semiautomated systems approach to the assessment of oxygen uptake during exercise. *Journal of Applied Physiology, 36,* 618–620.
72. Wilmore, J. H., & Norton, A. C. (1974). *The heart and lungs at work.* Schiller Park, IL: Beckman Instruments.
73. Wyndham, C. H., Strydom, N. B., Maritz, J. S., Morrison, J. F., Peter, J., & Potgieter, Z. U. (1959). Maximum oxygen intake and maximum heart rate during strenuous work. *Journal of Applied Physiology, 14,* 927–936.

Form OC 1

Assignments for $\dot{V}O_2Max$ Testing

Assignment

1. Calibrator

2. Performer

3. Performer's caretaker

4. Basic data recorder

5. Meteorologist

6. Oxygen recorder

7. Carbon dioxide recorder

8. Air volume recorder

9. Protocol controller

10. Starter/timer

Name

_____

_____

_____

_____

_____

_____

_____

_____

_____

_____

Form OC 2

F_EO_2 (%) and F_ECO_2 (%)[a]

Time	F_EO_2	F_ECO_2	Time	F_EO_2	F_ECO_2	Time	F_EO_2	F_ECO_2
1:15			6:15			11:15		
1:30			6:30			11:30		
1:45			6:45			11:45		
2:00			7:00			12:00		
M			M			M		
2:15			7:15			12:15		
2:30			7:30			12:30		
2:45			7:45			12:45		
3:00			8:00			13:00		
M			M			M		
3:15			8:15			13:15		
3:30			8:30			13:30		
3:45			8:45			13:45		
4:00			9:00			14:00		
M			M			M		
4:15			9:15			14:15		
4:30			9:30			14:30		
4:45			9:45			14:45		
5:00			10:00			15:00		
M			M			M		
5:15			10:15			15:15		
5:30			10:30			15:30		
5:45			10:45			15:45		
6:00			11:00			16:00		
M			M			M		

[a]An adjustment of 15–30 s may be necessary due to the delay through the mixing chamber and the drying tube of the analyzers; unaccounting for the delay would produce an error in O_2 of less than 2%.[26]

Form OC 3

Ventilation (V_E or V_I ATPS, STPD)

Time min:s	Air Meter Reading	Min Value $L \cdot min^{-1}$ ATPS	STPDcf =	Ventilation STPD (V_E or V_I) $L \cdot min^{-1}$
0:00				
1:00		0 – 1 =	× cf =	
2:00		1 – 2 =	× cf =	
3:00		2 – 3 =	× cf =	
4:00		3 – 4 =	× cf =	
5:00		4 – 5 =	× cf =	
6:00		5 – 6 =	× cf =	
7:00		6 – 7 =	× cf =	
8:00		7 – 8 =	× cf =	
9:00		8 – 9 =	× cf =	
10:00		9 – 10 =	× cf =	
11:00		10 – 11 =	× cf =	
12:00		11 – 12 =	× cf =	
13:00		12 – 13 =	× cf =	
14:00		13 – 14 =	× cf =	
15:00		14 – 15 =	× cf =	
16:00		15 – 16 =	× cf =	

Form **OC 4**

Maximal Oxygen Consumption

Name LYDIA GOULD Date 10 / 11 / 99 Time ____ a.m. ____ p.m. ____

Gender (M or F) F Age 21 y Wt 63.9 kg Ht ____ cm

Lab T_A 20.7 °C (closest 0.5) Air Meter T_A ____ °C P_B 750 torr

Relative Humidity 72 % P-H$_2$O ____ torr Fan: Yes ____ No X

Mode: TM X Bike ____ Seat Ht ____ Other ____ Time to Exhaustion ____

Time	Power or Stage[a]	F_EO_2 (%)	F_ECO_2 (%)	$\dot{V}_E$ or $\dot{V}_I$ STPD	True O_2 (%)	R	$\dot{V}O_2$ L·min^{-1}	ml·kg^{-1}·min^{-1}
0–1								
1–2								
2–3								
3–4								
4–5								
5–6								
6–7								
7–8								
8–9								
9–10								
10–11								
11–12								
12–13								
13–14								
14–15								
15–16								

[a]*Note:* The first complete whole min of running occurred between _____ min.

62.1 $\dot{V}O_2$ MAX

Form **OC 5**

Calculations for V̇O₂max Test Using Nomogram and Expired Air Volume

1. Convert $\dot{V}_E$ ATPS to $\dot{V}_E$ STPD:

   a. Get STPD CF from Table 5 or from Eqs. 5 and 6, with Table 6.

   STPD CF (Table 5) = ☐

   STPD CF (Eqs. 5 and 6 with Table 6) = [273 °K/(273 °K + T_A ☐ °C)]

   $\times$ [(P_B ☐ torr − P-H₂O ☐ (Table 6 torr)/760 torr]

   = (273 °K/ ☐ °K) $\times$ (☐ torr/760 torr)

   = ☐ $\times$ ☐ = ☐ CF

   b. Get $\dot{V}_E$ STPD (L/min) (from Eq. 6).

   $\dot{V}_E$ STPD (L/min) = $\dot{V}_E$ ATPS ☐ L/min $\times$ CF ☐ = ☐ L/min

2. Determine the R and true O₂ values from the nomogram in Figure 5.

   R from Fig. 5 = ☐   True O₂ from Fig. 5 = ☐ %

3. Get $\dot{V}O_2$ from Equation 1.

   $\dot{V}O_2$ (L/min) = V_E STPD ☐ L/min $\times$ true O₂ ☐ %

   = ☐ L/min

4. Get $\dot{V}O_2$ in units of ml/min from Equation 15.

   $\dot{V}O_2$ (ml/min) = ☐ L/min $\times$ 1000 = ☐ ml/min

5. Get relative oxygen consumption from Equation 16.

   $\dot{V}O_2$ ml/(kg $\times$ min) = ☐ ml/min divided by body weight ☐ kg

   = ☐ ml/(kg $\times$ min) or ml·kg⁻¹·min⁻¹

6. Get MET values from Equation 17.

   MET = ☐ ml/(kg $\times$ min) divided by 3.5 ml/(kg $\times$ min) = ☐ MET

Form OC 6

Comparisons Between Predictive and Direct Aerobic Tests

Maximal Oxygen Consumption (ml·kg⁻¹·min⁻¹)
Name of Test

Initials	Run/Walk	Step	Cycle	$\dot{V}O_2max$
1.				
2.				
3.				
4.				
5.				
6.				
7.				
8.				
9.				
10.				
11.				
12.				
13.				
14.				
15.				
16.				
17.				
18.				
19.				
20.				
21.				
M				

Chapter RB   Resting Blood Pressure

Numerous researchers have reported an inverse (negative) relationship between physical activity or fitness and morbidity (disease rate) or mortality (death rate), not only from coronary heart disease,[3,4,11,34,41,43,45] but from all causes.[4,5] Thus, physical activity and fitness are associated with a reduced risk of cardiovascular disease (CVD), and reduced deaths from CVD and all causes. In light of such evidence it seems prudent that the student of exercise physiology be knowledgeable about those tests that elucidate the cardiovascular system.

Blood pressure measurement is one of the most common clinical tests. It is recommended that all persons over 3 years of age should check their blood pressure annually.[46,47]

Because blood pressure screening or monitoring is such an important part of many physical fitness clinics, the technique of measuring blood pressure should be learned by many types of allied health personnel. Dr. H. K. Hellerstein, a renowned cardiologist, speaking as a member of the American Medical Association's Committee on Exercise, said, "Certainly every physical educator should know how to take blood pressure and record it."[21] Additionally, every physical educator should know how to interpret blood pressure.

Although the cause of hypertension (high blood pressure) in at least 90% of adults is unknown, it is associated with a high risk for future cardiovascular morbidity and mortality.[16] Hypertensives are more likely to accelerate atherosclerosis (narrowing of arteries) that may cause vascular occlusions and ruptures about 20 years earlier than in normotensives.[29] If there were obvious symptoms (e.g., pain, nausea) associated with high blood pressure, there would be less need to measure the actual pressure. However, high blood pressure may not be noticed outwardly until a fatal or near-fatal heart attack or stroke occurs. Thus, the primary clinical purpose of measuring blood pressure is to determine the potential risk of cardiovascular disease; if the pressure is high, then appropriate medications or lifestyle changes are recommended. Periodic monitoring of the blood pressure is done in order to check the efficacy of such recommendations.

Another purpose of measuring resting blood pressure is to establish a baseline by which to compare the effect of exercise on blood pressure. Thus, the effects of different types, intensities, or durations of exercise may be compared by noting their effects upon the baseline value. For example, blood pressure comparisons may be made between (1) isometric versus isotonic exercise, (2) different intensities of muscle contractions (e.g., 30% vs. 80% maximal contractions), and (3) short versus long durations of exercise.

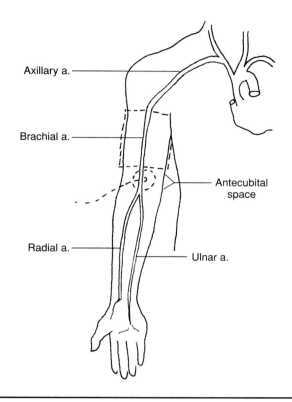

Figure 1 An internal view of the brachial artery and its origins and branches; the dotted diaphragm of the stethoscope is at the antecubital fossa (a = artery).

Physiological Rationale

High blood pressure is unhealthy; blood pressure, per se, is not unhealthy. Without blood pressure there would be no blood flow. Blood pressure is primarily dependent upon the volume of blood and the resistance of the blood vessels. The blood pressure that is commonly measured is that of the arteries. Thus, blood pressure may be defined for laboratory purposes as the force of blood distending the *arterial* walls. Typically, the brachial artery is sampled because of convenience and its position at heart level. The brachial artery (Fig. 1) is a continuation of the axillary artery and extends medially alongside the humerus; it gradually moves centrally as it nears the antecubital fossa (anterior

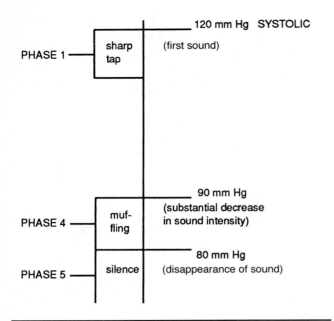

Figure 2 The three major phases of Korotkoff sounds when systolic pressure (1st phase) is 120 mm Hg, and diastolic pressures (fourth and fifth phases) are 90 and 80 mm Hg, respectively.

crease of the elbow), where it divides into the radial and ulnar arteries.[23]

Korotkoff Sounds

The determination of blood pressure in the typical laboratory setting is based upon the sounds made by the vibrations from the vascular walls. These sounds are referred to as Korotkoff sounds (named after their discoverer in 1905) (Fig. 2). In brief, when there is no blood flow (as when a tourniquet is applied), there will be no vibrations and thus no sound. Paradoxically, when there is completely nonobstructed flow of the blood, there is also no vibration and thus no sound; this is due to the streamlined flow of the blood. When blood flow is restricted by the application of a tourniquet or by any kind of pressure, and then gradually released, there will be a bolus of blood escaping at the peak point of blood pressure coinciding with left ventricular contraction (systole). This bolus of blood will cause vascular vibrations which result in a faint sound (phase 1); this is **systolic pressure.** As the restriction or pressure continues to be released, more blood escapes, causing even greater vibration and louder sounds. Phases 2 and 3 are not commonly used in recording blood pressures, and, therefore, have been deleted in Figure 2. More blood escapes as the cuff pressure continues to decrease. However, after phase three, as the blood flow becomes more streamlined due to less compression, there is a reduction of vibrations causing a muffling sound (phase 4). The fourth phase is sometimes difficult to distinguish. The American Heart Association describes it as

". . . a distinct, abrupt, muffling of sound (usually of a soft, blowing quality) . . .".[16] Identifying phase 4 is more difficult than phase 5.[15] When blood flow is completely streamlined there is a disappearance of sound (phase 5). The disappearance denotes **diastolic pressure,** the lowest pressure that exists in the arteries.

The Task Force on Blood Pressure Control in Children[46,47] recommends that both the point of muffling (phase 4) and the point of disappearance (phase 5) of the sound be recorded when taking blood pressure in children. Because of the frequency of these occurring simultaneously or fifth phase not occurring at all, the Task Force and the American Heart Association use the fourth phase to interpret children's norms and the fifth phase for all persons above 12 years of age. Occasionally, phase 4 should be used for adults whose sounds remain very faint to near zero levels.[49] Usually, the fourth phase is significantly higher than the fifth phase by about 5 mm of mercury (Hg).[10] Rarely do true diastolic pressures reach less than 40 mm Hg.[12] Thus, for any person whose sounds can be heard below this level, it seems logical to use the fourth phase instead of the fifth phase as the true diastolic pressure. Exercise technicians are encouraged to practice recording fourth phase in all persons because of the fourth phase's importance during exercise.

Pulse Pressure and Mean Pressure

Pulse pressure (PP) is the difference between systolic and diastolic pressures. It is used to calculate mean pressure (MBP). MBP is based upon the actual pressure that the arteries would sustain if blood flow were not pulsating. Because arterial blood pressure under resting conditions is at systolic level only about one-twentieth of the time during a cardiac cycle, mean pressure is always closer to diastolic pressure than it is to systolic pressure. Resting MBP is usually estimated as one-third the distance between fifth-phase diastolic pressure and systolic pressure[44] (Eq. 1), or, similarly, by multiplying the difference between SP and DP, that is, PP, by 0.33[51] (Eq. 2). MBP is typically between 90 and 100 mm Hg at rest.

$$MBP = (PP/3) + DP \qquad \text{Eq. 1}$$

where: $PP = SP - DP$

$$\text{Example: MBP (mm Hg)} = [(130 - 80) / 3] + 80$$
$$= (50/3) + 80$$
$$= 17 + 80$$
$$= 97 \text{ mm Hg}$$

or:

$$MBP = (0.33 \times PP) + DP \qquad \text{Eq. 2}$$

$$\text{Example: MBP (mm Hg)} = [0.33 \times (130 - 80)] + 80$$
$$= (0.33 \times 50) + 80$$
$$= 17 + 80$$
$$= 97 \text{ mm Hg}$$

Accuracy of Blood Pressure Measurements

Validity

The cuff method of measuring systolic and fifth-phase diastolic blood pressure is usually lower than the more accurate invasive method of measuring blood pressure by about 10 mm Hg (8%) and 5 mm Hg (6%), respectively; the fourth phase, however, is not significantly different from the invasive measurement of diastolic pressure.[44] Thus, the fourth phase appears to be the most valid indicator of diastolic pressure, although the fifth phase is commonly used for calculating mean pressures during a resting body state.

Reliability

The ability of the human ear to hear sounds is dependent upon the frequency (Hz) and pressure (decibels; dB) of the sounds. Unfortunately, Korotkoff sounds are neither of high frequency nor high decibel—both being less than the optimal hearing of the human ear.[35] Acceptable reliability coefficients can be obtained for the test-retest values of systolic ($r = .89$) and diastolic ($r = .83$) blood pressures.[a] The diastolic values of the fifth phase may be more repeatable than the fourth phase due to greater difficulty in determining muffling points versus disappearance points of fourth phase. In fact, one investigator encourages the use of fifth phase for this very reason, although it may not be hemodynamically justified for all persons.[31]

[a]Adams, G. M. (1968). Blood pressure reliability in the elderly. Unpublished raw data.

Method

Many types of instruments exist for measuring blood pressure. The original instrument in 1733, water in a glass tube, was used to measure the blood pressure of a horse.[2] Due to water's light weight (lower density) in comparison to mercury—the liquid now being used—a ladder was needed to enable the investigator to read the water column, which had risen about ten feet. Mercury, being nearly 14 times heavier than water, enables the measurement of blood pressure with a glass tube, which can be about one-fourteenth the length of the original water-filled glass tubes. If we still used water to measure human blood pressure, the tube would have to be a minimum of six feet tall, and the column of water would oscillate by more than one foot with each heartbeat.[22]

Due to the traditional use of mercury in blood pressure instrumentation, the unit of measure for blood pressure recordings is millimeters of mercury (mm Hg; Hg = hydrargyrum). Regardless of the type of blood pressure method or instrument, the unit of measure remains mm Hg. The graduations on the sphygmomanometer gauge are in 2-mm divisions and extend to 300 mm Hg.

The methods of blood pressure measurement may be divided into two categories—invasive and noninvasive.

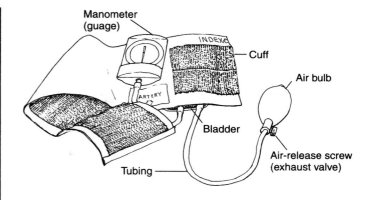

Figure 3 The main parts of an aneroid sphygmomanometer: gauge, tubing, cuff, bladder, air bulb, and air-release screw.

The *invasive* method is the more valid of the two methods and is usually reserved for clinical settings or precise research investigations. A thin, teflon tube, called an end-hole catheter or cannula, is connected on one end to a pressure transducer. The sensor end of the catheter is inserted into the brachial artery or ascending aorta while the transducer end is connected to a recorder. Although the invasive method is accurate for mean and diastolic pressures in the ascending aorta,[17] it is expensive, elaborate, and traumatic compared to the noninvasive method.

Two major methods are used to measure *noninvasive blood pressure*—cuff manometry and ultrasound Doppler. The cuff manometry method uses an instrument called a sphygmomanometer (sphygmo = pulse; pronounced sfig-mo-ma-nom-e-ter); it is more commonly referred to as a manometer. Both aneroid and mercury methods of manometry require a cuff with an air bladder; thus, the method is sometimes referred to as the cuff method (Fig. 3). The aneroid manometers use a metal bellows device that drives tiny gears that move the dial's pointers. Commercial electronic blood pressure instruments have not been endorsed by the American Heart Association, partly because of the difficulty in checking their accuracy and their infrequent use by health personnel. Unless special electronic sensors ("microphones") or recorders are used in conjunction with the cuffs, a stethoscope is required to auscultate the Korotkoff sounds; when this is done, the noninvasive method may be referred to as the **auscultatory method.** Surprisingly, experienced participants can sense their blood pressure fairly accurately while it is being auscultated.[13]

Procedures

Certain preparations, such as calibration and participant orientation, should be made in order to facilitate blood pressure measurement. **Calibration** of aneroid manometers, using a mercury manometer, should be done at six-month[29,30] to annual[25,47] intervals.

Calibration of Aneroid Sphygmomanometer

Assumption: The method of calibrating the aneroid sphygmomanometers assumes that the mercury sphygmomanometer is accurate. A good sphygmomanometer will not shift its indicating pointer or mercury column when the air-release screw is closed.

Zero

Most pointers on the dials of the aneroid sphygmomanometers are designed to rest at the zero marker when no air has been inserted into the bladder. However, some aneroid sphygmomanometers are not designed to return to the zero marker. Thus, the return of the indicator to zero is not an infallible criterion for accuracy in all aneroid manometers. Those that are designed to rest at zero should be returned to the manufacturer if they do not do so.

Range

Equipment: (1) Mercury sphygmomanometer, (2) a "Y" connector, the Y section of some stethoscopes may be used, (3) a short piece of surgical tubing (about four inches), (4) (optional) a can or bottle that approximates the circumference of a person's upper arm.

Configuration: (1) Wrap the cuff around the can or bottle; (2) connect the tube of the cuff's bladder to one end of the "Y" connector; (3) connect the tube of the mercury sphygmomanometer to another end of the Y; and (4) connect the tube of the aneroid dial to the third end of the Y connector (Fig. 4).

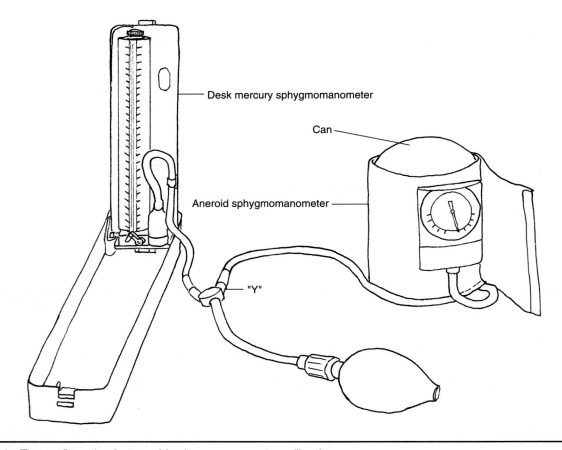

Figure 4   The configuration for aneroid sphygmomanometer calibration.

Procedure: (1) Inflate cuff's bladder until the aneroid dial reads 40 mm Hg; (2) read dial on mercury sphygmomanometer; (3) record actual mercury reading; (4) deflate bladder; (5) repeat same procedure at increments of 20 mm Hg; (6) devise a mathematical correction based upon the readings. If the discrepancy is greater than desired, then return the aneroid to the manufacturer.

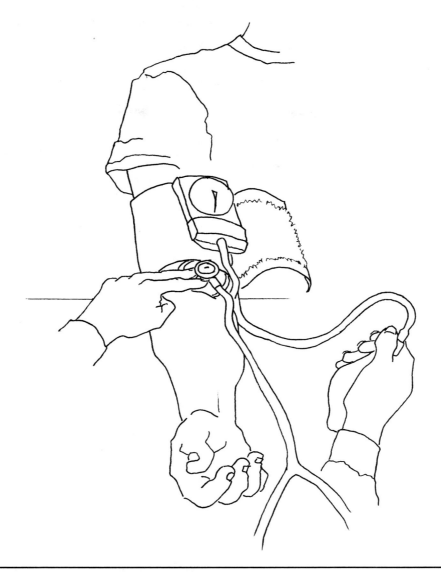

Figure 5 The position of the cuff (about 1 in. or 2.5 cm above the antecubital space) and diaphragm of the stethoscope.

Participant-orientation includes such preparatory rules that were suggested for the heart rate tests. Whereas those tests prescribed abstaining from smoking and caffeine for four hours prior to testing, the Joint National Committee on Detection, Evaluation, and Treatment of High Blood Pressure prescribes only a 30-min abstention.[26] A brief medical and family history concerning heart disease and hypertension is helpful. The subject should relax for at least five minutes in a comfortable environment prior to the blood pressure measurement.[16,26] Also, sleeveless shirts/blouses or loosefitting sleeves are recommended attire; if the sleeve appears to fit tightly around the subject's arm when the sleeve is rolled up, the shirt or sweater should be removed. The cuff and stethoscope should not be placed over cloth. A summary of the procedures for measuring blood pressure includes the following steps:

Procedural Steps

1. The participant should be in the seated position with the arm at heart level and resting on the armrest of a chair or on a table (Fig. 5).
2. The manometer should be clearly visible to the technician; mercury gauges should read so that the meniscus (top of mercury) is at eye level.
3. This step relates to subjects with suspected small or large arm circumferences. The technician measures the circumference of the subject's upper arm.
   a. The appropriate cuff size is selected based on the arm circumference guidelines in Table 1.
   b. Some cuffs have index lines that indicate if the cuff is too small or too large (Fig. 6).
4. The technician snugly places the blood pressure cuff so that the lower edge is approximately 2.5 cm (1 in.) above the antecubital space.[32]

Table 1 Guidelines for Type of Blood Pressure Cuff According to Limb Circumference (cir.)

Limb Size (cm)	Type of Cuff[a]	Bladder Size (cm)	
		Length	Width
Upper Arm Cir.			
32–42	Large Adult	33 or 42	15
24–32	Adult	24	12.5
18–26	Child	21.5	10
	(3–12 y)	18[b]	8[b]
	Ideal[c]	80% arm cir.	40–50% arm cir.
Thigh Cir.			
42–50	Thigh	37[b]	18.5[b]

[a]Other types of cuffs are: newborn and infant.
[b]Task Force, 1987.
[c]Frohlich et al., 1987.

a. The center of the bladder should be over the brachial artery.
b. Although some cuffs mark the location of the brachial artery, it may be helpful to palpate the brachial artery along the medial side of the antecubital space.[16]

5. The technician places the diaphragm, or bell,[16] of the stethoscope firmly, but not heavy enough to indent the skin, over the invisible brachial artery in the antecubital space.

6. After turning the air-release screw clockwise, the technician inflates the cuff to any of the three following levels:
   a. 160 mm Hg
   b. 20 mm Hg above expected or known BP
   c. 20–30 mm Hg above the disappearance of the radial pulse; this means that the technician inflates the cuff while palpating the subject's radial pulse, and that this procedure precedes the "official" measurement by 15–30 s.[16]

7. The technician turns the air-release screw counterclockwise so that the cuff pressure decreases at a rate of about 2–3 mm Hg[16,47] per heartbeat or 2–5 mm Hg per second.[39]

8. The technician listens carefully and mentally notes the first Korotkoff sound of two consecutive beats—systolic pressure (first phase), then fourth phase, then fifth phase at the nearest 2-mm mark on the manometer, respectively.

9. The technician continues listening for 10–20 mm Hg below the last sound heard to confirm disappearance.

10. The technician rapidly deflates the cuff.

11. The technician records the values in even numbers according to the accepted format: e.g., Systolic/Fourth Phase DP/Fifth Phase DP. Thus a hypothetical recording would appear as: 120/90/80 mm Hg.

12. The technician notes the presence or absence of auscultatory gaps and/or irregular pulse rhythm.

13. The technician repeats the measurement after 1–2 min, then averages the two readings unless they differ by

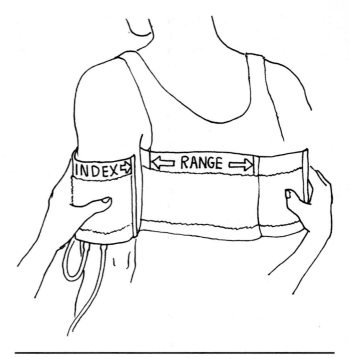

Figure 6 The cuff's index and range lines to determine the appropriate cuff size.

more than 5 mm Hg, in which case additional readings are made.[25,29] If more than two readings are necessary, average the two that are within 5 mm Hg.

Comments on Blood Pressure Procedures

Body and Arm Position

There is no *practical* difference in blood pressure measured in the seated position versus that measured in the supine position. However, *statistically,* there is a tendency for slightly higher values for systolic (6–7 mm Hg) and diastolic (1 mm Hg) in the supine position.[33,48] The standing position increases diastolic pressure but not systolic pressure.[19]

The sitting position should automatically place the subject's antecubital space of the arm at heart level. Blood pressures are higher if the arm is below the heart versus above the heart (nearly 1 mm Hg for each centimeter above or below heart level). Erroneously higher systolic and diastolic pressure values occur if the arm is allowed to hang at the subject's side rather than supported at heart level.[48]

For best exposure of the antecubital position, it helps to have the subject's palm upward with the thumb-side rotated outwardly (the anatomical position) and to have the arm nearly straight while resting on a platform (e.g., table). This provides the best contact with the brachial artery. The antecubital space should be left clear for the stethoscope's diaphragm.[6]

Various authorities recommend that the right arm be chosen for the blood pressure measurement.[7,47] This is partly because of the remote possibility that the genetic anomaly of coarctation (abnormal narrowing) between the aorta and subclavian artery will cause an elevated blood pressure. If the pressure in the right arm is normal, it is likely to be normal everywhere. However, higher right-arm values were not confirmed by some investigators,[10,18] nor did the investigators in the famous epidemiological study in Framingham, Massachusetts, measure blood pressure in the right arm.[27] In older patients, one group of investigators found that the systolic pressure in the right arm was not more than a few millimeters higher than in the left arm, and that the diastolic pressure was virtually the same in both arms.[20] The American Heart Association recommends that both arms be measured at the initial examination, and the arm with the higher pressure be measured in subsequent examinations.[16] Another consideration should be the comfort and convenience of both the technician and the subject.

Cuff Size

Special cuff sizes are available for small or large arms. Cuffs that are too small will overestimate blood pressure, whereas cuffs that are too large will underestimate blood pressure. The average overestimation by narrow cuffs is about 9 and 5 mm Hg for SP and DP, respectively.[37] The ideal cuff size is when the arm circumference is 2.6 times the size of the bladder width, or the bladder width is 40–50% of the arm circumference, and bladder length is 80% of arm circumference.[16]

Some cuff manufacturers print a criterion index line by which to determine proper cuff size (Fig. 6). For example, the cuff is placed so that the vertical arrow printed on the cuff is over the brachial artery. After the cuff encircles the arm, the index line should fall within the two horizontal range lines. These index lines can vary considerably among manufacturers. Thus lab personnel are encouraged to mark a line on the interior surface of the cuff at a distance of 32 cm from the standard cuff's left border.[37] Table 1 provides the proper guidelines for cuff size. Either the larger or smaller cuff may be used for overlapping values found in this table.

Controlling the Manometer and Stethoscope

No air spaces should be allowed between the skin and the diaphragm of the stethoscope. By not pressing heavily on the bell or diaphragm the technician can avoid turbulent blood flow induced by the diaphragm. Turbulence can lower the diastolic pressure reading, but is unlikely to distort systolic.[36] The technician should clear the cuff bladder's tubing away from the diaphragm because when they touch each other it sounds much like the Korotkoff sounds.

The technician should place the air bulb deep in the palm of the hand so that the thumb and index finger control the air-release screw. Often, technicians decrease the pressure too fast. Low systolic and high diastolic readings may occur when the rate of deflation is too fast.[16] Very slow deflation rates should be avoided in order to prevent prolonged discomfort, apprehensiveness, and fidgeting in the subject; all of which may increase the individual's blood

pressure. If the subject requires a repeated measurement for any reason, the pressure cuff should remain deflated for about 1–2 min between determinations; this will allow the blood in the venous circulation to return to normal.[16]

The meniscus level (the peak of the "hump") at the top of the column of mercury is the measuring point when using **mercury** manometers. The indicating pointer, of course, is used for the **aneroid** gauge. If using the mercury manometer the observer's eyes should be level with the meniscus in order to avoid parallax (angle distortion).

Results and Discussion

The interpretation of blood pressure is based upon the criteria that have been established by various professional medical groups. These criteria are established from large-scale studies that indicate the norms for that particular population and/or subpopulation (e.g., African Americans, males, females, children, etc.).

Blood pressure criteria are based upon the contribution of blood pressure to the risk of death due to cardiovascular disease. None of the authoritative study groups on blood pressure such as the American Heart Association,[1] the Task Force on Blood Pressure,[46,47] the Joint National Committee,[24–26] and the National High Blood Pressure Program[40] indicate that exceeding the criterion for systolic hypertension is more critical than exceeding the criterion for diastolic hypertension, or vice versa. The one exception to this may be the increased incidence of stroke with higher systolic pressures. Because blood pressure may be affected by nonpathological (nondisease) factors such as emotions, it is recommended that no one be classified as hypertense on the basis of only one day's measurements. A person should be classified as hypertense only when repeated,[16] or three,[46] measurements taken on separate occasions are over the established hypertension criteria.

Hypertension. The classification criteria listed in Table 2 are based on the Korotkoff sounds of the first and fifth phases. The criterion of 140/90 for what was formerly called borderline hypertension is now considered a legitimate criterion for hypertension.[1,24,26,50] All that is necessary to meet the criterion is for either systolic or diastolic pressure to reach the respective value, not necessarily both of them. When only one of the pressures exceeds the criterion it is sometimes referred to as *isolated* systolic (or diastolic) hypertension. Various authorities have suggested a category of high normal for younger persons with a blood pressure between 130–139/85–89.[26,28,46] Subdivisions of the hypertension category have been proposed, such as mild, moderate, severe, and very severe.[8,14,26] Age prevalence percentages are presented in Table 3.[26,40]

Average BP. The average values (125/82) listed in Table 2 are based on over 5000 men, ages 20–60+ y, who were tested at a fitness clinic.[42] These values are probably less

Table 2 Blood Pressure (mm Hg) Criteria for Various Categories

Category	Criteria (mm Hg)	
	Systolic	Diastolic (5th phase)
"Optimal"[26]	<120	<80
Average[43] (Active Men)	125	82
(Active Women)	119	78
High Normal[26]	130–139	85–89
Hypertension[26]		
Mild	140–159	90–99
Moderate	160–179	100–109
Severe	180–209	110–119
Very Severe	≥210	≥120
Hypotension	<90	<60
Shock	<80	<40

Sources: [26]Joint National Committee on Detection, Evaluation, & Treatment of High Blood Pressure. (1993). The Fifth report of the Joint National Committee on Detection, Evaluation, and Treatment of High Blood Pressure (JNC V). *Archives of Internal Medicine, 153*, 154–183; NIH Publication No. 93-1088. [43]Pollock, M. L., Wilmore, J. H., & Fox, S. M. (1978). *Health and fitness through physical activity.* Santa Barbara, CA: John Wiley & Sons.

Table 3 Age Prevalence Rates for Hypertension

	Percent
Total Adult Population[26]	25–33
Age-Specific Estimates[41]	
18–29 y	4
30–39	11
40–49	21
50–59	44
60–69	54
70–79	64
80+	65

[41]National High Blood Pressure Education Program Working Group. (1993). Report on primary prevention of hypertension. *Archives of Internal Medicine, 153,* 186–208.

Table 4 Percentile Norms for Blood Pressure in Active Men and Women Ages 20–39

	Men				Women			
%ile	Systolic		Diastolic		Systolic		Diastolic	
	AGES (y)				AGES (y)			
	20–29	30–39	20–29	30–39	20–29	30–39	20–29	30–39
99th	94	96	60	60	90	90	56	60
90	110	108	70	70	99	100	63	65
80	112	110	72	74	101	104	68	70
70	118	116	78	78	106	110	70	70
60	120	120	80	80	110	110	72	74
50	121	120	80	80	112	114	75	76
40	128	124	80	81	118	118	78	80
30	130	130	84	85	120	120	80	80
20	136	132	88	90	122	122	80	82
10	140	140	90	92	130	130	82	90
1st	158	168	110	110	141	160	90	110
n	367	1615			118	301		

Source: Data from Pollock, et al., *Health and Fitness Through Physical Activity,* 1978. Copyright © 1978 John Wiley & Sons, Inc., New York, NY.

than what would be found in the street population because they are men who have been tested at a fitness clinic, presumably with the intention of planning to exercise or to evaluate their existing exercise programs. The women's averages (119/78) are from the same investigators and include 914 active women the same ages as the men, that is, between 20 and 60+ years.

Optimal BP. The exact criteria for optimal SP and DP may not exist. For example, if the criteria were less than 120/80, then it would also have to consider symptoms displayed by the subject.[26] Thus the lowest blood pressure may be the best as long as symptoms such as lightheadedness, dizziness, and/or faintness (syncope) are absent.

Hypotension. There are no increased risks for cardiovascular disease in hypotensive persons; in fact, lower pressures

reduce the cardiovascular risk.[16] The hypotension criterion of 90 mm Hg in Table 2 is meant only for systolic pressure; there is no accepted criterion for diastolic pressure with respect to hypotension, although less than 60 mm Hg is unusual.[38] As with optimal blood pressure, hypotensive criteria really should be based upon symptoms. Thus, if an individual is experiencing dizziness, syncope, coldness, pallor, nausea, low urine output, and high arterial blood lactates when blood pressure decreases to a certain point, then that point should be the criterion for hypotension for that person.[9]

Norms are based on the average and standard deviation of blood pressures from a large population. In that respect they are similar to the Average category presented in Table 2. Norms for active persons of both sexes between the ages of 20 and 39 years are found in Table 4.[43] In general, women have lower blood pressures than men; younger persons have lower pressures than older persons.

References

1. American Heart Association. (1991). *1992 heart and stroke facts.* Dallas: American Heart Association.
2. Best, C. H., & Taylor, N. B. (1956). *The human body.* New York: Henry Holt & Co.
3. Blackburn, H., & Jacobs, D. R. (1988). Physical activity and the risk of coronary heart disease. *New England Journal of Medicine 319,* 1217–1219.
4. Blair, S. N., Kampert, J. B., Kohl, H. W., Barlow, C. E., Paffenbarger, R. S., & Gibbons, L. W. (1996). Influences of cardiorespiratory fitness and other precursors on cardiovascular disease and all-cause mortality in men and women. *JAMA, 276*(3): 205–210.
5. Blair, S. N., Kohl, H. W., Paffenbarger, R. S., Clark, D. G., Cooper, K. H., & Gibbons, L. W. (1989). Physical fitness and all-cause mortality. A prospective study of healthy men and women. *Journal of the American Medical Association, 262,* 2395–2401.
6. Boyer, J. (1976, December). Exercise and hypertension. *The Physician and Sportsmedicine,* pp. 35–49.
7. Burch, G. E. (1976). *Consultations in hypertension: A clinical symposium.* Rochester, NY: Pennwalt Prescription Products.
8. Cooper, E. S., & West, J. W. (1977). Hypertension and stroke. *Cardiovascular Medicine, 2,* 429–444.
9. daLuz, P. L., Weil, M. H., Liu, V. Y., & Shubin, H. (1974). Plasma volume prior to and following volume loading during shock complicating acute myocardial infarction. *Circulation, 49,* 98–105.
10. Das, B. C., & Mukherjee, B. N. (1963). Variation in systolic and diastolic pressure with changes in age and weight. *Gerontologia, 8,* 92–104.
11. Ekelund, L-G., Haskell, W. L., Johnson, J. L., Whaley, F. S., Criqui, M. H., & Sheps, D. S. (1988). Physical fitness as a predictor of cardiovascular mortality in asymptomatic North American men. The Lipid Research Clinics' Mortality Follow-Up Study. *New England Journal of Medicine, 319,* 1379–1384.
12. Engler, R. L. (1977). Historical and physical findings in patients with aortic valve disease. *The Western Journal of Medicine, 126,* 463–467.
13. Estes, S. B. (1977, May). Putting the cuff on hypertensive patients. *Patient Care,* 25.
14. Franklin, S. S., & Maxwell, M. H. (1977, March). Guide to prognosis in hypertension. *Hospital Medicine,* pp. 49–59.
15. Freis, E. D., & Sappington, R. F. (1968). Dynamic reactions produced by deflating a blood pressure cuff. *Circulation, 38,* 1085–1096.
16. Frohlich, E. D., Grim, C., Labarthe, D. R., Maxwell, M. H., Perloff, D., & Weidman, W. H. (1987). *Recommendations for human blood pressure determination by sphygmomanometers: Report of a special task force appointed by the steering committee, American Heart Association.* Dallas: National Center, American Heart Association.
17. Griffen, S. E., Robergs, R. A., & Heyward, V. H. (1977). Blood pressure measurement during exercise: A review. *Medicine and Science in Sports and Exercise, 29,* 149–159.
18. Harrison, E. G., Foth, G. M., & Hines, E. A. (1960). Bilateral indirect and direct arterial pressures. *Circulation, 22,* 419–436.
19. Hasegawa, M., & Rodbard, S. (1979). Effect of posture on arterial pressures, timing of the arterial sounds, and pulse wave velocities in the extremities. *Cardiology, 64,* 122–132.
20. Hashimoto, F., Hunt, W. C., & Hardy, L. (1984). Differences between right and left arm blood pressures in the elderly. *Western Journal of Medicine, 141,* 189–192.
21. Hellerstein, H. K. (1976, December). Exercise and hypertension. *The Physician and Sportsmedicine,* pp. 35–49.
22. Hill, A. V. (1927). *Living machinery.* New York: Harcourt, Brace, & Co.
23. Jackson, C. M. (Ed.). (1923). *Morris' human anatomy.* Philadelphia: P. Blakiston's Son & Co.
24. Joint National Committee on Detection, Evaluation, & Treatment of High Blood Pressure. (1984). The 1984 report of the Joint National Committee on Detection, Evaluation, and Treatment of High Blood Pressure (JNC V). *Archives of Internal Medicine, 44,* 1045–1057.
25. Joint National Committee on Detection, Evaluation, & Treatment of High Blood Pressure. (1988). The 1988 report of the Joint National Committee on Detection, Evaluation, and Treatment of High Blood Pressure (JNC V). *Archives of Internal Medicine, 148,* 1023–1038.
26. Joint National Committee on Detection, Evaluation, & Treatment of High Blood Pressure. (1993). The fifth report of the Joint National Committee on Detection, Evaluation, and Treatment of High Blood Pressure (JNC V). *Archives of Internal Medicine, 153,* 154–183.
27. Kannel, W. B., Philip, A. W., McGee, D. L., Dawber, T. R., McNamara, P., & Castelli, W. P. (1981). Systolic blood pressure, arterial rigidity, and risk of stroke. *Journal of the American Medical Association, 245,* 1225–1229.
28. Kaplan, N. M. (1976). Diagnosis and testing of the hypertensive patient. In G. Burch (Ed.), *Consultations in hypertension: A clinical symposium.* (pp. 6–11). New York: Pennwalt Prescription Products.
29. Kaplan, N. M. (1983). Hypertension. In N. Kaplan & J. Stannler (Eds.), *Prevention of coronary heart disease. Practical management of risk factors.* Philadelphia: W. B. Saunders.

30. Kaplan, N. M., Deveraux, R. B., Miller, H. S. (1994). Systemic hypertension. *Medicine and Science in Sports and Exercise, 26*(10), S268–S270.

31. King, G. E. (1969). Taking the blood pressure. *Journal of the American Medical Association, 209,* 1902–1904.

32. Kirkendall, W. M., Burton, A. C., Epstein, F. H., & Freis, E. D. (1967). Recommendations for human blood pressure determination by sphygmomanometry. *Circulation, 36,* 980.

33. Lategola, M. T., & Busby, D. E. (1975). Differences between seated and recumbent resting measurements of auscultative blood pressure. *Aviation, Space, & Environmental Medicine, 46,* 1027–1029.

34. Leon, A. S., Connett, J., Jacobs, D. R., & Rauramaa, R. (1987). Leisure time physical activity levels and risk of coronary heart disease and death: The multiple risk factor intervention trial. *Journal of the American Medical Association, 258,* 2388–2395.

35. Lightfoot, J. T., Tuller, B., & Williams, D. F. (1996). Ambient noise interferes with auscultatory blood pressure measurement during exercise. *Medicine and Science in Sports and Exercise, 28,* 502–508.

36. Londe, S., & Klitzner, T. S. (1984). Auscultatory blood pressure measurement—effect of pressure on the head of the stethoscope. *Western Journal of Medicine, 141,* 193–195.

37. Manning, D. M, Kuchirka, C., & Kaminski, J. (1983). Miscuffing: Inappropriate blood pressure cuff application. *Circulation, 68,* 763–766.

38. Milnor, W. R. (1968). Normal circulatory function. In V. B. Mountcastle (Ed.), *Medical physiology I* (pp. 118–133). St Louis: C. V. Mosby.

39. Moss, A. J., & Vigen, R. T. (1976). A new type sphygmomanometer valve. *Journal of the American Medical Association, 236,* 1880.

40. National High Blood Pressure Education Program Working Group. (1993). Report on primary prevention of hypertension. *Archives of Internal Medicine, 153,* 186–208.

41. Peters, R. K., Cady, L. D., Bischoff, D. P., Bernstein, L., & Pike, M. C. (1983). Physical fitness and subsequent myocardial infarction in healthy workers. *Journal of the American Medical Association 249,* 3052–3056.

42. Pollock, M. L., Wilmore, J. H., & Fox, S. M. (1978). *Health and fitness through physical activity.* Santa Barbara, CA: John Wiley & Sons.

43. Powell, K. E., Thompson, P. D., Caspersen, C. J., & Kendrick, J. S. (1987). Physical activity and the incidence of coronary heart disease. *Annual Review of Public Health, 8,* 253–287.

44. Robinson, T. E., Sue, D. Y., Huszczuk, A., Weiler-Ravell, D., & Hansen, J. E. (1988). Intra-arterial and cuff blood pressure responses during incremental cycle ergometry. *Medicine and Science in Sports and Exercise, 20,* 142–149.

45. Slattery, M. L., Jacobs, D. R., & Nichaman, M. Z. (1989). Leisure time physical activity and coronary heart disease death: The U.S. railroad study. *Circulation 79,* 304–311.

46. Task Force on Blood Pressure Control in Children. (1977). Report of the task force on blood pressure control in children. *Pediatrics 59* (Suppl.), 797–820.

47. Task Force on Blood Pressure Control in Children. (1987). Report of the task force on blood pressure control in children. *Pediatrics, 79,* 1–25.

48. Webster, J., Newnham, D., Petrie, J. C., & Lovell, H. G. (1984). Influence of arm position on measurement of blood pressure. *British Medical Journal, 288,* 1574–1575.

49. Walther, R. J., Tifft, C. P. (1985, March). High blood pressure in the competitive athlete: Guidelines and recommendations. *The Physician and Sportsmedicine,* pp. 93–114.

50. WHO/ISH. (1983). Guidelines for the treatment of mild hypertension. Memorandum from a WHO/ISH meeting. *Hypertension, 5,* 394–397.

51. Wilmore, J. H., & Costill, D. L. (1994). *Physiology of sport and exercise.* Champaign, IL: Human Kinetics.

Form RB 1

Individual Data for Resting Blood Pressure

Name: TOYA HART   Date: 11-1-99   Time: 2:30   a.m. ☐ p.m. ✓

Age: 23 y   Gender (M or F): F   Ht ☐ cm   Wt ☐ kg

Meteorological Data

Temperature (T) ☐ °C   RH ☐ % P_B ☐ torr

Blood Pressure Data

Arm circumference ☐ cm   Cuff Type: Large adult ☐ Adult ✓ Child ☐

Body Position: Seated ✓   Supine ☐   Standing ☐   Arm: Rt ✓ Left ☐

Auscultatory Method of Sphygmomanometry

Aneroid:

1st 118 / 4th 98 / 5th 78 mm Hg

Mercury:

1st ☐ / 4th ☐ / 5th ☐ mm Hg

$PP = SP$ [1st 118] $- DP$ [5th 78] $=$ 40 mm Hg

$MBP = [(SP$ [1st 118] $- DP$ [5th 78] $)/3] + DP$ [5th 78] mm Hg

$SP - DP$ (or PP)

$= ($ 40 $)/3 + DP$ [5th 78]

$(SP - DP)/3$

$=$ 13.3 $+ DP$ [5th 78] $=$ 91.3 mm Hg

Additional Measurement: 1st 118 / 4th 94 / 5th 82 mm Hg   1st ☐ / 4th ☐ / 5th ☐ mm Hg

Average of two measurements: 1st 118 / 4th 96 / 5th 80 mm Hg   %tile ☐ Table 4

Auscultatory gap: ☐ Yes ☒ No

Irregular pulse: ☐ Yes ☒ No

Form *RB 2*

Group Data for Resting Blood Pressure (mm Hg)

	MEN				WOMEN		
Initials	Systolic	Diastolic		Initials	Systolic	Diastolic	
		4th	5th			4th	5th
1.				1.			
2.				2.			
3.				3.			
4.				4.			
5.				5.			
6.				6.			
7.				7.			
8.				8.			
9.				9.			
10.				10.			
11.				11.			
12.				12.			
13.				13.			
14.				14.			
15.				15.			
16.				16.			
17.				17.			
18.				18.			
19.				19.			
20.				20.			
M				*M*			

Chapter EB   Exercise Blood Pressure

It is just as important to measure blood pressure at exercise as it is to measure heart rate. If only heart rate is measured, blood pressure is neglected as a contributor to the total power output of the heart. The consideration of both heart rate and blood pressure provides a better estimate of myocardial oxygen consumption than heart rate alone and the calculation of the rate-pressure product provides an indication of the heart's power output.[11,32]

The measurement of systolic pressure during progressive exercise may provide input toward diagnosing heart disease,[50] and, possibly, reveal potential problems in those persons who show exaggerated increases in exercise blood pressure despite being normotensive under a resting body state.[16,30,31] Conversely, decreases in systolic blood pressure despite increases in exercise intensity, may be clinically significant if accompanied by cardiac ischemia or angina (pain).[2]

The pulse pressure—the difference between systolic and diastolic pressure—provides the basis for calculating mean pressure at exercise. Lastly, the measurement of blood pressure during recovery from exercise may lead to the prevention of syncope in the performer.

Physiological Rationale

Numerous factors may affect blood pressure at exercise. These may include characteristics of the performers, such as their age, muscle mass, fitness level, and smoking status. Also, the type of exercise may affect blood pressure.[51] For example, weight lifting would be expected to increase blood pressure more than rhythmical aerobic exercise such as cycling or walking. Differences are found even among types of aerobic exercise; cycling, for example, elicits higher blood pressures than treadmill exercise.[27,42] Additionally, the exercise protocol itself may affect the rate of increase and absolute levels of blood pressure during exercise.

Blood pressure is mainly a function of cardiac output and peripheral resistance. In general, the increase in blood pressure during exercise is due to the increased cardiac output. Despite a decrease in peripheral resistance due to dilation of muscle arterioles, the increased cardiac output more than makes up for the decreased peripheral resistance.

Blood Pressure During Aerobic Exercise

Systolic pressure is expected to increase rather linearly,[4,48] and diastolic pressure changes very little, if at all, during progressive aerobic exercise (Fig. 1)[10,13,14] when measured by noninvasive sphygmomanometry.

Mean blood pressure (MBP) is calculated from pulse pressure (PP). At rest it may be estimated from the traditional calculation as one-third the distance from fifth-phase diastolic to systolic pressure. However, the mean pressure at exercise appears to be higher than that which is produced by the traditional equation. Thus, it may be more valid to use Equation 1, which uses one-half the distance between cuff-determined fifth-phase diastolic pressure and systolic pressure, as the mean pressure.[48]

$$\text{MBP (mm Hg)} = (SP - DP)/2 + DP \text{ or}$$
$$= (PP/2) + DP \qquad \text{Eq. 1}$$

The traditional calculation of mean pressure as one-third the distance between systolic and diastolic pressure appears to be justified also for estimating mean pressure during recovery from exercise.[48]

The Interaction of Heart Rate and Blood Pressure

As mentioned previously, the heart is affected by both its rate of pumping ($b\cdot min^{-1}$) and the force or resistance (mm Hg) it has to pump against. This power output of the heart is often referred to as either the **double product** or the **rate-pressure product (RPP)** because of the multiplication of the two factors, heart rate (HR) and systolic pressure (SP). The RPP, as calculated from Equation 2, is not meant to reflect differences in stroke volumes between individuals but is an accurate reflection of the myocardial oxygen requirement.[1,18] The product of HR and SP is divided by 100 in order to reduce the value to a convenient unit[47] and to agree closely with the oxygen consumption ($ml\cdot min^{-1}$) of the heart. The *rate* of myocardial fiber shortening is another important factor that is not included in the derived RPP.[21]

$$RPP = (HR \times SP)/100 \text{ or} \qquad \text{Eq. 2}$$
$$= HR \times SP \times 10^{-2}$$

where:

$$HR = \text{heart rate } (b\cdot min^{-1})$$
$$SP = \text{systolic pressure (mm Hg)}$$

For example, if the heart rate is 150 $b\cdot min^{-1}$ and systolic pressure is 200 mm Hg during exercise, then the RPP may be calculated as

$$(150 \times 200)/100 = 30,000/100 = 300$$

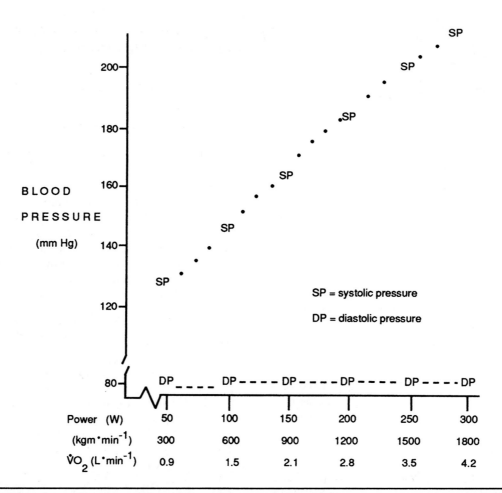

Figure 1 Relationship between systolic and fifth phase diastolic blood pressures versus exercise intensity in a typical 70-kg man.

Accuracy of Exercise Blood Pressure Measurements

Validity

The ability to measure exercise blood pressure accurately is complicated by the noise of the equipment and movement of the performer. Although the indirect noninvasive measurement of **systolic pressure** has been reported to be satisfactory,[41] it appears that the noninvasive cuff method of measuring systolic pressure underestimates the invasive direct measure of systolic pressure anywhere from 8 mm Hg[26,39] up to 11 mm Hg[48] or 15 mm Hg[26] during aerobic exercise.

One group of investigators[48] found that the intra-arterial **diastolic pressures** exceeded the noninvasive fourth and fifth phases for diastolic pressure by 5 and 13 mm Hg, respectively. This supports the use of the indirectly measured fourth phase as the most valid diastolic pressure during exercise. Their correlations between intra-arterial pressures and cuff pressures were .95 and .84 for systolic and diastolic (fourth phase) pressures, respectively. However, the fourth phase is not as clearly distinguishable as the fifth phase.

One group of reviewers recommended manual or automated sphygmomanometry to measure systolic pressure if the goal is to estimate the rate-pressure product.[22]

Reliability

Although various investigators have not supported high reliabilities in automated blood pressure methods,[5,6,35,44] including the measurement of diastolic blood pressure during recovery,[31] some have concluded that a few automated devices are a suitable alternative to human auscultatory methods.[22,36]

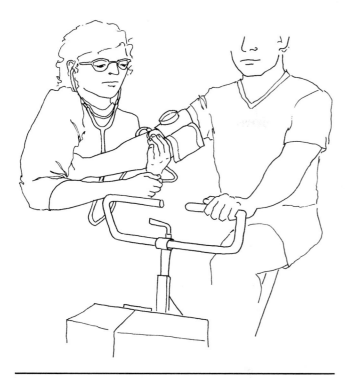

Figure 2 An appropriate position for the technician and performer while blood pressure is being measured at preexercise or during exercise.

Method

The measurement of blood pressure during exercise is one of the most common tests in an exercise laboratory. However, the technique is one of the most difficult to master, requiring many trials before the technician becomes confident. Although standards exist for measuring *resting* blood pressure, no such standards exist for *exercise* blood pressure.[22]

As expected, there are many similarities between the measurement of blood pressure at rest and at exercise. The differences include minor adjustments to the blood pressure technique and a more intense concentration on the fourth phase (muffling). During exercise it is not unusual for the vibrations to be heard even near zero levels[37] due to enhanced vasodilation at exercise.[19] Thus, fifth phase is not a valid indicator of diastolic pressure during exercise tests in many people. For this reason, the American Heart Association recommends the recording of fourth phase for exercise testing.[20]

If the subject tenses the arm while the technician is taking blood pressure, it will cause large oscillations in the aneroid pointer or the mercury column. Presumably, this is due to the change in upper arm circumference as the muscles contract. Thus, it is very important to promote muscle relaxation of the subject's arm (Fig. 2). Also, it is important to clear the antecubital space for the placement of the stethoscope's diaphragm. Sometimes the cuff will slide towards the elbow during exercise, or the bladder's rubber tubes will interfere with the antecubital space. Some researchers advise placing the cuff so that the tubing runs along the back of the upper arm rather than the front, especially during treadmill exercise.

Contraindicative Blood Pressure

Another consideration in measuring blood pressure at exercise is whether to perform the exercise test in the first place. Some authorities suggest that exercise testing is contraindicated (not recommended) if systolic is greater than 180 or diastolic greater than 100.[45] The American College of Sports Medicine (1995) takes a more liberal view by having no **absolute** contraindication criteria for blood pressure, but providing **relative** contraindicative criteria. This means that if resting systolic pressures are greater than 200 mm Hg or diastolic pressures are greater than 115 mm Hg, then the risk-benefit ratio must be evaluated before exercise testing.[2]

Protocol for Exercise Blood Pressure

Three separate protocols are presented in Table 1. In order to prescribe an appropriate exercise protocol, consideration should be given to the subject's fitness level. The prescription can be based upon prior tests of aerobic or physical power on the prospective performer. An exercise interval of 3 min should assure a steady state at each stage.[37] The exercise period starts at either 50, 75, or 100 W (300, 450, or 600 kg·m min^{-1}) depending upon the fitness level of the performer. Power levels are increased by 50 W after each 3-min time interval. Until the technician gains considerable confidence, repeated measures should be taken throughout the test; only the pressures measured at the last 30 s of each power interval, however, need to be recorded.

Summary of Procedures

The major differences in the technique for measuring blood pressure at exercise versus that at rest are the following: (a) the technician must support the exerciser's arm; (b) greater listening concentration is required due to the noise of the ergometer; and (c) the muffling point (fourth phase) is used often as the primary indicator of diastolic pressure at exercise.[48,52] The procedural steps for measuring blood pressure are as follows:

1. Obtain baseline blood pressures by measuring first-, fourth-, and fifth-phase pressures while the participant is resting on the cycle ergometer (or standing on the treadmill).
   a. With the cuff around the participant's arm, place that arm between your elbow and the side of your body (Fig. 2).
   b. Instruct the participant to relax the arm as much as possible.
   c. While taking the pressure, maintain the participant's arm in an extended position.

Table 1 Cycling Protocol for Exercise Blood Pressure

	Preexercise		
Seated on cycle ergometer			
	Exercise		
	Low-Power	**Moderate-Power**	**High-Power**
$\dot{V}O_2$max (L·min^{-1}) History	<2.1	2.1–2.9	>2.9
Time	**Power Prescription (W)**		
0:00–3:00	50	75	100
3:00–6:00	100	125	150
6:00–9:00	150	175	200
	Recovery		
9:00–12:00 Cool-down on ergometer	25	50	75
11:00–14:00	Seated in Chair		

Table 2 Comparative Blood Pressure Values at Submaximal Exercise, Maximal Exercise, and Recovery

	Systolic (mm Hg)	Diastolic (mm Hg)	
Submaximal Exercise		**4th Phase**	**5th Phase**
Cycling			
Normotense:	<200	~↑	↔ ~↑ ~↓
	10–18 per 50 W↑	7–11 per $\dot{V}O_2$ L·min^{-1}↑	
	30 per $\dot{V}O_2$ L·min^{-1}↑	~5 per 50 W↑	
Hypotense:	↓ with P increase		
	↓ >15 at given P		
Hypertense:	> normotense ↑		↑ >10–15
Treadmill			
Normotense:	7–10 per MET↑	↑ < cycling	
Hypertense:	>20 per MET↑		
Maximal Exercise			~↑
Normotense:			
General Population	150–250		
Young Adults:	150–250; 200		
Treadmill			
Active M (44 y)	190 ± 23		
Sedentary M (45 y)	185 ± 22		
Active W (42 y)	159 ± 19		
Sedentary W (48 y)	166 ± 23		
Hypertense:	220–230; ↑ >96	95; ↑ >15	
Hypotense:	↓ with P ↑; ↑ <33 from rest to max		
Recovery	Return to pre-exercise level within 5–8 min; possibly < pre-exercise up to 60–90 min		

Note: ~ = slight; ↑ = increase; ↔ = no change; ↓ = decrease; P = power level; M = men; W = women or watts.

d. Especially for treadmill exercise, tape or strap the stethoscope's diaphragm and the BP cuff to the performer's arm; you may need to remove the air bulb.
2. Use step #1 procedures for taking blood pressure during exercise, but allow cuff pressure to fall about 5–6 s per beat per second.[43]
3. Follow the exercise protocol for cycle ergometry (Table 1).
4. Record the blood pressure that was taken during the last 30 seconds of each exercise level.
5. Auscultatory heart rate may be taken during these times in order to calculate rate-pressure product.
6. Measure blood pressure during the last 30 s of the 3-min cool-down period while the performer pedals at 25, 50, or 75 W.

7. Measure blood pressure during the last 30 s of the 3-min recovery period while the subject is seated in a chair.
8. Graph blood pressures (mean pressure optional) on Form EB 3.

Results and Discussion

Various criteria and expectations for exercise blood pressure are presented in Table 2 for comparative purposes. The table is organized into submaximal and maximal levels of exercise intensity, in addition to recovery from exercise.

198 Exercise Blood Pressure EB-4

Blood Pressure at Submaximal Aerobic Exercise

Theoretically, **systolic pressure** is expected to increase somewhat linearly during aerobic cycling by approximately 10 mm Hg[38] or 15 mm Hg[4] for each 50 W (300 kg·m min^{-1}) increase in cycling power level. One group of investigators found a rate of increase of 27 mm Hg per 50 W based on a 30 mm Hg increase per liter increase in oxygen consumption on less active subjects monitored by intra-arterial catheter.[48]

During treadmill exercise one might expect a 7–10 mm Hg increase per MET increase.[3] It would be unusual for exercise heart rate to exceed systolic pressure in young adults. A hypertensive response in treadmill exercise may be indicated when systolic pressure increases at a rate greater than 20 mm Hg per MET,[17] or per 0.25 L·min^{-1} oxygen consumption. If systolic pressure fails to increase at all with progressive exercise, at worst, it may be a sign of coronary artery disease[50] and, at least, a warning sign.[1]

More controversy exists regarding **diastolic pressure** changes than systolic pressure changes during exercise. Part of this controversy may be attributed to the method of measuring diastolic pressure. One group concluded that the noninvasive fifth-phase diastolic pressure decreases slightly from rest to heavy cycling by only 3 mm Hg, but the fourth-phase cuff pressure and intra-arterial diastolic pressure increases from rest through maximal cycling by about 7–11 mm Hg per liter of oxygen consumed or about 4–6 mm Hg per 50 W.[48]

Some report actual decreases in diastolic pressure with progressive exercise in highly fit persons.[10,40] However, this decrease appears to be more characteristic of fifth phase than fourth phase. Others claim that a normal fifth-phase diastolic pressure response to exercise is one that does not increase by more than 10[16] to 15 mm Hg,[50] or that during treadmill exercise many healthy persons show slight increases in diastolic pressure of no more than 10 mm Hg during the first couple of minutes, followed by a progressive reduction into the peak exercise period.[12] Others reported a slight decrease or no change in diastolic pressure in healthy men during treadmill exercise.[53]

Blood Pressure at Maximal Aerobic Exercise

Quite often it is impossible to get a technically reliable blood pressure measurement while the performer is exercising at or near maximal intensity. In these cases, the blood pressure should be taken immediately after exercise with precautions taken to avoid postural syncope in the performer; usually, this would mean easy walking on the treadmill (or in-place) or easy pedalling on the ergometer. It is possible that by waiting to take blood pressure immediately after exercise, rather than during exercise, the peak blood pressure may be slightly underestimated.[28]

Maximal systolic pressure can be quite variable, ranging from 150 to 250 mm Hg in men and women,[10] with an average in a normal young person about 200 mm Hg.[24] This concurs with other investigators who found a maximal systolic pressure of 194 (±20) mm Hg for running on the treadmill.[15] Normotensive middle-aged persons reach maximal systolic pressures between 180 and 190 mm Hg.[11] If systolic blood pressure exceeds 240 mm Hg, it may indicate a susceptibility for developing resting hypertension.[33]

Sometimes during an exercise test, the blood pressure may reach a level that calls for termination of the test. A value greater than 260 mm Hg is a **relative** indication by ACSM for stopping the test,[2] and is the same value recommended by another investigator[17] as an **absolute** indicator for stopping the test. This is considerably higher than the 220 recommended by another researcher.[12] Ruptures have occurred in the blood vessels of experimental animals when systolic pressures were between 260 and 280 mm Hg.[25] Others suggest caution and consider it a hypertensive response if the systolic pressure exceeds 220 mm Hg.[9,12] Some consider the exercise response as hypertensive if the systolic pressure increases by more than 96 mm Hg from the resting level, and as hypotensive if the systolic pressure does not increase more than 33 mm Hg.[46]

Caution may be prudent when the subject's exercise **diastolic pressure** reaches 95 mm Hg.[9] However, the ACSM's (1995) relative indication for halting the test is when DP exceeds 115 mm Hg.[2]

Typical **mean** arterial pressures at maximal exercise are approximately 130 mm Hg, or may reach as high as 155 mm Hg.[10]

Blood Pressure During Recovery from Aerobic Exercise

Blood pressure often returns to the preexercise level within 5–8 min after the cessation of moderate exercise.[29,38,49] It is not unusual for systolic pressure to drop slightly lower than the preexercise systolic pressure.[7,23,24,34] For example, from the 5th to the 60th,[33] or up to the 90th min[7] of recovery from treadmill walking exercise, systolic blood pressure was slightly lower (8–12 mm Hg) than it was preceding exercise, possibly due to endorphin-like (opioid) effects.[8] Usually, recovery diastolic pressure is similar to preexercise. The return of blood pressure to resting levels is affected by the type, intensity, and duration of the original exercise in addition to the type of recovery. For example, it requires more than 3 min for blood pressure to return to normal after heavy cycling exercise (85% $\dot{V}O_2max$) if the cyclist recovers with unloaded pedalling at a slow rate.[48] However, if the performer were to stand upright immediately after the same exercise, it is quite possible that blood pressure would drop rapidly and drastically. Venous pooling of blood in the legs would reduce the blood flow to the brain and possibly lead to syncope.

Table 3 Comparative Values for the Rate-Pressure Product (RPP) at Maximal Exercise

Rate-Pressure Product (RPP; HR × SP/100)			
Men[46]	268–398	Active Men[11]	341 ± 45
Women[46]	240–348	Active Women[11]	281 ± 37

Rate-Pressure Product (RPP)

The classifications in Table 3 are rate-pressure products at maximal exercise in men and women of a wide age range.[11,46] The data from Bruce and his colleagues categorize the men (n = 2634) and women (n = 238) into active and sedentary groups.[11]

References

1. American College of Sports Medicine. (1991). *Guidelines for exercise testing and prescription.* Philadelphia: Lea & Febiger.
2. American College of Sports Medicine. (1995). *ACSM's Guidelines for exercise testing and prescription.* Philadelphia: Williams & Wilkins.
3. American Heart Association. (1975). *Exercise testing and training of individuals with heart disease or at high risk for its development: A handbook for physicians.* New York: Author.
4. Andersen, K. L., Shephard, R. J., Denolin, H., Varnauskas, E., & Masironi, R. (1971). *Fundamentals of exercise testing.* Geneva, Switzerland: World Health Organization.
5. Barker, W. F., Hediger, M. L., Katz, S. H., & Bowers, E. J. (1984). Concurrent validity studies of blood pressure instrumentation. *Hypertension, 6,* 85–91.
6. Becque, M. D., Katch, V., Marks, C., & Dyer, R. (1993). Reliability within subject variability of $\dot{V}E$, $\dot{V}O_2$, heart rate and blood pressure during submaximum cycle ergometry. *International Journal of Sports Medicine, 14,* 220–223.
7. Bennett, T., Wilcox, R. G., & MacDonald, I. A. (1984). Postexercise reduction of blood pressure in hypertensive men is not due to an acute impairment of baroreflex function. *Clinical Science, 67,* 97–103.
8. Boone, J. B., Levine, M., Flynn, M. G., Przza, F. Y., Kubitz, E. R., & Andres, F. F. (1992). Opioid receptor modulation of postexercise hypotension. *Medicine and Science in Sports and Exercise, 24,* 1108–1113.
9. Boyer, J. (1976, December). Exercise and hypertension. *The Physician and Sportsmedicine,* pp. 35–49.
10. Brooks, G. A., & Fahey, T. D. (1984). *Exercise physiology: Human bioenergetics and its application.* New York: John Wiley & Sons.
11. Bruce, R. A. (1977). Current concepts in cardiology: Exercise testing for evaluation of ventricular function. *The New England Journal of Medicine, 296,* 671–675.
12. Chung, E. K. (1983). *Exercise electrocardiography—A practical approach.* Baltimore, MD: Waverly Press.
13. Clarke, D. H. (1975). *Exercise physiology.* Englewood Cliffs, NJ: Prentice-Hall.
14. deVries, H. A. (1986). *Physiology of exercise for physical education and athletics.* Dubuque, IA: Wm. C. Brown.
15. Dishman, R. K., Patton, R. W., Smith, J., Weinberg, R., & Jackson, A. (1987). Using perceived exertion to prescribe and monitor exercise training heart rate. *International Journal of Sports Medicine, 8,* 208–213.
16. Dlin, R. A., Hanne, N., Silverberg, D. S., & Bar-Or, O. (1983). Follow-up of normotensive men with exaggerated blood pressure response to exercise. *American Heart Journal, 106,* 316–320.
17. Dressendorfer, R. H. (1980, July). ACSM workshop manual, 110.
18. Edington, D. W., & Cunningham, L. (1975). *Biological awareness.* Englewood Cliffs, NJ: Prentice-Hall.
19. Frohlich, E. D., Grim, C., Labarthe, D. R., Maxwell, M. H., Perloff, D., & Weidman, W. H. (1987). *Recommendations for human blood pressure determination by sphygmomanometers: Report of a special task force appointed by the steering committee, American Heart Association.* Dallas: National Center, American Heart Association.
20. Frohlich, E. D., Grim, C., Labarthe, D. R., Maxwell, M. H., Perloff, D., & Weidman, W. H. (1988). Recommendations for human blood pressure determination by sphygmomanometers: Report of a special task force appointed by the steering committee. *Hypertension, 11,* 210A–222A.
21. Gianelly, R. E., Goldman, R. H., Treister, B., & Harrison, D. C. (1967). Propranolol in patients with angina pectoris. *Annals of Internal Medicine, 67,* 1216–1224.
22. Griffin, S. A., Robergs, R. A., & Heyward, V. H. (1997). Blood pressure measurement during exercise: A review. *Medicine and Science in Sports and Exercise, 29,* 149–159.
23. Hannum, S. M., & Kasch, F. W. (1981). Acute postexercise blood pressure response of hypertensive and normotensive men. *Scandinavian Journal of Sport Science, 3,* 11–15.
24. Hayberg, J. M., Montain, S. J., & Martin, W. H. (1987). Blood pressure and hemodynamic responses after exercise in older hypertensives. *Journal of Applied Physiology, 63,* 270–276.
25. Hellerstein, H. K. (1976, August). Exercise tests inadequate for cardiac patients. *The Physician and Sportsmedicine,* pp. 58–62.

26. Henschel, A., De la Vega, F., & Taylor, H. L. (1954). Simultaneous direct and indirect blood pressure measurements in man at rest and work. *Journal of Applied Physiology, 6,* 506–512.

27. Hermansen, L., Ekblom, B., & Saltin, B. (1970). Cardiac output during submaximal and maximal treadmill and bicycle exercise. *Journal of Applied Physiology, 29,* 82–86.

28. Hollingsworth, V., Bendick, P., & Franklin, B. (1988). Validity of postexercise arm ergometer blood pressures? *Medicine and Science in Sports and Exercise, 20,* (Suppl. 2), Abstract #435, S73.

29. Hyman, A. S. (1971). Cardiorespiratory endurance. In ACSM (Eds.), *Encyclopedia of sport sciences and medicine* (pp. 1067–1070). New York: MacMillan.

30. Jette, M., Landry, F., Sidney, K., & Blumchen, G. (1988). Exaggerated blood pressure response to exercise in the detection of hypertension. *Journal of Cardiopulmonary Rehabilitation, 8,* 171–177.

31. Jette, M., Landry, F., Tiemann, B., & Blumchen, G. (1991). Ambulatory blood pressure and Holter monitoring during tennis play. *Canadian Journal of Sport Science, 16,* 40–44.

32. Jorgensen, C. R. (1972). Physical training and myocardial function. *New England Journal of Medicine, 287,* 104–105.

33. Kaplan, N. M., Deveraux, R. B., & Miller, H. S. (1994). Systemic hypertension. *Medicine and Science in Sports and Exercise, 26*(10): S268–S270.

34. Kaufman, F. L., Hughson, R. L., & Schaman, J. P. (1987). Effect of exercise on recovery blood pressure in normotensive and hypertensive subjects. *Medicine and Science in Sports and Exercise, 19,* 17–20.

35. LaBarthe, D. R. (1976). New instruments for measuring blood pressure. *Drugs, 11,* (Suppl. I), 48–51.

36. Lightfoot, J. T., Tankersley, C., Rowe, S. A., Freed, A. N., & Fortney, S. M. (1989). Automated blood pressure measurements during exercise. *Medicine and Science in Sports and Exercise 21,* 698–707.

37. Lightfoot, J. T., Tuller, B., & Williams, D. F. (1996). Ambient noise interferes with auscultatory blood pressure measurement during exercise. *Medicine and Science in Sports and Exercise, 28,* 502–508.

38. Michael, E. D., Burke, E. J., & Avakian, E. V. (1979). *Laboratory experiments in exercise physiology.* Ithaca, NY: Mouvement Publications.

39. Morehouse L. E., & Miller, A. T. (1976). *Physiology of exercise.* St. Louis: C. V. Mosby Co.

40. Nagle, F. J. (1975, May). Conducting the progressive exercise test. Symposium at the 22nd Annual American College of Sports Medicine Convention, New Orleans.

41. Nagle, F. J., Naughton, J., & Balke, B. (1966). Comparison of direct and indirect blood pressure with pressure-flow dynamics during exercise. *Journal of Applied Physiology, 21,* 317–320.

42. Niederberger, M., Bruce, R., Kusumi, F., & Whitkanack, S. (1974). Disparities in ventilatory and circulatory responses to bicycle and treadmill exercise. *British Heart Journal, 36,* 377–382.

43. Nieman, D. C. (1995). *Fitness and sports medicine: A health-related approach.* Palo Alto, CA: Bull Publishing.

44. O'Brien, E., Fitzgerald, D., & O'Malley, K. (1985). Blood pressure measurement: Current practice and future trends. *British Medical Journal, 290,* 729–733.

45. Pollock, M. L., Wilmore, J. H., & Fox, S. M. (1978). *Health and fitness through physical activity.* Santa Barbara, CA: John Wiley & Sons.

46. Pyfer, H. R., Mead, W. F., Frederick, R. C., & Doane, B. L. (1976). Exercise rehabilitation in coronary heart disease: Community group programs. *Archives of Physical Medicine and Rehabilitation, 57,* 335–342.

47. Robinson, B. F. (1967). Relation of heart rate and systolic blood pressure to the onset of pain in angina pectoris. *Circulation, 35,* 1073–1083.

48. Robinson, T. E., Sue, D. Y., Huszczuk, A., Weiler-Ravell, D., & Hansen, J. E. (1988). Intra-arterial and cuff blood pressure responses during incremental cycle ergometry. *Medicine and Science in Sports and Exercise, 20,* 142–149.

49. Ruddell, H., Berg, K., Todd, G. L., McKinney, M. E., Buell, T. C., & Eliot, R. S. (1985). Cardiovascular reactivity and blood chemical changes during exercise. *Journal of Sports Medicine, 25,* 111–119.

50. Sheps, D. S., Ernst, J. C., Briese, F. W., & Myerburg, R. J. (1979). Exercise-induced increase in diastolic pressure: Indicator of severe coronary artery disease. *The American Journal of Cardiology, 43,* 708–712.

51. Tuxen, D. V., Sutton, J., Upton, A., Sexton, A., McDougal, D., & Sale, D. (1983). Brainstem injury following maximal weight lifting attempts [Abstract]. *Medicine and Science in Sports and Exercise, 15,* 158.

52. Walther, R. J., & Tifft, C. P. (1985, March). High blood pressure in the competitive athlete: Guidelines and recommendations. *The Physician and Sportsmedicine,* pp. 93–114.

53. Wolthius, R. A., Froelicker, V. F., Fischer, J., & Triehwasser, J. H. (1977). The response of healthy men to treadmill exercise. *Circulation, 55,* 153–157.

Form EB 1

Individual Data for Exercise Blood Pressure

Name: _Toya Hart_   Date: _11-8-99_   Time: ___ a.m. ___ p.m.

Age: _23_ y   Gender (M or F): _F_   Ht: _173_ cm   Wt: _63.6_ kg

Temperature (T): _21.8_ °C   RH: _46_ % P_B: _749_ torr

Mode (check): Bike ___   Other ___   Bike Model ___   Seat Ht ___

Prior Test Score(s): $\dot{V}O_2max$ ___ L·min⁻¹   ___ L·min⁻¹

Time	Power W	Systolic Pressure ✓ (SP)	Diastolic Pressure 4th Phase (DP-4th)	5th Phase ✓ (DP-5th)	Pulse Pressure (PP)	Heart Rate (HR)	Rate-Pressure Product (RPP)
Preexercise (on bike)		120	84	80	40	101	121.2
Exercise		120	80	70			
2:30–3:00	50	~~88~~	~~80~~	~~80~~	50	101	145.2
5:30–6:00	100	136	80	76	60	155	20.8
8:30–9:00	150	148	84	80	68	173	256.0
Recovery: Cool-Down							
11:30–12:00	25	122	84	80	42	127	154.7
In Chair Recovery							
14:30–15:00	0	120	80	80	40	101	121.2

Mean Blood Pressure (MBP)

Body State	Time	Pulse Pressure (PP)	PP/3 or /2	+ DP	= MBP
Preexercise		40	/3 = 13.3	+ 80	= 93.3
Exercise	8:30–9:00	68	/2 = 34	+ 80	= 114
Recovery	11:30–12:00	42	/3 = 14	+ 80	= 94
Recovery	14:30–15:00	40	/3 = 13.3	+ 80	= 93.3

MAP = (DBP + ⅓ PP) = MBP
PP = SBP - DBP
RPP = HR × SBP / 100

Form *EB 2*

Group Data for Exercise Blood Pressure

Power (W)	50			75			100			125			150			175			200		
							Blood Pressure (mm Hg; 1st, 4th, and 5th phases)														
Initials	1st	4th	5th	1st	4th	5th	1st	4th	5th	1st	4th	5th	1st	4th	5th	1st	4th	5th	1st	4th	5th
1.																					
2.																					
3.																					
4.																					
5.																					
6.																					
7.																					
8.																					
9.																					
10.																					
11.																					
12.																					
13.																					
14.																					
15.																					
16.																					
17.																					
M																					

Form *EB 3*

Graph of Blood Pressure (BP) before, during, and after Cycling

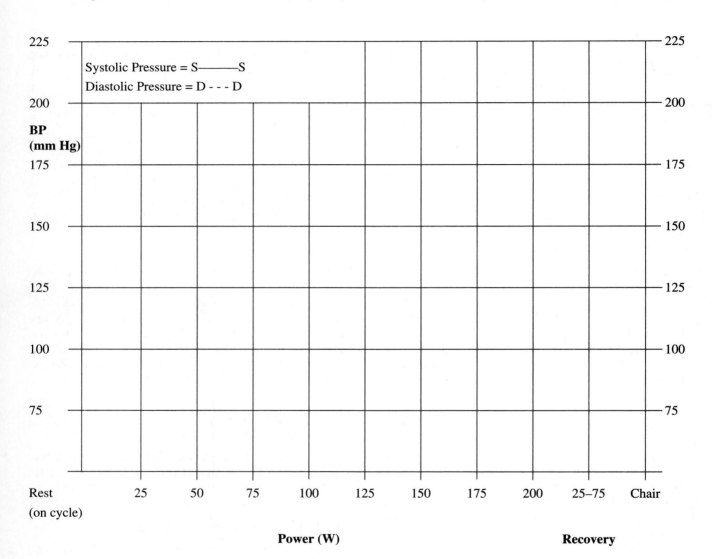

Systolic Pressure = S———S
Diastolic Pressure = D - - - D

BP (mm Hg) axis: 225, 200, 175, 150, 125, 100, 75

X-axis: Rest (on cycle), 25, 50, 75, 100, 125, 150, 175, 200, 25–75, Chair

Power (W)   **Recovery**

Chapter RE — Resting Electrocardiogram

The diagnosis of the electrocardiogram (ECG) is one of the most important and accurate evaluations of the quantity and quality of heartbeats. Although 4 million electrocardiograms may have been interpreted by computer in the United States in 1975, that still leaves 76 million that were interpreted by the human brain.[9] An Englishman was the first (1887) to record electrical current from the human body's surface,[1,2] but it was a Dutchman, Willem Einthoven, who received the Nobel Prize in 1924 for his 1901 "elektrokardiograph" (EKG) because of his more sophisticated instrument and his publications on electrocardiography.[4]

Physiological Rationale

The rationale for the ECG is based upon the heart's generation of an electrical current (force or voltage) which is then transferred to the skin through the body's salty fluid medium. The voltage from an ordinary flashlight battery is about 1500 times greater than the skin's voltage.[10] The electrodes (leads), which are placed on the skin, transfer this current from the skin to the electrocardiograph (the machine), where it is then recorded on special graph paper (electrocardiogram). Generally, when the current moves from the negative electrode to the positive electrode an upright deflection (positive wave) occurs on the graph paper. When the current moves from the positive electrode to the relatively negative electrode, a downward deflection or negative wave is recorded. When there is no movement of the current or when it is moving perpendicular to the two electrodes, the tracing is termed isoelectric; this means that there is neither a positive nor negative deflection, thus remaining at baseline (Fig. 1).[15]

The descriptions of the basic ECG waves and segments are presented in Table 1 and Figure 2. Einthoven arbitrarily assigned alphabetical letters to the waves of the ECG, starting with the middle of the alphabet to avoid confusion with vitamins.

To interpret the electrocardiogram, one must first understand the meaning of the graph paper when it is being recorded upon at standard operating speed (25 mm·s⁻¹). A magnified section of ECG paper is presented in Figure 3. The bold vertical lines divide the graph into 5-mm or 0.2-s sections. Each thin vertical line represents 1 mm or 0.04 s. The horizontal lines represent voltages; the divisions between the bold lines represent 5 mm or 0.5 mv. The thin horizontal lines divide the graph into 1-mm or 0.1-mv sections.

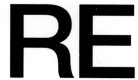

Calibration of Electrocardiograph

The grid lines enable the technician to calibrate the electrocardiograph during the recording of each lead at rest and immediately prior to the ECG exercise test. This is done by pressing the calibration button (1.0 mv) while the paper is moving. The rectangular deflection wave should be 10 mm (1 cm) high; if it is not, then the sensitivity control should be adjusted until a 10-mm wave is elicited. The 10-mm deflection should not shift more than 3.7 mm toward baseline when the button is held for 3.2 s.

Method

The technician should work calmly and unhurriedly; this will relax the subject and provide an adequate rest period prior to the recording. While attaching the electrodes, the technician should set the subject at ease by a calm, informal, yet professional manner. The technician need not interpret the tracing during testing unless an exercise ECG test immediately follows. In general, save interpretation for a later time when it can be studied carefully.

Lead Nomenclature, Sites, and Skin Preparation

Leads may be classified anatomically into six limb (extremity) leads and six chest (precordial) leads. Also, they may be classified electronically, as bipolar standard (limb) leads or unipolar (augmented and chest) leads.

Bipolar Standard Leads (I, II, and III)

Bipolar leads represent the difference in electric potential between two sites and are recorded in the frontal plane (anterior surface of thorax). The negative electrode is placed on the right arm (RA; medial wrist). The positive electrodes are on the left arm (LA; medial wrist) and leg (LL; medial lower leg just above ankle) for leads I and II, respectively. The left arm is relatively negative to the positive left leg in lead III. The ground electrode is placed on the right leg (RL). Table 2 summarizes the standard lead configuration.

Augmented Extremity Leads (aVR, aVL, and aVF)

All modern electrocardiographs automatically record unipolar augmented leads. The term *augmented* means that the amplitude of the waves is 50% greater than an older

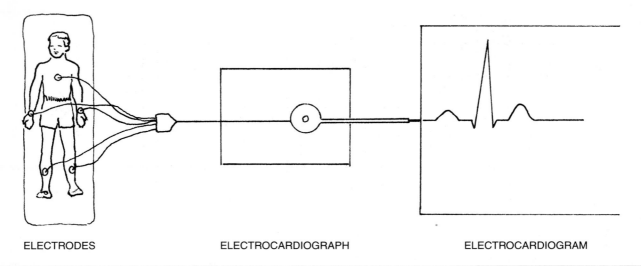

ELECTRODES　　　　　ELECTROCARDIOGRAPH　　　　　ELECTROCARDIOGRAM

Figure 1　Interfacing the heart with the ECG: The electrical currents from the heart are amplified by the electrocardiograph and recorded as the electrocardiogram.

Table 1 Basic ECG Waves, Complexes, Intervals, and Segments

Waves
P: The small, dome-shaped positive wave that represents the stimulus for atrial contraction; depolarization; atrial activation.
Q: A little negative wave that initiates depolarization, the stimulus for contraction, of the ventricles.
R: The large, triangular-shaped positive wave of ventricular depolarization.
S: The negative wave of ventricular depolarization.
T: A medium-sized, dome-shaped positive wave representing repolarization of the ventricles; the stimulus for the ventricles to relax.

Complex
QRS: The three waves of ventricular depolarization; the beginning of the Q-wave to the end of the S-wave.

Intervals
Q–T: Ventricular systole; the beginning of the Q-wave to the end of the T-wave.

Segment
ST: This horizontal line represents the early phase of ventricular repolarization; normally it is isoelectric, meaning that it is at baseline; the end of the S-wave to the beginning of the T-wave; sensitive to ischemia.

PR: The end of the P-wave to the beginning of the Q-wave; technically, this segment should be called the P-Q segment.

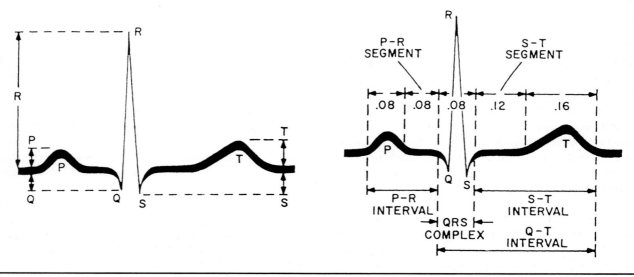

Figure 2　The basic waves and segments with their criteria for measuring: (a) Wave voltage amplitudes (mV) and (b) Interval or segment durations (s).

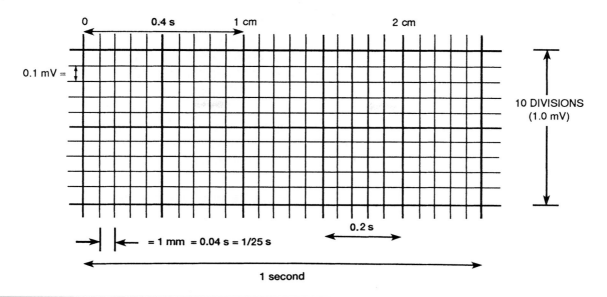

Figure 3 Magnified section of typical ECG paper.

Table 2 Standard Limb Lead Configuration and Sites

Lead	Site	Electrode Abbreviation	Electrode Color
I	Right (–) and left (+) arms	RA – LA	RA = white
			LA = black
II	Right arm (–) and left leg (+)	RA – LL	LL = red
			RL = green
III	Left arm (–) and left leg (+)	LA – LL	Chest = brown
Ground	Right leg	RL; G	

technique would produce. These three added limb leads essentially augment the three standard leads by connecting the standard leads to a common central lead and then viewing the current over the right (aVR) or left (aVL) shoulder or from the left leg (aVF).[4]

Chest Leads

These are often referred to as the unipolar precordial leads; the six leads are named from V_1 to V_6. In addition to Figure 4, Table 3 describes the sites for the six chest electrodes (V_{1-6} leads). Chest electrodes are positioned vertically relative to intercostal spaces (between ribs) and horizontally according to the sternum, clavicle, and axilla (armpit). The technician locates the chest electrode positions by firmly palpating the subject's chest along the vertical border of the sternum.

Electrode Site Preparation

The inner surfaces of the wrists and ankles are preferred for leads I, II, and III because of the relative absence of hair. The electrode site is wiped with an alcohol pad; light rubbing will help remove dry skin, dirt, and/or oil, which all act as insulators to current and thus are poor conductors of electricity.

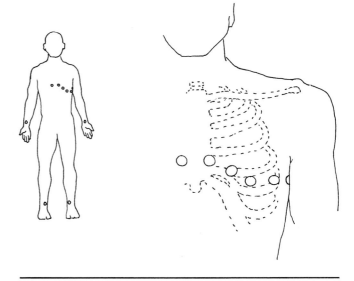

Figure 4 The typical electrode placement for the 12-lead system for resting ECG; for the exercise ECG, the limb electrodes are placed on the torso.

Table 3 Sites for Chest Precordial Electrodes

Chest Lead	Anatomical Site
V_1	4th intercostal space at *right* sternal margin
V_2	4th intercostal space at *left* sternal margin
V_3	Midpoint between V_2 and V_4
V_4	5th intercostal space at mid-clavicular line
V_5	Same horizontal level as V_4 at left anterior axillary line
V_6	Same horizontal level as V_4 and $_5$ at left mid-axillary line

Electrocardiograph Procedures

Einthoven's original 1901 electrocardiograph required five people to operate and was so large that it occupied two rooms. A subject's hands and left foot were placed into three buckets of a salt solution serving as electrodes. Since that time many types of electrocardiographs have been manufactured. Although electrocardiograph procedures may differ with different brands, the following procedures apply to most single-channel (one-lead-at-a-time) electrocardiographs. A multi-channel ECG tracing is depicted in Figure 5.

1. Turn on *power switch*. Only a few seconds of warmup is required due to the solid-state nature of electrocardiographs.
2. Turn lever of *amplifier* to On only after the person is connected to all limb (extremity; RA, LA, LL, and G) leads. Turning the amplifier on prior to these attachments will cause the stylus to swing wildly and possibly damage it.
3. *Print* the participant's name and the date on the ECG paper.
4. *Record* by shifting the Run lever to 25 so the paper will move at a speed of 25 mm/s; some machines can go to 50 mm/s but that is not the standard speed.
5. *Center* the ECG tracing with the Stylus Position control knob.
6. *Darken or lighten* the ECG tracing by adjusting the Stylus Heat screw with a screwdriver or strong fingernail.
7. *Standardize* the recording by pressing the Calibration-STD button. After the technician gains experience, the standardization process may be recorded while taking the actual ECG recordings of each lead. The standard deflection is placed between the T and P waves of two different cardiac cycles.
8. *Record* the 12 leads by rotating the Lead Selector knob; record for approximately 5 s at each lead except for lead II (the standard lead), which should be recorded for 12 s; lead II can then be used to calculate resting heart rate.
9. The vertical time lines enable the technician to calculate resting heart rate accurately. The 1-mm or 0.04-s vertical lines represent a minute rate of

1500 mm/min. Thus, if the number of millimeters from the peak of one R wave (spike) to the next cardiac cycle's R peak is 22 mm, then heart rate may be calculated from Equation 1 as follows:[5]

$$\text{HR (b/min)} = 1500 \, / \, \text{R-R mm} \qquad \text{Eq. 1}$$
$$= 1500 \, / \, 22$$
$$= 68 \text{ b/min to closest whole beat}$$

10. Technician pays particular attention to rate, rhythm, and ST segment.

Results and Discussion

The Surgeon General and others have declared that daily moderate physical activity is protective against cardiovascular disease and all-cause mortality.[3,13] Clinical exercise physiologists often administer ECG tests to high-risk persons in the United States who may be following the advice of the Surgeon General's *Physical Activity and Health* report[13] to increase their physical activity level. Three of the most basic variables encountered on an electrocardiogram are (1) heart rate, (2) heart rhythm, and (3) ST depression.

Heart Rate

Although the criteria for a normal resting ECG vary slightly with different investigators, those in Table 4[7] may serve as an appropriate guide. Persons with resting heart rates over 100 b·min^{-1} are in a state of tachycardia, whereas those with resting heart rates less than 60 b·min^{-1} are in bradycardia. Further divisions of bradycardia may be designated arbitrarily as depicted in Table 5.[8] However, sinus bradycardia often does not indicate a clinically abnormal state. Although Table 5 indicates that rates between 40 and 49 b·min^{-1} are categorized as moderate bradycardia,[8,14] reports[8] of trained distance runners having heart rates during waking hours of 43 (±5 b·min^{-1}) indicates a bradycardiac condition that is associated with normality.

The seated heart rates for men and women from the ages of 18 to over 65 y are presented in Table 6.[6] Because heart rate is not known to differ with age in adult persons, the original table has been reduced to a single age group. In general, the average man's heart rate (ranging from 66–71 b·min^{-1}) is slightly less than the average woman's (69–73 b·min^{-1}) heart rate. Although the original table of the YMCA publication attaches fitness categories to each heart rate range, this table simply provides non-qualitative categories such as "low," "average," and "high," based upon the original statistical separations that used qualitative categories such as "excellent" and "poor".

Heart Rhythm

When the rhythm of heart rate is irregular it is often referred to as arrhythmia. Usually ventricular premature beats

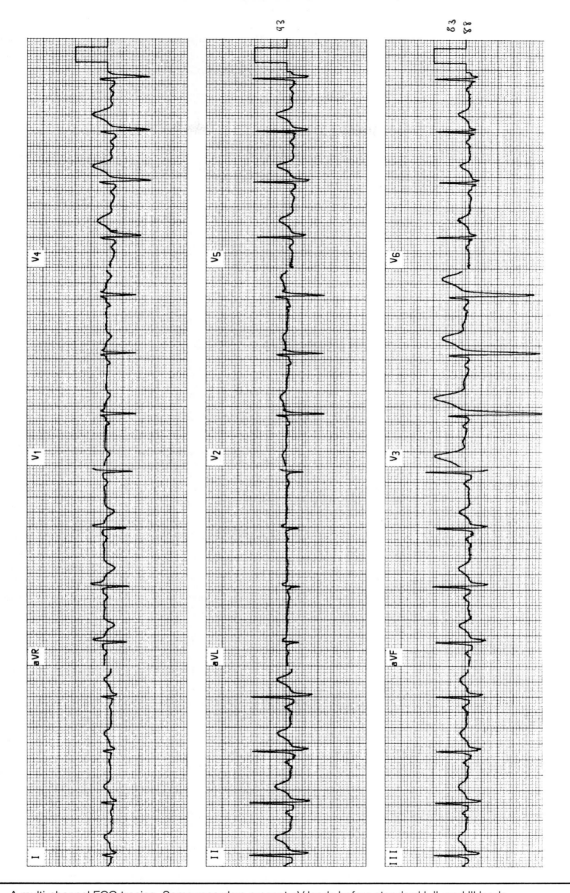

Figure 5 A multi-channel ECG tracing. Some recorders present aV leads before standard I, II, and III leads.

Table 4 Criteria for Normal in the Resting ECG

Component		Criteria	
HR	60–100 b·min^{-1}; regular sinus rhythm		
Waves	Amplitude (mV)	Polarity (+, –, or iso^a)	Duration (s)
P	<2–3	+: I, II, aVF, V_{2-6}	<0.11
Q		–: I–III, aVR, V_{5-6}	≤0.03
QRS (R)^b	<30 in II and V_5	+: 2 of 3 std leads	0.05–0.12
	>5 sum: I–III		
	>5: $V_{1\&6}$		
	>7: $V_{2\&5}$		
	>9: $V_{3\&4}$		
T	<5: I–III	+: I, II; –: aVR; often: III	
	<10: V_{1-6} -leads	+: V_{3-6} (not notched)	
Interval	Amplitude	Polarity	Duration
P-R (Q)		Isoelectric	0.12–0.20
Q-T		Mixed interval (+, –, iso)	0.30–0.43
Segment			
ST	0.0 relative to T-P segment	Isoelectric +: often $V_2 - V_4$	0.10–0.16

Note: ^{a}iso = isoelectric; baseline.
^{b}axis = –30° to +90°
Source: Data from Goldman, 1967. *Principles of Clinical Electrocardiography,* Lange Medical Pub., Los Altos, CA.

Table 5 Clinical Types of Bradycardia

Bradycardia Type	Heart Rate
Mild	50–59
Moderate	40–49
Severe; Pathologic	<40

Source: Based on statements by Kammerling, J. M. (1988). Sinus node dysfunction. In D. P. Zipes & D. J. Rowlands (Eds.), *Progress in cardiology: Arrhythmias, Part II* (p. 210). Philadelphia: Lea & Febiger.

Table 6 Summary of YMCA Norms for Resting Heart Rate (HR) in Men and Women Ages 18 to 65$^+$ y

Heart Rate Category	Heart Rates (b·min^{-1})	
	Men	Women
Low	49–57	54–60
Moderately Low	58–63	61–65
< Average	64–67	66–69
Average	68–71	70–73
> Average	72–76	74–78
Moderately High	77–83	79–84
High	84–98	85–99

Source: Based on data from Table in Chapter 4 of Golding, L. A., Myers, C. R., & Sinning, W. E. (1989). *Y's way to physical fitness: The complete guide to fitness testing and instruction.* Human Kinetics. Champaign, IL.

or contractions (VPB or VPC or PVC) are of greater concern than premature atrial (supraventricular) contractions (PAC). One hierarchy of VPB severity ranges from an absence of severity if no VPB occur in one hour, to a high severity if more than 30 VPB per hour occur; also, the severity increases if the form of the VPB is multiform (varying shape), then repetitive couplets (e.g., bigeminy), then to ventricular tachycardia (>3 consecutive VPB).[11]

ST Depression

The ST portion of the ECG is a segment that is often used to diagnose heart disease. It is measured from the baseline (isoelectric), which can be defined as a "line connecting two consecutive P-Q junctions."[12] If the whole segment is more than 1 mm below the isoelectric line, it could indicate ischemic heart disease. The final diagnosis should be that of a cardiologist.

References

1. Adrian, R. H., Channell, R. C., Cohen, L., & Noble, D. (1976, July). The Einthoven string galvanometer and the interpretation of the T-wave of the electrocardiogram. *Physiological Society,* pp. 67–70.

2. Besterman, E., & Creese, R. (1979). Waller—Pioneer of electrocardiography. *British Heart Journal, 42,* 61–64.

3. Blair, S. N., Kampert, J. B., Kohl, H. W., Barlow, C. E., Macera, C. A., Paffenbarger, R. S., & Gibbons, L. W. (1996). Influences of cardiorespiratory fitness and other precursors on cardiovascular disease and all-cause mortality in men and women. *JAMA, 276,* 205–210.

4. Brailey, A. G. (1978). Basic electrocardiography. In P. K. Wilson (Ed.), Cardiac rehabilitation and adult fitness (pp. 69–83). Cited in *Emphasie, 5* (2).

5. Fisher, A. G., & Jensen, C. R. (1990). *The scientific basis of athletic conditioning.* Philadelphia: Lea & Febiger.

6. Golding, L. A., Myers, C. R., & Sinning, W. E. (1989). *Y's way to physical fitness: The complete guide to*

Chapter EE Exercise Electrocardiogram

The Exercise ECG Test is popularly known as the **stress test.** Less intimidating names are the **Graded Exercise Test (GXT)** or the **Exercise Tolerance Test (ETT).** Whatever the name, the Exercise ECG Test incorporates many characteristics that have been discussed in some of the previous tests. For example, it includes the measurements of heart rate, blood pressure, and, sometimes, oxygen consumption. The primary distinction of this test over other tests is the recording of the electrical conductivity of the heart—the **electrocardiogram (ECG).** The Exercise ECG Test has the advantage over some other evaluations of the cardiovascular system in that it is noninvasive, nonradiative, and relatively inexpensive.

There are at least three objectives in taking the electrocardiogram during the exercise test: (1) to assure the safety of the performer during exercise testing and training, (2) to measure accurate heart rates, and (3) to diagnose the performer or patient for cardiovascular disease.

The first two objectives—safety and accurate heart-rate recordings—may be accomplished by nonmedical personnel. However, the Exercise ECG may not be warranted for all asymptomatic—no cardiovascular disease (CVD) symptoms—and apparently healthy persons. The American College of Cardiology and the *American Heart Association Guidelines* state that the Exercise ECG Test is not warranted unless "healthy" people have two or more major risk factors—smoking, hypertension, hypercholesterolemia, and family history of CVD.[4] The American College of Sports Medicine (1995) does not consider the clinical exercise ECG test a prerequisite if apparently healthy persons of any age perform only moderate exercise ($\leq 60\%$ $\dot{V}O_2max$) during recreation or testing.[6] Some believe that the exercise ECG is beneficial for all persons because it provides a baseline by which to compare possible future exercise ECG tests.

The third objective—diagnosis of cardiovascular disease—is the primary responsibility of the physician, who may seek input from the allied health staff, which may include a clinical exercise physiologist and/or exercise technologist. Thus, the ECG Exercise Test often is an interdisciplinary test between medical and nonmedical personnel. Although it is not within the role of an exercise laboratory technician to serve as a cardiologist, it is important for the technician to understand the basic concepts of electrocardiography and to recognize the most critical ECG abnormalities encountered in exercise testing.[33] The Exercise ECG Test is often the precursor test for angina (chest pain) patients to one or more of the following expensive tests: (1) angiography, which requires an X-ray-visible dye to be injected into the coronary arteries, (2) exercise scintigraphy, whereby radionuclide thallium allows the blood flow to be followed in the myocardium, and (3) echocardiography, which provides views of the heart produced by ultrasound waves.

Physiological Rationale

The exercise electrocardiogram is more apt to reveal latent (previously hidden) cardiovascular problems than the resting electrocardiogram.[23] For example, 10.2% of 7,023 normal resting ECG exams were deemed abnormal on maximal treadmill ECG tests.[18] Of those persons with known coronary heart disease, 30% may not be revealed by resting ECG, but if an exercise ECG is administered, 80% of these will be revealed.[41]

Method

The Exercise ECG Test is usually preceded by a resting electrocardiogram in order to screen subjects for whom exercise may be contraindicated and to enhance the interpretation of the exercise electrocardiogram. The Exercise ECG Test always includes measurements of heart rate and blood pressure periodically throughout the test. Often a prediction of aerobic power ($\dot{V}O_2max$) is made on the basis of heart rate or exercise duration. Sometimes the rate of perceived exertion (RPE) scale is used to monitor the performer's perception of the exercise intensity. Thus, the methodology of the Exercise ECG Test may be categorized into (a) exercise protocol; (b) the measurement of blood pressure, heart rate, and RPE; (c) and the recording of the ECG.

Exercise Protocol

Although the first popular Exercise ECG Test used a step bench,[40] the most common protocols for these tests use either cycle ergometers or treadmills. However, with the invention of an electronic stair ergometer and subsequent oxygen consumption prediction equations,[54] it is possible that step ergometry may again become a popular mode of ergometry in Exercise ECG Tests.

Table 1 Sample of a Continuous-Progressive Protocol for Cycle Ergometry

Time min	Force[a] N	W	Power[a] N·m·min⁻¹	Total Work kJ	Energy kcal·min⁻¹	Total Energy kcal
0–1	5	25;	1500	1.5	3.0	3.0
1–2	5	25;	1500	3.0	3.0	6.0
2–3	10	50;	3000	6.0	4.5	10.5
3–4	10	50;	3000	9.0	4.5	14.5
4–5	15	75;	4500	13.5	6.0	20.5
5–6	15	75;	4500	18.0	6.0	26.5
6–7	20	100;	6000	24.0	7.5	34.0
7–8	20	100;	6000	30.0	7.5	41.5
8–9	25	125;	7500	37.5	9.0	50.5
9–10	25	125;	7500	45.0	9.0	59.5
10–11	30	150;	9000	54.0	10.5	70.0
11–12	30	150;	9000	63.0	10.5	80.5
12–13	35	175;	10500	73.5	12.0	92.5
13–14	35	175;	10500	84.0	12.0	104.5
14–15	40	200;	12000	96.0	14.0	118.5
15–16	40	200;	12000	108.0	14.0	132.5
16–17	45	225;	13500	121.5	16.0	148.5
17–18	45	225;	13500	135.0	16.0	164.5
18–19	50	250;	15000	150.0	17.5	182.0
19–20	50	250;	15000	165.0	17.5	199.5

[a]Force applicable for mechanically braked ergometers; power is based on 50 rpm on Monark® ergometer.

Cycling Protocols

The protocol for the Exercise ECG Test is usually a continuous and progressive type. *Continuous,* as opposed to *intermittent,* is a term used to characterize a test in which the performer does not stop exercising until the end of the test. *Progressive* simply means that the exercise intensity is graded; that is, it increases at periodic intervals.

Continuous-progressive protocols can be subdivided into two types based upon submaximal or maximal exercise. Submaximal tests often are targeted to a specified percent maximal heart rate reserve (e.g., 85% HRRmax) or to symptom-limited endpoints. If the performer is healthy and willing, however, it is preferable to perform a maximal test. In general, the continuous protocol provides either 3- or 4-min periods at each power level if the power increments are 50 W or greater; less time (1 or 2 min) is needed if the power increments are 25 W or less (see Table 1).[37] A recovery period of 2–4 min should be allotted for no-load or minimal-load cycling.

Treadmill Protocols

The treadmill ergometer is the most popular ergometer for ECG stress testing.[17,53] Table 2[6] and Figure 1[5] summarize several popular treadmill protocols. Table 3 and other summaries[6,14,42,49,55] of exercise protocols are available. The Bruce (also see Table 4) and Balke protocols are the most popular for exercise tests in apparently healthy persons.[52] The original **Bruce** test lacked a good warmup at stage 1 for low-fit persons; however, the modified Bruce test remedied this by providing a 0% or 5% slope instead of a 10% slope at stage 1.[44] The Balke and the Taylor protocols were designed originally for Maximal Oxygen Consumption

Tests. The **Balke** protocol may be delimiting due to leg fatigue in some persons and is sometimes modified from 3.3 mph to 3.0 mph for women.[50] The **Ellestad** protocol[7] has an endpoint at 95% of age-predicted maximal heart rate.[24] As with the original Bruce test, the first stage of the Ellestad test may be too difficult for older or poorly fit persons. The **Naughton,**[46] or similar **Stanford,**[6] protocol is flexible and time efficient in that the first stage is chosen so that all persons can complete a minimum of 1.5 stages. For example, if the performers are likely to complete stage 4, then they may begin at stage 3. The **Harbor** protocol increases the power continuously by a ramp method,[56] or uniform amount, each minute; the increase depends on the performer's fitness. The performer usually reaches $\dot{V}O_2$max in about 10 min. For all protocols, a recovery period of 2–4 min should be allotted for walking at 2–3 mph at 0% grade.[5]

Indirect Oxygen Consumption

The approximate **oxygen cost** and MET for each stage of various protocols is presented in Table 2,[6] and again for the Bruce test in Table 4.[5] The oxygen cost at steady state for any protocol can be predicted, without actually measuring it, from ACSM equations for either walking (Eq. 1) or running (Eq. 2).[6]

Walk: $\dot{V}O_2$ (ml·kg⁻¹·min⁻¹)
$$= [3.5 + (0.1 \times v)] + (v \times \% \times 1.8) \qquad \text{Eq. 1}$$

Run: $\dot{V}O_2$ (ml·kg⁻¹·min⁻¹)
$$= [3.5 + (0.2 \times v)] + (v \times \% \times 0.9) \qquad \text{Eq. 2}$$

where: v = velocity in meters per minute (m·min⁻¹)
% = grade or slope

Table 2 The Oxygen Cost and MET for Various Stages of Four Treadmill Protocols

Treadmill Protocols

O₂ Cost ml/kg/min	Mets	Balke-Ware Grade at 3.3 mph 1-min stages	Ellestad 3/2/3 min stages mph	Ellestad \gr	Bruce 3 min stages mph	Bruce gr	Stanford Grade at 3 mph 3-min stages	Stanford Grade at 2 mph 3-min stages	Mets
		26	6	15	5.5	20			
		25							
		24			5.0	18			16
		23	5	15					15
		22							
56.0	16	21							14
52.5	15	20							13
49.0	14	19							
45.5	13	18							
42.0	12	17	5	10	4.2	16	22.5		12
38.5	11	16					20.0		11
35.0	10	15					17.5		10
31.5	9	14					15.0		9
28.0	8	13					12.5		8
24.5	7	12	4	10	3.4	14			
21.0	6	11					10.0	17.5	7
17.5	5	10	3	10	2.5	12	7.5	14	6
14.0	4	9					5.0	10.5	5
10.5	3	8							
7.0	2	7							
3.5	1	6							
		5	1.7	10	1.7	10	2.5	7	4
		4			1.7	5	0.0	3.5	3
		3			1.7	0			2
		2							1
		1							

Adapted from fig. 5-3 on pp. 92 and 93 of American College of Sports Medicine. (1995). *ACSM's guidelines for exercise testing and prescription.* © American College of Sports Medicine. Reprinted by permission.

For example, if a performer walks through stage 2 of the Bruce test at 2.5 mph (4.0 kph), or 72.4 m·min⁻¹, at 12% slope, then the oxygen cost can be calculated according to Equation 1 as follows:

$$\dot{V}O_2 = [3.5 + (0.1 \times 72.4 \text{ m·min}^{-1})] + (72.4 \times 0.12 \times 1.8)$$
$$= [3.5 + (7.24)] + 15.6$$
$$= 10.74 + 15.6$$
$$= 25.80 \text{ ml·kg}^{-1}\text{·min}^{-1}$$

The equivalent **MET** value may be calculated by dividing the oxygen cost by the one-MET value— 3.5 ml·kg⁻¹·min⁻¹ (Eq. 3).

$$\text{MET} = \dot{V}O_2 \div 3.5 \qquad \text{Eq. 3}$$

Therefore the MET value of a performer walking at 72.4 m·min⁻¹ on a 12% grade is

$$\text{MET} = 25.80 \div 3.5 = 7.4 \text{ MET}$$

The **maximal oxygen consumption ($\dot{V}O_2$max)** for the Bruce test may be estimated from various regression equations, or from Table 4, or from the nomogram in Figure 2.[5]

Treadmill regression equations have been derived from the endurance times associated with the Bruce, Balke,[1,15,28] and Balke-modified protocols.[29] The regression equation for the Bruce test is selected based on its suitability for the performer—men or women,[15,16] or young men.[36]

Men:
$$\dot{V}O_2\text{max (ml·kg}^{-1}\text{·min}^{-1}) = (2.94 \times \text{min}) + 7.65 \quad \text{Eq. 4}$$

Women:
$$\dot{V}O_2\text{max} = (2.94 \times \text{min}) + 3.74 \qquad \text{Eq. 5}$$

Young Men:
$$\dot{V}O_2\text{max} = (3.62 \times \text{min}) + 3.91 \qquad \text{Eq. 6}$$

where: min = time to exhaustion in Bruce test; decimal min

For example, if a woman completed stage 2, a total time of 6 min, on the Bruce test, then her $\dot{V}O_2$max based on Equation 5 is calculated as follows:

$$\dot{V}O_2\text{max} = (2.94 \times 6.0) + 3.74$$
$$= 17.64 + 3.7$$
$$= 21.34 \text{ ml·kg}^{-1}\text{·min}^{-1}$$

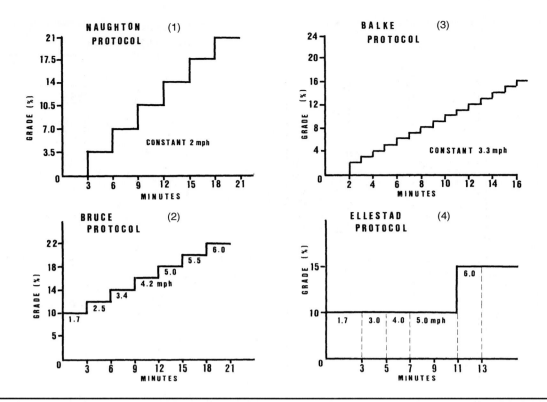

Figure 1 Four popular treadmill protocols: (1) Naughton, (2) Bruce, (3) Balke, and (4) Ellestad. From the American College of Sports Medicine, *Guidelines for Exercise Testing and Prescription,* 1986. Copyright © Lea and Febiger Publishers. Malvern, PA. Reprinted by permission.

Table 3 Summary of Four Common Treadmill Protocols

Protocol	Stages #	Speed Range mph	Grade Range %	Stage Time min/stage	Total Time min[a]
Bruce[b]	7	1.7–6.0	10–22	3	21
Balke[7]	22	3.3	2–22	1	22
Naughton (original)	13	1.0–2.0	0–22	2	30
Ellestad[24]	6	1.7–6.0	10; 15	2–3	13+

Notes: [a]Only if performer can continue to the end of the protocol.
[b]Bruce protocol for *clinical* testing may include two preliminary 3-min stages at 1.7 mph at 0% and 5% grade.

Table 4 Original[a] Bruce Test Stages and Corresponding METs and Maximal Oxygen Consumption ($ml \cdot kg^{-1} \cdot min^{-1}$)

Stage	mph	$km \cdot h^{-1}$	$m \cdot min^{-1}$	MET	$\dot{V}O_2max$[b]	Time (min)
1	1.7	2.7	45.6	5	17.5	3
2	2.5	4.0	72.4	7	24.5	6
3	3.4	5.5	91.1	10	35.0	9
4	4.2	6.8	112.6	13	45.5	11:45
5	5.0	8.0	134.0	16	56.0	15
6	5.5	8.8	147.4	19	66.5	17:40
7	6.0	9.7	160.8	22	77.0	21

Note: [a]The modified versions start at either 0% or 5% slope.[44]
[b]Assumes completion of given stage.

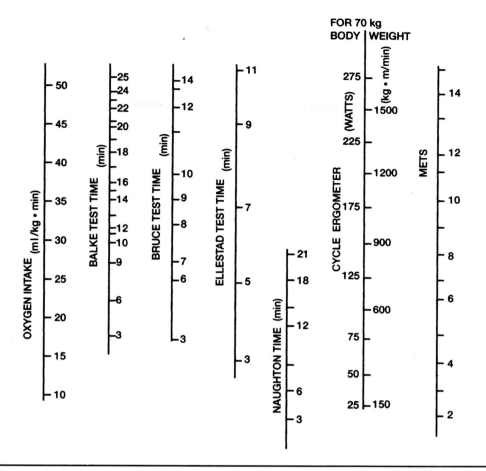

Figure 2 An estimate of exercise intensity is made by drawing a horizontal line from the time on a given exercise protocol to oxygen consumption or MET level. From the American College of Sports Medicine, *Guidelines for Exercise Testing and Prescription,* Fig. 2–4, p. 26, 1986. Copyright © Lea and Febiger Publishers. Malvern, PA. Reprinted by permission.

Accuracy of the Exercise ECG and Predictive $\dot{V}O_2$max Test

The terms sensitivity and specificity are often used to evaluate the effectiveness of Exercise ECG Tests. *Sensitivity* is the percentage of coronary heart disease (CHD) patients who have abnormal exercise tests. This percentage is around 60–75%. Unfortunately, this also means that 25–40% of those with CHD would not be detected by an exercise ECG test. *Specificity* is the percentage of healthy persons who have normal exercise tests; this percentage is around 90%, meaning that 10% of all normals would have abnormal tests.[20] Exercise test performers are labeled *positive* if the ECG reveals problems in the conduction pathway and/or dynamics of the heart. *Negative* tests mean that no problems were apparent during the test; that is, nothing indicative of heart disease was found.

The validity of the treadmill predictive tests is quite high based upon the reported correlations between maximal oxygen consumption and treadmill time. For example, Bruce found a correlation of .90 with a standard error of estimate less than 2 ml·kg^{-1}·min^{-1}.[15] Others report correlations from .88 to .97 with standard errors of about 3 ml·kg^{-1}·min^{-1}.[8] A correlation of .797 was found between the Bruce-predicted treadmill test and the 1.5-mile run; the Bruce predictions were significantly higher than the 1.5-mile run predictions of maximal oxygen consumption.[30]

The advantage of using the ACSM steady-state equations (1 and 2) for the terminal exercise stage to predict $\dot{V}O_2$max is that they can be applied to any protocol. However, the terminal oxygen cost usually overestimates the performer's $\dot{V}O_2$max.[27] A more accurate prediction (*SEE* = 4.4 ml·kg^{-1}·min^{-1}) may be made if the ACSM value is corrected as follows in Equation 7:[27]

$$\dot{V}O_2\text{max(ml·kg}^{-1}\text{·min}^{-1}) = (0.869 \times \text{ACSM } \dot{V}O_2) - 0.07 \qquad \text{Eq. 7}$$

For example, if a performer's ACSM oxygen cost at the terminal stage is calculated from Equation 2 as 40.05 ml·kg^{-1}·min^{-1}, then that person's $\dot{V}O_2$max calculated from Equation 7 is

$$\dot{V}O_2\text{max(ml·kg}^{-1}\text{·min}^{-1}) = (0.869 \times 40.08) - 0.07$$
$$= 34.82 - 0.07$$
$$= 34.75$$

The maximal oxygen consumption may also be estimated by consulting Table 4, which relates maximal oxygen consumption to the time to exhaustion on the Bruce test. The nomogram in Figure 2 may be used for the Bruce test and other protocols to predict maximal oxygen consumption and MET by drawing a horizontal line from the termination time (min) to $\dot{V}O_2$ and MET.[5]

Measurement of Blood Pressure, Heart Rate, and RPE

Blood Pressure

The American College of Sports Medicine recommends that blood pressure be measured with the subject in the supine, sitting, and standing positions prior to exercise.[5] Presumably, these measures are taken under relaxed conditions. Additional resting measures may be taken when the performer is prepared to exercise while seated on the cycle ergometer, standing on the treadmill, or in front of the step bench. These latter measurements are referred to as the anticipatory or preexercise measures.

At exercise the blood pressure should be taken during the last minute of each stage or interval of the exercise protocol.[6] In recovery, it should be taken immediately after exercise, especially if the final exercise measurement was cancelled due to extraneous movement of the performer. Recovery blood pressures are usually taken at 1–2 min intervals. The first few measurements of recovery blood pressure may be taken during *active* recovery (e.g., low-intensity cycling or walking slowly on the treadmill or in-place), and subsequent measurements may be made while the person is *passive* (e.g., seated in a chair) until the pressure returns nearly to baseline.

Heart Rate

Calibrated **cardiotach** monitors can be useful to estimate the heart rate of the exerciser. Ideally, EKG simulators can be used to check the accuracy of the cardiotach.

Heart rate can be calculated from the **electrocardiogram** itself. Heart rate can be calculated by taking the average distance for one cardiac cycle (one R-wave to the next R-wave) and dividing it into 1500. For example, 1500 divided by 9.0 mm results in a heart rate of 167 b·min⁻¹ (often abbreviated as bpm). By measuring the horizontal distance (mm) between eleven normal cardiac cycles (first to eleventh R-spike), the heart rate at exercise can be calculated from Equation 8.

$$HR\ (b \cdot min^{-1}) = 60\ s \div (0.1 \times 10\text{-R-R mm} \times 0.04) \quad \text{Eq. 8}$$

where: 60 s = 1 min
10-R-R mm = distance of 10 cardiac cycles
0.1×10-R-R = average R-R interval; mm
0.04 = time (s) elapsing for each mm

The equation may be simplified by multiplying the two constants, 0.1 and 0.04, and then using the product 0.004 to divide into 60 s. Thus Equation 8 becomes:

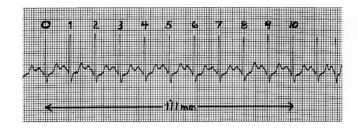

Figure 3 An actual ECG strip used to calculate heart rate.

Table 5 Rapid Estimation of Heart Rate from the Number (#) of 5-mm Vertical Lines

Boxes (# from R-R)	mm	Time (s)	Heart Rate b·min⁻¹
1	5	0.20	300
2	10	0.40	150
3	15	0.60	100
4	20	0.80	75
5	25	1.00	60

$$HR\ (b \cdot min^{-1}) = 60\ s \div (0.004 \times 10\text{-R-R mm}) \quad \text{Eq. 9}$$

For example, in Figure 3 the distance for ten cardiac cycles (11 R spikes) during exercise is measured as 111 mm. The following calculation provides an exercise heart rate of 135 b·min⁻¹:

$$\begin{aligned} HR\ (b \cdot min^{-1}) &= 60\ s \div (0.004 \times 111\ mm) \\ &= 60\ s \div 0.444 \\ &= 135\ b \cdot min^{-1} \end{aligned}$$

Another method of calculating heart rate uses the 3-s black marks at the top of ECG paper. By multiplying the number of R-waves (to closest tenth of a cycle) in a 6-s interval by ten, the bpm is produced (Eq. 10).

$$b \cdot min^{-1} = \#\ of\ R\text{-waves in }6\ s \times 10 \quad \text{Eq. 10}$$

The technician can make a rapid estimation of heart rate by memorizing the heart rate that is related to each **5-mm box**.[26] First, count the number of 5-mm boxes—indicated by bold vertical lines at every fifth vertical line (0.20 s)—from the first R-wave to the second. Then relate the number of boxes listed in Table 5 to the heart rate or simply divide the number of 5-mm boxes into 300. For example, the ECG in Figure 3 shows slightly over two boxes between R-waves. Therefore, the heart rate has to be between 150 and 100 b·min⁻¹. The more exact rate is found by dividing 2.2 boxes into 300, thus 136 b·min⁻¹.

"Rulers" to measure heart rate are often provided free by electrocardiograph manufacturers or drug companies. The index line or arrow is placed on an R-spike, then the rate is read at the appointed cardiac cycle—usually three for resting rates, ten for exercise rates.

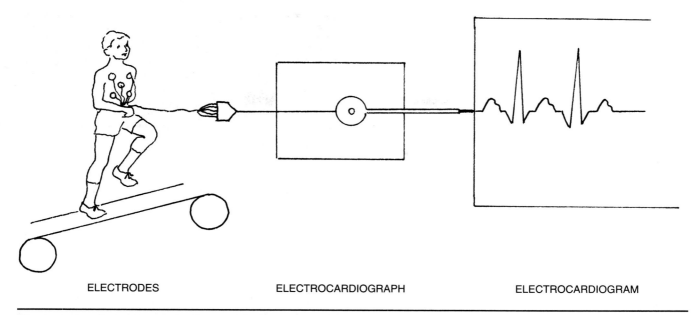

| ELECTRODES | ELECTROCARDIOGRAPH | ELECTROCARDIOGRAM |

Figure 4 Interfacing the heart with the ECG. The electrical currents from the heart are transferred from the skin by the electrodes, amplified by the electrocardiograph, and then recorded as the electrocardiogram.

Rate of Perceived Exertion (RPE)

The revised RPE scale with ratio properties may be more suitable for determining subjective symptoms associated with breathing, aches, and pains.[12] Prior to the Exercise ECG Test, the performer should be instructed as to the meaning of the RPE scale. A large RPE poster should be prominently placed or held so that the exerciser has no trouble viewing the RPE scale. Hand signals may be necessary if the performer is using a respiratory valve.

The Electrocardiogram

The basic concept of exercise electrocardiography is depicted in Figure 4. The methods of electrocardiography are dependent upon the objectives of the test and the selected electrocardiograph and lead system.

Electrocardiographic Equipment

Electrocardiograph and Monitor. The electrocardiograph is the recording machine, whereas the paper recording itself is the electrocardiogram. Prior to today's technology, some tests used a single-channel ECG recorder with or without a monitor. Original monitors were the "bouncing-ball" type, which left only a readable trace for a fraction of a second; newer monitors enable persisting or "freezing" traces, and some can retrieve cycles from memory (Fig. 5). Expensive electrocardiographs and monitors are available that display three to twelve channels nearly simultaneously instead of one. They may include an ECG analysis system and an interface with the treadmill or ergometer.

Leads and Cable. The lead/cable system for the Exercise ECG Test has improved tremendously since Einthoven's

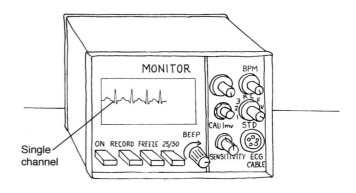

Figure 5 An example of an electrocardiograph with a single-channel display monitor.

original system for resting electrocardiograms that required a person to maintain both hands and the left foot in three buckets of salt solution. The popular Master ECG Step Test from the 1930s to 1960s was a more portable system but still required the person to carry relatively thick and heavy cables while exercising. In fact, the system was so cumbersome that the person's movements made it impossible to take a readable recording during exercise; only after the exerciser stopped would the tracing be made. Today the electrodes and cables are very lightweight. Present electrodes come preprepared with electrolyte solution and are disposable.

ECG Procedures

The procedures for administering the Exercise ECG Test are concerned with the (1) safety of the participant, (2) application of the electrodes, and (3) ECG protocol.

Table 6 Cardiovascular Disease (CVD) Risk Factors

Positive Risk Factor	Criteria
Age[a]	Men >45 y; Women >55 y
Family History	Premature CVD death or MI[b] in parents or siblings: Men—before 55 y Women—before 65 y
Smoking	Current smoker
High Cholesterol	>200 mg/dl (>5.2 mmol/L)
Diabetes	Insulin dependent (ID) >30 y of age; non-ID >35 y of age
Very Sedentary	Sitting nearly all day

Note: [a]These age criteria are 5 y greater than those for physician exam and supervision.
[b]MI = myocardial infarction.
Adapted from Table 2-2, p. 18 of American College of Sports Medicine. (1995). *ACSM's guidelines for exercise testing and prescription.* © ACSM.; Indianapolis, IN 46206-1440.

Safety

Probably the most effective way to assure a safe Exercise ECG Test is to choose a healthy person to perform the test. The American College of Sports Medicine provides guidelines regarding who needs an exercise test before being cleared for exercise, or who needs physician supervision during the exercise test.[6] For **vigorous** (>60% $\dot{V}O_2max$) exercise, men over 40 years of age and women over 50 who have more than one risk factor for coronary artery disease (Table 6) need to be medically evaluated by a physician prior to exercise testing and be physician supervised during the exercise test.[6] Thus, both age and health-status criteria—such as being apparently healthy, or at higher risk, or diseased—are important considerations with respect to test supervision. For example, maximal treadmill tests of over 24,000 men and women produced nearly 1100 abnormal exercise tests. Of these, men and women who were apparently healthy had lower abnormality rates than those at higher cardiovascular disease (CVD) risk and those with CVD. Secondly, the abnormal rate increased exponentially with age, regardless of health status.[34] For **submaximal,** or **moderate,** (≤60% $\dot{V}O_2max$) exercise testing, apparently healthy persons, meaning those without symptoms or disease or no more than one risk factor, of any age may participate without prior medical examination or physician-supervised exercise test.[6,14]

The safety of the participant is partially dependent upon proper interpretation of the electrocardiogram. The risks associated with Exercise ECG Tests are often classified into morbidity and mortality—morbidity referring to injury or traumatic event and mortality referring to death. A morbidity rate of less than 0.1% and no mortality occurred in more than 15,000 mainly coronary patients who performed the exercise test.[16] Also, morbidity and mortality rates of 2.4 and 1, respectively, per 10,000 tests occurred in a survey of 170,000 exercise tests.[51] These rates from physician-supervised tests do not differ from nonphysician-

Table 7 Absolute and Relative Indications for Termination of an Exercise Test

Absolute Indications for Stopping the Test

1. Acute MI or suspicion of myocardial infarction (MI).
2. Onset of moderate-to-severe angina (chest pain).
3. Drop in systolic blood pressure (SBP) with increasing power level accompanied by signs or symptoms or drop below standing resting SBP.
4. Serious arrhythmias [e.g., second- or third-degree atrioventricular (AV) block, sustained ventricular tachycardia or increasing premature ventricular contractions (PVC), atrial fibrillation with fast ventricular response] (Fig. 6).
5. Signs of poor perfusion (blood flow), including pallor, cyanosis, or cold and clammy skin.
6. Unusual or severe shortness of breath.
7. Central nervous system symptoms, including ataxia (incoordination), vertigo (dizziness), visual or gait problems, or confusion.
8. Technical inability to monitor the ECG.
9. Performer's request.

Relative Indications for Stopping the Test

1. Pronounced ECG changes from baseline (>2 mm of horizontal or downsloping ST-segment depression, or >2 mm of ST-segment elevation (except in lead aVR) (Fig. 7).
2. Any chest pain that is increasing.
3. Physical or verbal manifestations of severe fatigue or shortness of breath (dyspnea).
4. Wheezing.
5. Leg cramps or intermittent claudication (grade 3 on 4-point scale).
6. Hypertensive response (SBP >260 mm Hg; DBP >115 mm Hg).
7. Less serious arrhythmias such as supraventricular tachycardia.
8. Exercise-induced bundle branch block that cannot be distinguished from ventricular tachycardia.

From American College of Sports Medicine. (1995). *ACSM's guidelines for exercise testing and prescription,* 5th ed., p. 97, table 5–4, © 1995 American College of Sports Medicine.

supervised tests, such as those supervised by exercise physiologists,[33] ideally, ACSM-certified exercise physiologists. Thus, with proper supervision, the exercise test is not very risky. Proper supervision also means that the ECG monitor should be observed at all times by at least one technician. Thus, it is important that the technician know how to interpret the ECG that is being viewed on the monitor or paper.

The safety of the performer is enhanced if the technician and supervisor of the Exercise ECG Test are familiar with the criteria for stopping the test. It is not within the scope of this manual to explain all of the criteria listed by the American College of Sports Medicine,[6] but they are presented in Table 7 so that interested students will be inspired to learn more about them by taking other courses or workshops. Simulated ectopic beats (e.g., premature ventricular contractions; PVC) are presented in Figure 6. An example of ST-depression, a common indicator of myocardial ischemia, is presented in Figure 7.

Electrode Application

The procedures for applying electrodes can be simple or complex, depending upon the number of electrodes. A Mason-Likar modification[38] of the classic twelve-lead (ten

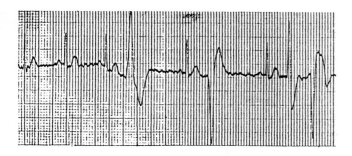

Figure 6 Premature ventricular contractions of a multifocal nature.

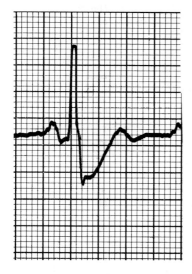

Figure 7 An example of severe ST-depression (6–7 mm) in an elderly man.

electrodes) resting electrocardiogram is often used for the exercise test hookup.[5] However, the electrodes typically placed on the arms and legs in the resting ECG are placed instead on the upper torso when using the Mason-Likar configuration for the exercise test (Figs. 4 and 8). The right arm (RA; white) negative electrode is placed just below (~2 cm) the distal end of the clavicle at the infraclavicular fossa. The left arm (LA; black) positive electrode is placed similarly below the left clavicle, avoiding muscle masses. The left (LL; red) and right leg (RL; green) electrodes are placed just superior to the left and right anterior superior iliac spines, respectively, at the level of the navel[11] at the anterior axillary line.[39] Precordial unipolar chest leads are applied at the same sites as those for the resting ECG.

A simple three-electrode lead system may be used that is somewhat similar to the V_5 unipolar and the CM5 bipolar lead systems[9,10,19,48] and Holland's[32] configurations. The RA electrode is placed on the person's manubrium, and the LA and RL electrodes are placed at the left V_5 and right side of the chest, respectively; the ECG selector

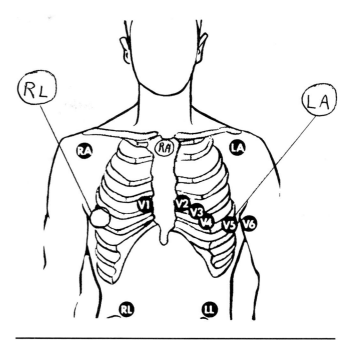

Figure 8 The Mason-Likar and CM-5 lead sites.

switch is at lead 2. These less sensitive,[5] but simpler and effective bipolar lead systems are often used in testing asymptomatic persons; it reduces the time and expense of electrode placement.

In order to avoid muscle and outside electrical interference (artifact), the skin of the person at each electrode site should be prepped before the electrode is applied. Three steps to prepping the skin are: (1) scrubbing the site with alcohol, (2) shaving the skin with a razor if hairs are visible, and (3) abrading the skin lightly with fine-grain sandpaper, emery cloth, or a special abrading pad. A final wiping of the skin with alcohol is sometimes performed. The alcohol swab, sandpaper, and razor must be discarded after their use on one person.

The ECG Protocol

The technician records the ECG while the subject is at rest, exercise, and recovery. The person's name, date, body position or exercise stage should be labeled appropriately on the ECG strip.

Resting and/or Pre-Exercise ECG. Ideally, a resting twelve-lead ECG should be taken before administering the exercise ECG test. It should be required for subjects who are at greater risk based on their history or risk factor analysis. Although some laboratories include a pre-exercise hyperventilation recording, some authorities do not recommend it because of reducing the tests specificity (i.e., the ability to detect true normals).[22] After taking the resting ECG, a pre-exercise recording should be taken while the performer is seated on the cycle or standing on the treadmill.

Table 8 ECG Criteria for an Abnormal Exercise Test

1. Exercise-induced ST-depression or elevation of ≥ 1 mm relative to the Q-Q line, lasting ≥ 0.06 s[a] from the J-point (Fig. 7).
2. Ventricular tachycardia ("V-tach"; ≥ 3 consecutive PVC) or >30% frequency of PVC.
3. Exercise-induced left or right bundle branch block (delayed and abnormal spread of excitation).
4. Sustained supraventricular tachycardia.
5. R-on-T PVC.
6. Exercise-induced second- or third-degree heart block.
7. Postexercise U-wave inversion (possible faulty repolarization of septum).
8. Inappropriate bradycardia (slow heart rate).

Note: [a]1995 ACSM "Guidelines; 1986 "Guidelines" = 0.08 s.
American College of Sports Medicine, *"Guidelines for Exercise Testing and Prescription"*, 1986, Lea and Febiger 200 Chesterfield Pkwy Malvern PA 19355-9725. Reprinted by permission.

Exercise and Recovery ECG. During exercise and recovery, the ECG is monitored constantly, but a tracing may be recorded only at each stage of the test; more frequent recordings may be made if so indicated. The exercise recording usually is taken for the last 10–15 s of each stage. A recording should be taken immediately after the last stage of exercise. A recording should be taken during active recovery at 1 or 2 min, and at passive recovery at the 5th min of postexercise. The participant should not be released from monitoring until all subjective and physiological symptoms have returned to normal.

Results and Discussion

Persons performing the Exercise ECG Test can be evaluated according to their fitness and symptoms. The symptom of special concern in this chapter is the ECG. The interpretation of the performer's fitness can be made through a variety of sources, many found in the chapters for Aerobic Fitness in *Exercise Physiology Laboratory Manual.*

ECG Interpretation

The Exercise ECG Test in epidemiological studies has demonstrated that asymptomatic men with abnormal tests have 10 to 15 times the risk of coronary artery disease than those with normal exercise tests.[20]

Table 8 presents ECG criteria for abnormality in exercise testing that have been endorsed by the American College of Sports Medicine,[5] whereas the following list provides the typical changes associated with exercise:[6]

1. Small changes in the shape and amplitude of the P wave.
2. P wave moves closer to the T wave, forming before the T wave reaches baseline at high heart rates.
3. Q wave increase.
4. Slight decrease in R wave amplitude.

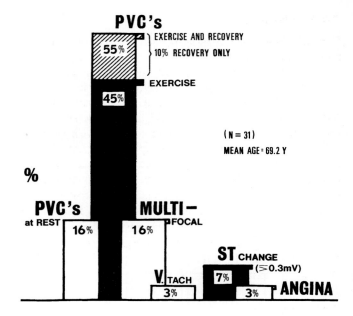

Figure 9 Comparison of abnormal ECG responses at rest and during the exercise/recovery period. (Based on data from Ambe et al., 1973.)

5. Likely increase in T wave amplitude.
6. Slightly shorter QRS duration.
7. J-point (end of S wave and start of T wave) depression.
8. Shorter Q-T interval.

Arrhythmia

It is not abnormal for healthy persons to have an occasional skipped beat during the day.[45] Prevalence of these premature ventricular contractions (PVC) may vary with the age of the population and the duration of the monitoring. Prevalency may be as high as 80% with 24-h monitoring of a population[a] or as low as 50% in a young cohort,[13] or about 5% in only a 2-min monitoring of middle-aged men,[21] or nearly 3% incidence in the typical time it takes for administering a resting ECG.[47]

The chances of recording ECG abnormalities during exercise is greater than at rest.[2,35,43] During maximal exercise testing in normal men, the younger men averaged close to 30% incidence of PVC, while the middle-aged men averaged close to 43%.[25] Forty-four percent of normal men in another study experienced PVC during maximal exercise.[43] Figure 9 illustrates that only 16% of the elderly persons showed premature ventricular contractions at rest, but 55% showed PVC during the exercise and recovery period.[2]

---

[a]Personal communication, Nov. 2, 1984, SWACSM Convention, Las Vegas, NV.

S-T Segment

During ischemia, the affected myocardial fibers are slow in reestablishing normal polarity, thus changing the S-T segment[31] and, possibly, increasing the number of ectopic beats.[55] S-T segment depression in a true-positive test probably will not be evident unless a major coronary artery is 60% occluded.[14] True-positive ST-depression, indicating myocardial ischemia, is best noted by the lateral leads, I, V_4, V_5, and V_6[22] with 1.0 mm of displacement continuing for 0.06 s (i.e., 60 ms).[6] The American Association of Cardiovascular and Pulmonary Rehabilitation[3] considers a moderate risk, especially in persons with cardiac symptoms, to be an exercise-induced ST-depression between 1–2 mm, whereas a higher risk is greater than 2 mm. If clinically significant S-T segment depression occurs, then a follow-up thallium-imagery technique is usually advised to validate the positive stress ECG test.

References

1. Alexander, J. F., Liang, M. T. C., Stull, G. A., Serfass, R. C., Wolfe, D. R., Ewing, J. L. (1984). A comparison of the Bruce and Liang equations for predicting V̇O₂max in young adult males. *Research Quarterly for Exercise and Sport, 55,* 383–387.

2. Ambe, K. S., Adams, G. M., & deVries, H. A. (1973). Exercising the aged [Abstract]. *Medicine and Science in Sports, 5,* 63.

3. American Association of Cardiovascular and Pulmonary Rehabilitation. (1994). *Guidelines for cardiac rehabilitation programs.* Champaign, IL: Human Kinetics.

4. American College of Cardiology/American Heart Association Subcommittee on Exercise Testing. (1986). Guidelines for exercise testing: A report of the American College of Cardiology/American Heart Association Task Force on Assessment of Cardiovascular Procedures. *Journal of American College of Cardiology, 8,* 725–738.

5. American College of Sports Medicine. (1986 & 1991). *Guidelines for exercise testing and prescription.* Philadelphia: Lea & Febiger.

6. American College of Sports Medicine. (1995). *ACSM's Guidelines for exercise testing and prescription.* Philadelphia: Williams & Wilkins.

7. Balke, B., & Ware, R. W. (1959). An experimental study of physical fitness of Air Force personnel. *U.S. Armed Forces Medical Journal, 10,* 675.

8. Baumgartner, T. A., & Jackson, A. S. (1988). *Measurement for evaluation in physical education and exercise science.* Dubuque, IA: Wm. C. Brown.

9. Blackburn, H. (1969). *Measurement in exercise electrocardiography.* Springfield, IL: Charles C Thomas.

10. Blackburn, H., Taylor, H. L., Vasquez, C. L., & Puchner, T. C. (1966). The electrocardiogram during exercise. *Circulation, 34,* 1034–1043.

11. Boone, T., & Zwiren, L. (1993). Surface anatomy for exercise programming. In ACSM (Eds.), *Resource manual for guidelines for exercise testing and prescription.* Philadelphia: Lea & Febiger.

12. Borg, G. A. V. (1982). Psychophysical bases of perceived exertion. *Medicine and Science in Sports and Exercise, 14,* 377–381.

13. Brodsky, M., Wu, D., Denes, P., Kanakis, C., & Rosen, K. (1977). Arrhythmias documented by 24-hour continuous electrocardiographic monitoring in 50 male medical students without apparent heart disease. *The American Journal of Cardiology, 39,* 390–395.

14. Brooks, G. A., & Fahey, T. D. (1987). *Fundamentals of human performance.* New York: Macmillan.

15. Bruce, R. A. (1972). Multi-stage treadmill test of submaximal and maximal exercise. In American Heart Association's Committee on Exercise (Eds.), *Exercise testing and training of apparently healthy individuals: A handbook for physicians* (pp. 32–34). New York: American Heart Association.

16. Bruce, R. A. (1974). Methods of exercise testing. *The American Journal of Cardiology, 33,* 715–720.

17. Chung, E. K. (1983). *Exercise electrocardiography: Practical approach.* Baltimore, MD: Williams & Wilkins.

18. Cooper, K. H. (1977). The treadmill re-examined. *American Heart Journal, 94,* 811–812.

19. Costill, D. L., Branam, G. E., Moore, J. C., Sparks, K., & Turner, C. (1974). Effects of physical training in men with coronary heart disease. *Medicine and Science in Sports, 6,* 95–100.

20. Council on Scientific Affairs. (1981). Indications and contraindications for exercise testing. *Journal of the American Medical Association, 246,* 1015–1018.

21. Crow, R. S., Pineas, R. J., Dias, V., Taylor, H. L., Jacobs, D., Blackburn, H. (1975). Ventricular premature beats in a population sample. *Circulation, 51,* (Suppl.), III-211–III-215.

22. Dubach, P., & Froelicher, V. F. (1991). Recent advances in exercise testing. *Journal of Cardiopulmonary Rehabilitation, 11,* 29–38.

23. Duda, M. (1984). Basketball coaches guard against cardiovascular stress. *The Physician and Sportsmedicine,* pp. 193–194.

24. Ellestad, M. H. (1980). *Stress testing. Principles and practice.* Philadelphia: F. A. Davis.

25. Faris, J. V., McHenry, P. L., Jordan, J. W., Morris, S. N. (1976). Prevalence and reproducibility of exercise-induced ventricular arrhythmias during maximal exercise testing in normal men. *The American Journal of Cardiology, 37,* 617–622.

26. Fisher, A. G., & Jensen, C. R. (1990). *The scientific basis of athletic conditioning.* Philadelphia: Lea & Febiger.

27. Foster, C., Crowe, A. J., Daines, E., Dumit, M., Green, M. A., Lettau, S., Thompson, N. N., & Weymier, J. (1996). Predicting functional capacity during treadmill

testing independent of exercise protocol. *Medicine and Science in Sports and Exercise, 28,* 752–756.

28. Foster, C., Jackson, A. S., Pollock, M. L., Taylor, M. M., Hare, J., Sennett, S. M., Rod, J. L., Sarwar, M., & Schmidt, D. H. (1984). Generalized equations for predicting functional capacity from treadmill performance. *American Heart Journal, 107,* 1229–1234.

29. Frid, D. J., Ellefsen, K., Porcari, J., Ward, A., Ockene, I., & Rippe, J. (1988). Estimating $\dot{V}O_2max$ from a modified Balke treadmill protocol: Validation in a young healthy population. *Medicine and Science in Sports and Exercise, 20,* (Suppl.), Abstract #3, S1.

30. Ginder, J. (1984). *The Bruce vs. Cooper predictive tests for aerobic power in prospective fire fighters.* Unpublished Master's project, California State University, Fullerton.

31. Goldman, M. J. (1967). *Principles of clinical electro-cardiography.* Los Altos, CA: Lange Medical Publications.

32. Holland, G. J., Heng, M. K., & Weber, F. (1988). Conducting and interpreting exercise tests for asymptomatic adults. *Cardiovascular Reviews and Reports, 9,* 54–63.

33. Knight, J. A., Laubach, C. A., Butcher, R. J., & Menapace, F. J. (1995). Supervision of clinical exercise testing by exercise physiologists. *The American Journal of Cardiology, 75,* 390–391.

34. Kohl, H. W., Gibbons, L. W., Gordon, N. F., & Blair, S. N. (1990). An empirical evaluation of the ACSM Guidelines for Exercise Testing. *Medicine and Science in Sports and Exercise, 22,* 533–539.

35. Kosowsky, B. D., Lown, B., Whiting, R., & Guiney, T. (1971). Occurrence of ventricular arrhythmias with exercise as compared to monitoring. *Circulation, 46,* 826–832.

36. Liang, M. T. C., Alexander, J. F., Stull, G. A., & Serfass, R. C. (1982). The use of the Bruce equation for predicting $\dot{V}O_2max$ in healthy young men. [Abstract]. *Medicine and Science in Sports and Exercise, 14,* 129.

37. Luft, V. C., Cardus, D., Lim, T. P. K., Anderson, E. C., & Howarth, J. L. (1963). Physical performance in relation to body size and composition. *Annals of New York Academy of Science, 110,* 795–808.

38. Mason, R. E., & Likar, I. (1966). A new system of multiple-lead exercise electrocardiography. *American Heart Journal, 71,* 196.

39. Mason, R. E., Likar, I., Biern, R. D., & Ross, R. S. (1967). Multiple-lead exercise electrocardiography. *Circulation, 336,* 517–525.

40. Master, A. M., & Oppenheimer, E. J. (1929). A simple exercise tolerance test for circulatory efficiency with standard tables for normal individuals. *American Journal of Medical Sciences, 177,* 223–243.

41. McArdle, W. D., Katch, F. I., & Katch, V. L. (1991). *Exercise physiology: Energy, nutrition, & human performance.* Philadelphia: Lea & Febiger.

42. McArdle, W. D., Katch, F. I., & Katch, V. L. (1994). *Essentials of exercise physiology.* Philadelphia: Lea & Febiger.

43. McHenry, P. L., Morris, S. N., Kavalier, M., & Jordan, J. W. (1976). Comparative study of exercise-induced ventricular arrhythmia in normal subjects and patients with documented coronary artery disease. *The American Journal of Cardiology, 37,* 609–616.

44. McInnis, K. J., & Balady, G. J. (1994). Comparison of submaximal exercise responses using the Bruce vs modified Bruce protocols. *Medicine and Science in Sports and Exercise, 26,* 103–107.

45. Misner, J. E., Bloomfield, D. K., & Smith, L. (1975). Periodicity of premature ventricular contractions (PVC) in healthy, active adults. [Abstract]. *Medicine and Science in Sports, 7,* 72.

46. Naughton, J. (1977). Stress electrocardiography in clinical electrocardiographic correlations. In J. C. Rios (Ed.), *Cardiovascular Clinics, 8,* 127–139. Philadelphia: F. A. Davis.

47. Okajuma, M., Scholmerich, P., & Simonson, E. (1960). Frequency of premature beats. *Minnesota Medicine,* p. 751.

48. Phibbs, B. P., & Buckels, L. J. (1975). Comparative yield of ECG leads in multistage stress testing. *American Heart Journal, 90,* 275–276.

49. Pollock, M. L., Bohannon, R. L., Cooper, K. H., Ayres, J. J., Ward, A., White, S. R., & Linnerud, A. C. (1976). A comparative analysis of four protocols for maximal treadmill stress testing. *American Heart Journal, 92,* 39–46.

50. Pollock, M. L., Foster, C., Schmidt, D. H., Hellman, C., Linnerud, A. C., & Ward, A. (1982). Comparative analysis of physiological responses to three different maximal graded exercise test protocols in healthy women. *American Heart Journal, 103,* 363.

51. Rochmis, P., & Blackburn, H. (1971). Exercise tests: A survey of procedures, safety, and litigation experience in approximately 170,000 tests. *Journal of the American Medical Association, 217,* 1061–1066.

52. Stuart, R. J., & Ellestad, M. H. (1980). National survey of exercise stress testing facilities. *Chest, 77,* 94.

53. Thacker, S. B., & Berkelman, R. L. (1988). Public health surveillance in the United States. *Epidemiological Reviews, 10,* 164.

54. Van Oosbree, P., Dennehy, C., & Ben-Ezra, V. (1988). Predicting $\dot{V}O_2$ on the stairmaster. *Medicine and Science in Sports and Exercise, 20,* Abstract #335, S56.

55. Wasserman, K., Hansen, J. E., Sue, D. Y., Whipp, B. J., & Casaburi, R. (1994). *Principles of exercise testing and interpretation.* Philadelphia: Lea & Febiger.

56. Whipp, B. J., Davis, J. A., Torres, F., & Wasserman, K. (1981). A test to determine parameters of aerobic function during exercise. *Journal of Applied Physiology, 50,* 217–221.

Chapter LV Lung Volumes

Evaluation of respiratory function is important for early diagnosis and management of pulmonary diseases such as emphysema, chronic bronchitis, asthma, and pneumonia. The pulmonary tests essentially involve the determination of various lung volumes and airflow rates. The influence of the environment, lifestyle, and age may be evaluated by periodically testing the lungs for deterioration or improvement.

The measurement of each of the four lung volumes serves to demonstrate the physiology of respiration and to test for respiratory disease. The vital capacity, a composite of three lung volumes, has been used frequently, along with its timed components (1 s and 3 s), for diagnosing lung disease.[31]

Physiologically, the four lung volumes are nonoverlapping divisions of the lungs at different stages of breathing (Fig. 1). For example, the **inspiratory reserve volume (IRV)** is the volume of air that can be inspired maximally at the end of a normal inspiration. The volume of air in a normal breath is the **tidal volume (TV or V_T)**. The volume of air that can be expired maximally after a normal expiration is the **expiratory reserve volume (ERV)**. The **residual volume (RV)** is the volume of air remaining in the lungs after a maximal expiration. The **vital capacity (VC)**, an overlapping volume, is a sum of three different lung volumes (Eq. 1).

$$VC \text{ (ml or L)} = IRV + TV + ERV \qquad \text{Eq. 1}$$

Vital Capacity and Forced Expiratory Volume

The vital capacity test is one of the oldest[18] and most common respiratory tests. It provides an indirect indication of the size of the lungs, although it is not a complete measure of the entire lung size because it does not account for residual volume. It is often measured in fitness and/or health clinics in order to assess the effects of smoking, disease, or environment, or as a part of the hydrostatic weighing test for body composition. Restrictive lung diseases (e.g., fibrosis, pneumonia, and pulmonary vascular disease) and chest wall stiffness or respiratory muscle weakness (often associated with natural aging) may reduce the vital capacity.

Large vital capacities have been associated with potentially high aerobic performances. In general, vital capacity is related to three uncontrolled characteristics: (1) age, (2) height, and (3) gender. The older a person becomes, the less elastic become both the thoracic cage and respiratory muscles. The reduced expansion of the chest restricts lung expansion, which, along with reduced respiratory muscle

VC (mL or L) = IRV + TV + ERV

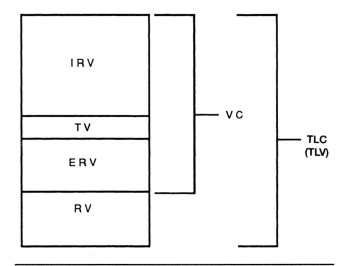

Figure 1 The four lung volumes (IRV, TV, ERV, RV), vital capacity (VC), and total lung volume (TLV) or capacity (TLC).

strength, reduces vital capacity. The taller one is, the greater is the vital capacity; this is basically a function of lung size, taller people having larger lungs. Chest circumference is not as closely related to lung size because chest muscle hypertrophy has little or nothing to do with lung size. Finally, with respect to gender, men have larger lungs than women, even when corrected for body size.

The measurement of vital capacity (VC) simply requires that an individual blow as large a breath of air as possible into a spirometer. If the person is asked to exhale as fast as possible, the VC is termed more appropriately the Forced (or fast) Vital Capacity (FVC). If volumes are measured at various time intervals, such as at 1.0 s or 3.0 s, then these components of VC are referred to as Forced Expiratory Volumes ($FEV_{1.0}$ or $_{3.0}$, respectively). These timed volumes can be helpful in evaluating late-phase obstructive lung diseases such as emphysema, bronchitis, and asthma. The only air volume that remains in the person's lungs after such a maximal effort is the residual volume, a volume that normally cannot be exhaled. Thus, the person expels three of the four components of the total lung volume—the inspiratory reserve volume (IRV), the tidal volume (TV), and the expiratory reserve volume (ERV)—when performing the vital capacity test.

Method

The equipment and procedures for measuring the four lung volumes and vital capacity have many similarities. Depending upon the type of equipment, some of these measures can be taken sequentially without changing the instrumentation. Many of the procedures described here are those recommended by the American Thoracic Society's Committee on Proficiency Standards.[2]

Equipment and Procedures for Measuring Vital Capacity

Vital capacity can be measured easily with an automated electronic spirometer such as the Vitalometer®[7] Its features are similar to most other wet spirometers in that its container (body) is filled with distilled water. A hollow tube runs through the middle and extends above the water level at one end and connects to an outside respiratory hose at the other end (Fig. 2). A lightweight plastic bell with an open bottom is inside the body of the 9-liter container. By enclosing the hollow tube, the bell will rise when a person exhales through the external respiratory hose. This causes the attached chain on a pulley to move the volume indicators (pointers) of the vitalometer. A *red* pointer on a circular scale indicates the vital capacity value. The *black* pointer indicates the designated *timed volumes* (0.5, 0.75, 1, 2, 3 s). A disadvantage of the vitalometer is that it fails to meet the American Thoracic Society's requirement of providing a digital or graphic recording.[2]

The vital capacity can be measured with 9.0- or 13.5-liter spirometers (Fig. 3), whose distinguishing features include the rotating drum (kymograph or ventilograph) and the container for carbon dioxide absorbent (e.g., barium hydroxide lime). The bell's counterbalanced chain passes over a pulley and is attached to a pen that records all respiratory movements on the spirogram (chart paper) of the kymograph. The kymograph or drum can rotate at slow (32 mm·min^{-1}), moderate (160 mm·min^{-1}), or fast (1920 mm·min^{-1}) speeds.

Regardless of the instrument being used to measure vital capacity, the methods are very similar. The pretest preparations should ensure that the equipment is ready for use and is properly sanitized and calibrated, in addition to ensuring that the subject is prepared.

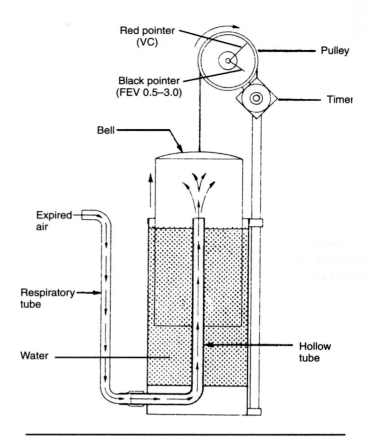

Figure 2 A schematic diagram of an automated wet spirometer (e.g., Vitalometer®), showing the upward movement of the bell as the subject exhales through the respiratory tube into the water-filled container.

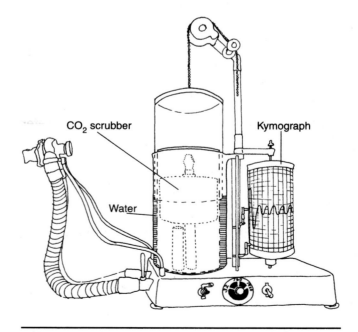

Figure 3 A wet spirometer with the kymograph for recording lung volumes. It includes a two-way breathing valve and a container of CO_2 "scrubber."

Calibration of Respiratory Instruments

Manufacturers should testify that their instruments meet the recommendations of the American Thoracic Society.[2] To assure accurate volumes of spirometers or pneumotachs, the technician should pump air through the instrument using a calibrated syringe ($\geq$3 L).

The residual volume analyzers require the test (calibrated) gases—oxygen, nitrogen, helium, or carbon dioxide.

Preparation

Ideally, persons should not have exercised within 12 hours of pulmonary function testing.[11] This is partly because the vital capacity has been shown to be reduced temporarily after exercise.[22] For example, both vital capacity and $FEV_{1.0}$ may be decreased significantly at the 5th and 10th min but not at the 30th min after varying intensities of exercise.[29] It is customary to measure lung volumes while the person is in the seated position. The standing position, which gives slightly greater volumes than sitting,[33] is recommended because the norms presented later are based on the standing position.[19,26,27]

Individuals should wear a noseclip if they are inexperienced in the vital capacity test or if the data are to be used for research. The technician should ask the person if it is possible to breathe with the mouth closed when wearing the noseclip. If the person can still breathe, the noseclip should be readjusted until he/she cannot breathe when the mouth is closed. It is possible to perform valid tests of vital capacity in experienced persons by simply having them pinch the nose with the fingers during the test.

In order to ensure that the person knows exactly what to do, the technician and performer should rehearse the commands and practice the breathing maneuvers. The technician should demonstrate the maneuvers;[2] the technician need not use the spirometer.

Measuring FVC and $FEV_{1.0-3.0}$ Using the Vitalometer

1. In preparation for the test, the bell of the vitalometer should be pushed to its lowest position. The indicator pointers—red and black—should be turned clockwise to the starting position (300–400 mL). The timing knob should be set at the 1.0-s position in order to measure $FEV_{1.0}$.
2. The performer holds the respiratory tube at the junction of the mouthpiece and tube.
3. The performer inhales as deeply as possible (maximal inspiration) without inhaling *from* the respiratory tube.
4. At the point of maximal inspiration, the performer places the mouthpiece into the mouth and exhales as much air as possible and as fast as possible. The entire exhalation should last about 5 s[16] to 10 s[2], although most persons will expire their entire VC within 4 s.[14,17]

Technicians should give verbal encouragement such as Go, All the way out, Keep going, Looking good, Push, and Gut it out!

5. The technician reads and records the red (VC) and black ($FEV_{1.0}$) pointers to the closest 50 mL (or 0.05 L).
6. The bell automatically returns nearly to the starting position after the performer removes his/her mouth from the breathing tube; if it does not, the technician should press gently down on the bell so that it does.
7. Repeat the test three times; the *best* value is used for interpretive purposes.
8. After three trials with the timer at 1.0 s, the participant performs three trials at 3.0 s in order to measure the $FEV_{3.0}$.
9. The technician thanks the participant for such cooperation and effort, in addition to mentioning that it is possible that the abdominal muscles will be slightly sore on the next day.

The breathing maneuver for measuring vital capacity when using the 9.0- or 13.5-L respirometer is the same as that using the vitalometer. It may be more convenient, however, to measure vital capacity with the subject seated if the measurement is made sequentially from the other lung volume measurements. The techniques for making the measurement on the respirometer follow.

Measuring FVC and $FEV_{1.0-3.0}$ Using the Respirometer

1. The participant places the mouthpiece into the mouth.
2. The technician places the pen of the respirometer at the lower portion of the spirogram, making sure that there is enough space for the pen excursion for the expiratory capacity.
3. The technician switches the rotating drum to the slow speed (32 mm per min; 1 min between vertical lines).
4. After a few normal breaths by the participant, the technician requests him/her to perform the vital capacity maneuver that has been rehearsed—maximal inspiration followed by maximal expiration.
5. When the participant is nearly at the peak of the inspiratory capacity, the technician switches to the moderate (160 mm per min; 12 s between vertical lines) or fast (1920 mm/min; 1 s between vertical lines) speed.
6. The participant removes the mouthpiece and relaxes while the technician flushes the respirometer a few times (manually lifts and lowers the bell).
7. The test is repeated three times.
8. The technician calculates the vital capacity and the $FEV_{1.0}$ and $_{3.0}$ from the spirogram.

Expiratory Reserve Volume, Tidal Volume, and Inspiratory Reserve Volume

The measurement of lung volumes from the 9.0- or 13.5-L respirometer can be done while testing the vital capacity. In

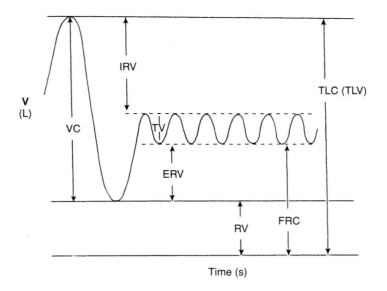

Time (s)

Figure 4 Spirogram of lung volumes and vital capacity (VC): TV = tidal volume, IRV = inspiratory reserve volume, ERV = expiratory reserve volume, RV = residual volume, FRC = functional residual capacity, TLC = total lung capacity or volume.

fact, the tidal volume, expiratory reserve volume, and inspiratory volume may be measured from the spirogram obtained by performing the ventilatory maneuvers just prior to the VC test. It is simply a matter of calculating the respective volumes based upon the diagram presented in Figure 4.

The vitalometer was not designed to measure lung volumes other than vital capacity. However, reasonable estimates of expiratory reserve volume may be made with the vitalometer by following these steps:

1. The technician inserts a three-way stopcock at some point between the subject's mouthpiece and the respiratory tube of the vitalometer; the stopcock may be eliminated if proper timing of the mouthpiece insertion is practiced.
2. The technician turns the stopcock so that the direction of airflow is not toward the vitalometer.
3. The participant places the mouthpiece of the valve into his or her mouth and breathes normally.
4. The technician instructs the participant to pause momentarily at the end of a normal tidal volume.
5. At the end-tidal pause, the technician turns the stopcock so that air is directed from the subject to the vitalometer.
6. After the technician turns the valve of the stopcock, the participant exhales maximally.
7. At the end of the maximal exhalation, the value is read at the red pointer.
8. The technician returns the bell and pointer to the starting position.
9. The participant removes the mouthpiece and relaxes during step 8.
10. The entire test procedure is repeated two more times.

Residual Volume (RV)

The residual volume is the only lung volume that cannot be measured directly; it is also the most complicated and expensive method. Depending upon the chosen method and instrumentation, the reader may have to consult additional sources.[4,8,9,10,13,36,37]

Residual volume may vary daily by about 5% in either direction for healthy individuals.[8] The standard error of measurement is about 100 ml based upon a review of traditional methods,[36] and about 125 ml when using a simplified method.[37] Contrary to vital capacity, residual volume has been shown to increase temporarily after exercise,[15] and it should not be measured for at least 30 min after exercise.[5]

Traditional methods to measure residual volume require expensive gas analyzers. One method requires a nitrogen or oxygen analyzer and is called the **nitrogen washout** method. The two **helium dilution methods** (multiple breath and single breath) require a helium analyzer.

Nitrogen Washout

The rationale for using the nitrogen washout method of estimating residual volume is based upon the measurement of the functional residual capacity (FRC). This is because residual volume cannot be measured directly but can be derived by subtracting the known expiratory reserve volume (ERV) from the FRC (Eq. 2).

$$RV \text{ (ml)} = FRC - ERV \qquad \text{Eq. 2}$$

Oxygen (O_2) Dilution

The O_2 dilution method eliminates the need for a nitrogen or helium analyzer but requires rapid-responding carbon dioxide and oxygen analyzers.[37] Fortunately, the analyzers are fairly common in exercise physiology laboratories. This simplified method's reliabilities range from $r = .96$[32] to $.99$,[37] with a validity coefficient of $.92$.[37]

The procedures for the oxygen dilution technique of reaching nitrogen equilibrium by using only oxygen and carbon dioxide analyzers is conceptualized by Equation 3.

$$RV = \frac{\text{bag } VO_2 \times N_2 \%}{79.8 - N_2 \%} \qquad \text{Eq. 3}$$

where:

VO_2 = initial volume of oxygen in bag
$N_2\%$ = $100\% - (O_2\% + CO_2\%)$; represents the $N_2\%$ in mixed air in the bag at the point of equilibrium
79.8 = assumed percentage of nitrogen in air

For example, if the initial volume of oxygen in the anaesthesia bag is 5 L and the percentages of oxygen and carbon dioxide are 75% and 5% respectively, then the calculation of residual volume is as follows:

$$RV(L) = \frac{5.0 \times \left[100 - (75 + 5)\right]}{79.8\% - \left[100 - (75 + 5)\right]}$$
$$= (5.0 \times 20\%)/(79.8\% - 20\%)$$
$$= 100/59.8 = 1.67 \text{ L}$$

Several preparations are necessary before measuring the residual volume using the simplified method. The vital capacity of the subject must be measured prior to the RV test. In addition, the technician should set up the instrumentation as follows: (a) attach a 5-L anaesthesia bag to a two-way syringe stopcock; (b) attach the other end of the bag to a three-way breathing valve that can be opened to room air or the bag; (c) flush the bag with oxygen about three times; (d) fill the bag with a volume of oxygen that is 80–90% of the subject's vital capacity.

Procedures for the Simplified Method of the RV Test

1. The technician fills a small anaesthesia bag to an accurately measured volume of oxygen; for example, manually push the bell of a spirometer that has been filled with 100% oxygen so the oxygen flows into the bag, and then calculate the amount taken from the spirometer.

2. The participant, wearing a noseclip and in the sitting position, breathes normally via the mouthpiece attached to the three-way breathing valve opened to room air. If the main purpose of measuring RV is subsequently to measure body density by underwater weighing, then RV should be measured in the bent-over sitting position.

3. The technician instructs the participant to perform a maximal expiration after a normal breath.

4. At the end of the maximal expiration the technician turns the three-way valve open to the 5-L bag of oxygen.

5. The technician instructs the participant to breathe deeply (but not vacuating the bag) five to seven times at about one breath per 2 s.

6. Following the five to seven breaths, the technician instructs the participant to exhale to maximal expiration.

7. The technician turns the valve to close the 5-L bag, thus opening the valve to room air.

8. The technician thanks the participant and removes the noseclip.

9. The participant removes his or her mouth from the mouthpiece.

10. The technician removes about 1 L of air from the bag; the remaining contents are analyzed using the carbon dioxide and oxygen analyzers.

11. The technician uses Equation 3 to find residual volume.

12. The technician repeats the procedure until readings are within 200 ml (a strict criterion may be 100 ml) of each other; the average of these is the subject's RV.

13. The technician corrects the volume to BTPS using Equation 9 (or Eq. 8 with Table 1).

14. The total lung volume (TLV) or capacity (TLC) can be derived easily from a combination of lung volumes or capacities that are now known.

$$TLC = FRC + IC \qquad \text{Eq. 4}$$
$$TLC = RV + VC \qquad \text{Eq. 5}$$

Calculations and Corrections for Lung Volumes and Vital Capacity

Certain calculations are made in order to correct respiratory volumes to conventional units of measure. Additionally, simple calculations are necessary in some instances in order to allow for easier interpretation of the norms; an example of the latter is the conversion of the FEV values to a percentage of the VC value.

Correction of Lung Volumes to Conventional Volumes

The final recorded respiratory lung volumes always should be expressed in terms of BTPS, where the BT represents normal body temperature, the P represents the barometric pressure at the test site, and the S represents the saturation level of the air volume. For example, the vital capacity value (liters or milliliters) that is read on the spirometer is in terms of ATPS. The ATPS abbreviation means that the volume of ambient (A) air is at laboratory temperature and pressure and is saturated with water vapor. In other words, the air that is expired from the subject's lungs decreases from the typical body temperature of 37 °C to 33 °C at the mouth exit[24] to that of the laboratory or spirometer temperature, usually 20–25 °C. The air remains saturated because of the water surrounding the bell of the spirometer. The barometric pressure is read from the laboratory barometer.

Table 1 Correction Factors (CF) for Converting ATPS Volumes (100% RH) to BTPS Volumes at ~760 torr

Ambient T (°C)	CF	Ambient T (°C)	CF
20	1.102	29	1.051
21	1.096	30	1.045
22	1.091	31	1.039
23	1.085	32	1.032
24	1.080	33	1.026
25	1.075	34	1.020
26	1.068	35	1.014
27	1.063	36	1.007
28	1.057	37	1.000

Table 2 Water Vapor Pressure ($P-H_2O$) at 100% Saturation at Given Temperatures (T)

°C	T °K	$P-H_2O$ torr	°C	T °K	$P-H_2O$ torr
20	293	18	31	304	34
21	294	19	32	305	36
22	295	20	33	306	38
23	296	21	34	307	40
24	297	22	35	308	42
25	298	24	36	309	45
26	299	25	37	310	47
27	300	27	38	311	50
28	301	28	39	312	52
29	302	30	40	313	55
30	303	32			

Source: Data from Comroe, J. H., Forster, R. E., Dubois, A. B., Briscoe, W. A., & Carlsen, E. (Eds), p. 10, 323, 1962; Chicago: Year Book Medical Publishers, p. 10, 323, 1962.

Because of the temperature difference between the air in the lungs (body) and that of the air being measured in the ambient environment (spirometer), a correction must be made. Because air molecules expand at higher temperatures, it is logical to expect the BTPS values to be higher than ATPS volumes (unless under unusually hot conditions whereby the ambient temperature is over 37 °C). The correction factors presented in Table 1 were derived from Equation 6, which accounts for both the expansion of gas and the increase of water vapor pressure due to the increase of temperature. Table 1 should serve all laboratory pressures because the differences are extremely small. The correction factors range from 1.0 (no correction) at 37 °C to about 1.1 at 20 °C. The correction factors are then used to multiply the ATPS volume in order to obtain the BTPS volume.[9]

$$\text{BTPS CF} = \frac{273 \; °K + T_B \; °C}{273 \; °K + T_A \; °C} \qquad \text{Eq. 6}$$
$$\times \frac{P_B - P-H_2O_A}{P_B - P-H_2O_B}$$

where:

BTPS CF = the correction factor for respiratory volumes
T_B = body temperature (assumed to be 37 °C at rest)
T_A = ambient (environmental or spirometric) temperature
P_B = laboratory barometric pressure
$P-H_2O_A$ = vapor pressure of water at the T_A
$P-H_2O_B$ = vapor pressure of water at T_B (assumed, 47 torr)

The vapor pressure of water ($P-H_2O$) at 100% saturation and at temperatures between 20 °C and 40 °C may be found by referring to Table 2. The water vapor pressure at other saturation percentages (RH%) can be found by using Equation 7 in conjunction with Table 2. Equation 7 simply calls for the multiplication of the water vapor pressure (torr) at 100% relative humidity (RH%) by the %RH at the ambient temperature. When using wet (water-filled) spirometers, however, the air is always 100% saturated; thus there is no need to use the equation or table. However, if using dry spirometers (e.g., bellows-type air meters) then

the equation or table must be used. As relative humidity decreases, the water vapor pressure also decreases at any given temperature. Thus, an RH decrease causes an increase in the magnitude of the correction factor because of a greater difference between the ambient (A) water pressure and the lung (B) water pressure. As temperature increases at any given relative humidity, the water pressure increases, thus reducing the difference between the BTPS and ATPS conditions.

$$P-H_2O_A \text{ (torr)} = RH\% \times 100\% \; P-H_2O_A \qquad \text{Eq. 7}$$

For example, if the ambient relative humidity (RH%) is 50% and the temperature is 25 °C, then the following calculation provides the water vapor pressure at ambient conditions:

$$P-H_2O_A \text{ (torr)} = 50\% \times 24 \text{ torr (Table 2)}$$
$$= 12 \text{ torr}$$

If a person is tested under extremely humid ambient conditions, or if a wet spirometer is used, whereby the temperature is 25 °C at 100% RH and the barometric pressure is 758 torr, then by inserting the proper values into Equation 6 and making the following calculations we could find the BTPS correction factor:

$$\text{BTPS CF (torr)} = \frac{273 \; °K + 37 \; °C}{273 \; °K + 25 \; °C}$$
$$\times \frac{758 \text{ torr} - 24 \text{ torr}}{758 \text{ torr} - 47 \text{ torr}}$$
$$= (310 \; °K / 298 \; °K) \times (734 \text{ torr} / 711 \text{ torr}) =$$
$$1.04 \times 1.03 = 1.07 \text{ (same as Table 1)}$$

Thus, by simply finding the respiratory correction factor (CF) and then multiplying the ATPS volume by that factor, one may calculate the BTPS volume (V_{BTPS}) (Eq. 8).

$$V_{BTPS} \text{ (L)} = CF \times V_{ATPS} \qquad \text{Eq. 8}$$

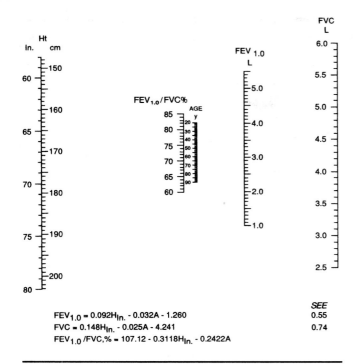

$$FEV_{1.0} = 0.092H_{In.} - 0.032A - 1.260$$
$$FVC = 0.148H_{In.} - 0.025A - 4.241$$
$$FEV_{1.0}/FVC,\% = 107.12 - 0.3118H_{In.} - 0.2422A$$

SEE
0.55
0.74

Figure 5 Nomogram for predicting vital capacity (VC), Forced Expiratory Volume in 1.0 s (FEV₁) and FEV₁/FVC% (BTPS), in **men** between the ages of 20–29 y.
From J. F. Morris, "Spirometry in the Evaluation of Pulmonary Function", in *The Western Journal of Medicine*, 125, (2), fig. 2, p. 114, 1976. Copyright © 1976 California Medical Association.

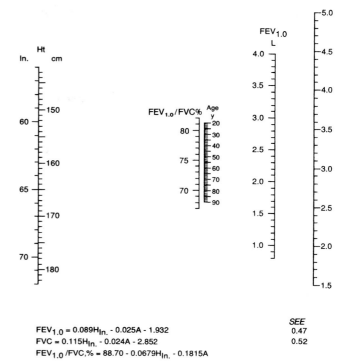

$$FEV_{1.0} = 0.089H_{In.} - 0.025A - 1.932$$
$$FVC = 0.115H_{In.} - 0.024A - 2.852$$
$$FEV_{1.0}/FVC,\% = 88.70 - 0.0679H_{In.} - 0.1815A$$

SEE
0.47
0.52

Figure 6 Nomogram for predicting vital capacity (VC), forced expiratory volume in 1.0 s (FEV₁), and FEV₁/FVC% (BTPS) in **women** between 20–90 y of age.
From J. F. Morris, "Spirometry in the Evaluation of Pulmonary Function", in *The Western Journal of Medicine*, 125, (2), fig. 3, p. 115, 1976. Copyright © 1976 California Medical Association.

For example, if the vital capacity value on the wet spirometer (or vitalometer) reads 5.40 L and the ambient temperature is 22 °C, then by referring to Table 1 or by using Equation 6 (use only the equation for dry spirometers) the BTPS correction factor is found to be 1.09. Then by using Equation 8 the following calculation is made to get the respiratory volume (V_{BTPS}):

$$V_{BTPS} (L) = 1.09 \times 5.40 = 5.89 \text{ L}$$

The equation (6) for the correction of the volume of air in the spirometer (V_A) to the volume of air in the lungs (V_B) can be summarized by Equation 9:

$$V_{BTPS} = V_{ATPS} \times \frac{310}{273 + T_A} \times \frac{P_B - P\text{-}H_2O}{P_B - 47}$$

Eq. 9

In summary, the BTPS volume reflects the actual environmental condition of the lungs, whereas the ATPS volume reflects the environmental condition at the test site. The only difference in calculating the CF for dry versus wet conditions is that the dry condition requires the use of Table 2 with Equation 7. In other words, the lower RH% must be accounted for so as to increase the CF.

Calculations to Facilitate the Interpretation of Scores

The largest observed vital capacity and forced expiratory volume can be interpreted more meaningfully if the expected scores are known (Predicted VC or PVC and Predicted FEV or PFEV, respectively). It is also meaningful to know what percentage of the predicted score (%P) is represented by the observed vital capacity (VC_{obs}). Both the predicted and observed respiratory volumes should be presented in BTPS terms.

The predicted value of vital capacity may be approximated from the appropriate nomogram[26] for gender (Fig. 5 for men; Fig. 6 for women) or calculated from the regression equations (Equations 10 for men and 11 for women). The standard errors of estimates are 0.74 and 0.52 L, respectively.[26,27] These equations give values that are virtually identical to other equations published elsewhere.[1,23] The values may be multiplied by 0.85 for African Americans and Asians.[1] If the decimals are ignored in the equations, the answer will be in units of milliliters; thus, the equations will predict the vital capacity within 740 or 520 ml for two-thirds of the population at any given height (Ht) and age for each gender, respectively.

Men: VC_{BTPS} (L) = 0.148 Ht (in.) or 0.058 Ht
(cm) – 0.025 Age – 4.241   Eq. 10

Women: VC_{BTPS} (L) = 0.115 Ht (in.) or 0.045 Ht
(cm) – 0.024 Age – 2.852   Eq. 11

For example, a 46-year-old man who is 69 in. (175 cm) tall would be expected to have a vital capacity of 4.82 L based upon the following calculations:

$$VC_{BTPS} \text{ (L)} = (0.148 \times 69 \text{ in.}) - (.025 \times 46 \text{ y})$$
$$- 4.241 = 10.21 - 1.15 - 4.241 = 4.819 \text{ L}$$

or using cm: (0.058×175.26)

$$- (0.025 \times 46) - 4.241$$
$$= 10.17 - 1.15 - 4.241 = 4.79$$

Equation 12 is used to calculate the percent of predicted.

$$\%P = (VC_{obs}/PVC) \times 100 \qquad \text{Eq. 12}$$

Thus, if the 46-year-old man in the previous example had an observed vital capacity measure of 6.00 L, then the percent predicted (%P) would be calculated as follows:

$$\%P = (6.00/4.82) \times 100$$
$$= 1.24 \times 100$$
$$= 124\%$$

The expected or predicted values for Forced Expiratory Volumes in 1.0 s for men and women can be found from the respective nomograms in Figures 5 and 6 or from their predictive equations. As with the prediction equation for vital capacity, the prediction equations (Equations 13 and 14) for the forced expiratory volume in 1 s ($PFEV_1$) considers the gender, age, and height of the person.[26] The standard errors of the estimates are 0.55 for men and 0.47 for women.

Men: $PFEV_1$ (L) = 0.092 Ht (in.) or 0.036 Ht
(cm) – 0.032 Age – 1.260   Eq. 13

Women: $PFEV_1$ (L) = 0.089 Ht (in.) or 0.035 Ht
(cm) – 0.025 Age – 1.932   Eq. 14

Results and Discussion

As in previous chapters, the focus of attention when discussing the results of the tests is on the interpretation of the test scores. As noted earlier, the tests for the four lung volumes are of physiological significance and when interpreted in conjunction with vital capacity and FEV tests add a clinical significance.

Respiratory Lung Volumes

Some typical values for three respiratory volumes,[8] have been converted to percentages of vital capacity and total lung volume in Table 3. As long as a person's respiratory values are normal, they are not good predictors of fitness or performance in a standard environment; this is especially true when such values are adjusted for body size, gender, and age. The approximated percentages for IRV, TV, and

ERV are based on the assumption that the percentages do not vary with total lung volume. Absolute values for residual volume and total lung volume in a typical 20- to 30-year-old man and woman are presented also in Table 3. A slightly higher value for residual volumes in adult men (1300 ml) has been reported.[28]

Vital Capacity

Over twenty different "norms" are commonly used by various labs.[2] The valid interpretation of vital capacity should consider the person's age, height, gender, and smoking status. The norms that are presented in Figures 5 and 6 are based on nearly 1000 nonsmoking men and women.[27] The nonsmoking normative values are equivalent to an improvement of lung function that represents a 10-year decrease in age[25] compared to some traditional norms that included smokers.[18] This is attributed to destruction of the pulmonary tissues and consequent degrees of chronic obstructive pulmonary disease (COPD) in those persons with cigarette addiction. The investigators in the famous epidemiological heart study in Framingham, Mass., found that the vital capacity and the FEV_1 were associated with living capacity; thus, the lower the VC or $FEV_1\%$, the greater the risk of death.[3]

The vital capacities for a typical man and woman between the ages of 20 and 30 years are 4.8 L and 3.2 L respectively.[8] The highest vital capacity for a female measured in our laboratory was 5.98 L in a former swimmer who was predicted to be 3.99 based upon her age of 31 years and her height of 5.5 ft (~168 cm). This observed value represented 150% of her predicted value. One of the highest men's %PVC was 132% by a 48-year-old who was predicted to have a VC of 4.77 L, but had an observed value of 6.32 L.

In general, an individual's measured vital capacity (BTPS) should be a minimum of 80% of the predicted value in order to be considered normal.[26] Percentages between 100% and 120% would be considered good, and those above 120% could be classified as high. The vital capacity and FEV_1 criteria for various degrees of ventilatory impairment—restrictive and obstructive—are presented in Table 4. Because the FEV_1/VC has been shown to decrease linearly through the course of chronic obstructive lung disease,[31] the table's criteria are expressed three ways: (1) the observed VC percent of predicted FVC, (2) the observed FEV_1 percent of predicted FEV_1, and (3) FEV_1 percent of observed VC. With respect to FEV_1/VC, normal persons should be able to exhale more than 80% of their vital capacity in 1 s (FEV_1); 94% during the first 2 s (FEV_2); and 97% during the first 3 s (FEV_3). A decrease in pre-exercise FEV_1 versus post-exercise FEV_1 of 10% or greater following strenuous exercise might suggest exercise-induced bronchospasm.[20,21,30,34] This bronchospasm in most chronic asthmatics and many allergic persons is usually maximal between 5 and 15 min after exercise.

Table 3 Typical Respiratory Lung Volumes (%VC; %TLV mL) and Capacities (mL)

Lung Volume	%VC	%TLV		Absolute Volumes (mL)			Capacities	
				Men	Women		Men	Women
IRV	65	52	IRV	3100	1900	VC	4800	3200
TV	10	8	TV	400–500	350–450	IC	3600	2400
ERV	25	20	ERV	1200	900	FRC	2400	1800
RV		20	RV	1200	1000			
			TLV	6000	4200			

From J. F. Morris, "Spirometry in the Evaluation of Pulmonary Function", in *The Western Journal of Medicine,* 125, (2), table 2, p. 116, 1976. Copyright © 1976 California Medical Association.

Table 4 Degrees of Restrictive or Obstructive Lung Disease Based on VC/PVC[b], FEV_1/$PFEV_1$,[c] and FEV_1/VC[c]

Subjective Degree	Percentage
Normal	>80
Mild; borderline[a]	65–80; 70–79
Moderate	50–64
Severe	35–49
Very Severe	<35

From J. F. Morris, "Spirometry in the Evaluation of Pulmonary Function," in *The Western Journal of Medicine, 125,* (2), Table 2, p. 116, 1976. Copyright © 1976 California Medical Association.
[a]Note: Mahler's (1993) lower criterion for normal.
[b]VC may be normal in some *obstructive* patients.[1]
[c]FEV_1 may be normal, and FEV_1/FVC may be normal or increased in some *restrictive* patients.[1]

References

1. American College of Sports Medicine. (1995). *ACSM's Guidelines for exercise testing and prescription.* Philadelphia: Williams & Wilkins.
2. American Thoracic Society. (1987). Standardization of spirometry—1987 update. *American Review of Respiratory Disease, 136,* 1285–1298.
3. Ashley, F., Kannel, W. B., Sorlie, P. D., & Masson, R. (1975). Pulmonary function: Relation to aging, cigarette habit, and mortality. *Annals of Internal Medicine, 82,* 736–745.
4. Brown, L. K., & Miller, A. (1987). In A. Miller (Ed.), *Pulmonary function tests* (Chapter 5). Orlando, FL: Grune & Stratton.
5. Buono, M. J., Constable, S. H., Morton, A. R., Rotkis, T. C., Stanforth, P. R., & Wilmore, J. H. (1981). The effect of an acute bout of exercise on selected pulmonary function measurements. *Medicine and Science in Sports and Exercise, 13,* 290–293.
6. Cissik, J. H., & Louden, J. A. (1979, April/May). Measurement precision of screening spirometry in normal adult men. *Cardiovascular Practice (CVP), 63,* 65–68.
7. Collins, Warren E. (1976). *The timed vitalometer.* Braintree, MA: Author.
8. Comroe, J. H., Forster, R. E., Dubois, A. B., Briscoe, W. A., & Carlsen, E. (1962). *The Lung.* Chicago: Year Book Medical Publishers.
9. Consolazio, C. F., Johnson, R. E., & Pecora, L. J. (1963). *Physiological measurements of metabolic functions in man.* New York: McGraw-Hill.
10. Cooper, C. B. (1995). Determining the role of exercise in patients with chronic pulmonary disease. *Medicine and Science in Sports and Exercise, 27,* 147–157.
11. Cordain, L., Tucker, A., Moon, D., & Stager, J. M. (1990). Lung volumes and maximal respiratory pressures in collegiate swimmers and runners. *Research Quarterly for Exercise and Sport, 61,* 70–74.
12. Darling, R. C., Cournand, A., & Richards, D. W. (1940). Studies on the intrapulmonary mixture of gases. III. An open circuit method for measuring residual air. *Journal of Clinical Investigation, 19,* 609–618.
13. Enright, P. L., & Hyatt, R. E. (1987). *Office spirometry.* Philadelphia: Lea & Febiger.
14. Gaensler, E. A. (1951). Analysis of the ventilatory defect by timed capacity measurements. *The American Review of Tuberculosis, 64,* 256–278.
15. Girandola, R., Wiswell, R., Mohler, J., Romero, G., & Barnes, W. (1977). Effects of water immersion on lung volumes: Implications for body compositional analysis. *Journal of Applied Physiology, 43,* 276–279.
16. Goldman, A. L. (1979, April/May). Standardization of spirometry. *Cardiovascular Practice (CVP),* 35–39.
17. Hodgkin, J. E., Balchum, O. J., Kass, I., Glaser, E. M., Miller, W. F., Haas, A., Shaw, D. B., Kimbel, P., & Petty, T. L. (1975). Chronic obstructive airway diseases—current concept in diagnosis and comprehensive care. *JAMA, 232,* 1243.
18. Hutchinson, J. (1846). On capacity of lungs and on respiratory functions with view of establishing a precise and easy method of detecting disease by spirometer. *Tr. Med.-Chir. Society of London, 29,* 137.
19. Kory, R. C., Callahan, R., Boren, H. G., & Syner, J. C. (1961). The Veterans Administration-Army cooperative study of pulmonary function. *American Journal of Medicine, 30,* 243–258.
20. Kyle, J. M., Walker, R. B., Hanshaw, S. L., Leaman, J. R., & Frobase, J. K. (1992). Exercise-induced

bronchospasms in the young athlete: Guidelines for routine screening and initial management. *Medicine and Science in Sports and Exercise, 24,* 856–859.

21. Mahler, D. A. (1993). Exercise-induced asthma. *Medicine and Science in Sports and Exercise, 25,* 554–561.

22. Maron, M., Hamilton, L., & Maksud, M. (1979). Alterations in pulmonary function consequent to competitive marathon running. *Medicine and Science in Sports and Exercise, 11,* 244–249.

23. Miller, A. (1986). *Pulmonary function tests in clinical and occupational lung disease.* Orlando, FL: Grune & Stratton.

24. Miller, M. R., & Pincock, A. C. (1986). Linearity and temperature control of the Fleisch pneumotachograph. *Journal of Applied Physiology, 60,* 710–715.

25. Mohler, S. R. (1981). Reasons for eliminating the "age 60" rule. *Aviation, Space, and Environmental Medicine, 52,* 445–454.

26. Morris, J. F. (1976). Spirometry in the evaluation of pulmonary function. *The Western Journal of Medicine, 125,* 110–118.

27. Morris, J. F., Koski, A. Johnson, L. C. (1971). Spirometric standards for healthy nonsmoking adults. *American Review of Respiratory Disease, 103,* 57–68.

28. National Academy of Sciences. (1958). *Handbook of respiration.* Philadelphia: W. B. Saunders.

29. O'Krory, J. A., Loy, R. A., & Coast, J. R. (1992). Pulmonary function changes following exercise. *Medicine and Science in Sports and Exercise, 24,* 1359–1364.

30. Scoggin, C. (1985). Exercise-induced asthma. *Chest, 87* (Suppl.), 48S–49S.

31. Sobol, B. J., & Emirgil, C. (1977). Clinical significance of pulmonary function tests. *Chest, 72,* 81–85.

32. Thorland, W. G., Johnson, G. O., Cisar, C. J., & Housh, T. J. (1987). Estimation of minimal wrestling weight using measures of body build and body composition. *International Journal of Sports Medicine, 8,* 365–370.

33. Townsend, M. C. (1984). Spirometric forced expiratory volumes measured in the standing versus the sitting posture. *American Review of Respiratory Disease, 130,* 123–124.

34. Virant, F. S. (1992). Exercise-induced bronchospasm—Epidemiology, patho-physiology, and therapy. *Medicine and Science in Sports and Exercise, 24,* 851–855.

35. Wasserman, K., Hansen, J. E., Sue, D. Y., Whipp, B. J., & Casaburi, R. (1994). *Principles of exercise testing and interpretation.* Philadelphia: Lea & Febiger.

36. Wilmore, J. H. (1969). A simplified method for determination of residual lung volume. *Journal of Applied Physiology, 27,* 96–100.

37. Wilmore, J. H., Vodak, P. A., Parr, R. B., Girandola, R. N., & Billing, J. E. (1980). Further simplification of a method for determination of residual lung volume. *Medicine and Science in Sports and Exercise, 12,* 216–218.

Form *LV 1*

Individual Data for FVC, FEV$_{1.0}$ and $_{3.0}$

Name [   ] Date [   ] Time [   ] a.m. [   ] p.m. [   ]

Age [   ] y Gender (M or F) [   ] Ht [   ] cm Wt [   ] kg

Smoker:
now _____
past _____
never _____

Temperature (T) [   ] °C P_B [   ] torr RH (dry spirometer) [   ] %; wet $\underline{100\%}$

Correction Factor (CF) [   ] (Table 1 wet; 100% RH) [   ] (Table 2; Eqs. 7 & 9)

Vital Capacity (ATPS) Trial: #1 [   ] mL #2 [   ] mL #3 [   ] mL (circle highest)

VC (BTPS) = CF [   ] × VC (ATPS) [   ] mL = [   ] mL; ÷ 1000 = [   ] L

Predicted VC (PVC)

Men: PVC = (0.148 × [   ] in.) or (0.058 × [   ] cm) − (0.025 × [   ] y) − 4.241

= [   ] − [   ] − 4.241 = [   ] L

(0.148 × in. or 0.058 × cm) − (0.025 × y)

Women: PVC = (0.115 × [   ] in.) or (0.045 × [   ] cm) − (0.024 × [   ] y) − 2.852

= [   ] − [   ] − 2.852 = [   ] L

(0.115 × in. or 0.045 × cm) − (0.024 × y)

% PVC = (VC$_{obs}$BTPS [   ] /PVC [   ]) × 100 = [   ] %

FEV$_{1.0}$
ATPS Trial: #1 [   ] mL #2 [   ] mL #3 [   ] mL (circle highest)

FEV$_1$ BTPS = CF [   ] FEV$_1$ × ATPS [   ] mL = [   ] mL; ÷ 1000 = [   ] L

Men: PFEV$_1$ = (0.092 × [   ] in.) or (0.036 × [   ] cm) − (0.032 × [   ] y) − 1.260

= [   ] − [   ] − 1.260 = [   ] L

(0.092 × in. or 0.036 × cm) − (0.032 × y)

Women: PFEV$_1$ = (0.089 × [   ] in.) or (0.035 × [   ] cm) − (0.025 × [   ] y) − 1.932

= [   ] − [   ] − 1.932 = [   ] L

(0.089 × in. or 0.035 × cm) − (0.025 × y)

%PFEV$_1$ = (FEV$_{1obs}$BTPS [   ] /PFEV$_1$ [   ]) × 100 = [   ] %

FEV$_{3.0}$
ATPS Trial: #1 [   ] mL #2 [   ] mL #3 [   ] mL (circle highest)

FEV$_3$BTPS = CF [   ] × [   ] FEV$_3$ATPS = [   ] mL; ÷ 1000 = [   ] L

%FEV$_3$ of VC BTPS = (FEV$_3$ BTPS [   ] mL /VC BTPS [   ] mL) × 100 = [   ] %

Form *LV 2*

Individual Data for Residual Volume

Name ☐ Date ☐ Time ☐ a.m. ☐ p.m. ☐

Age ☐ y   Gender (M or F) ☐   Ht ☐ cm   Wt ☐ kg

Temperature (T) ☐ °C   RH 100%

P_B ☐ torr   Correction Factor (CF) ☐   VC ☐ L (BTPS)

80% × VC = ☐ L; 90% × VC = ☐ L   Initial VO_2 (bag) ☐ L

Oxygen % in Bag	Carbon Dioxide % in Bag
Trial #1:	
Trial #2:	
Trial #3:	

$$RV (L) = \frac{VO_2 \boxed{} L \times [100\% - (O_2 \boxed{} \% + CO_2 \boxed{} \%)]}{79.8\% - [100\% - (O_2 \boxed{} \% + CO_2 \boxed{} \%)]}$$

$$= \frac{\boxed{} L \times \boxed{} \%}{79.8\% - \boxed{} \%} \quad \frac{VO_2 \times [100\% - (O_2\% + CO_2\%)]}{[100\% - (O_2\% + CO_2\%)]}$$

$$= \boxed{} L \quad \frac{VO_2 \times [100\% - (O_2\% + CO_2\%)]}{\boxed{}} = \boxed{} L$$

$$(79.8\% - \%)$$

238   Lung Volumes   LV-12

Form *LV 3*

Group Data for Lung Volumes, Vital Capacity, and $FEV_{1.0}$ and $_{3.0}$

Initials   **Volumes and Capacities (BTPS; ml)**

Men	IRV	TV (V_T)	ERV	RV	VC	FEV_1	FEV_3
1.							
2.							
3.							
4.							
5.							
6.							
7.							
8.							
9.							
10.							
Mean							

Women	IRV	TV (V_T)	ERV	RV	VC	FEV_1	FEV_3
1.							
2.							
3.							
4.							
5.							
6.							
7.							
8.							
9.							
10.							
Mean							

Chapter ER Exercise Respiration

Support for exercise testing is based on the nonlinear relationship between functional capacity and symptoms.[21] Thus, it is not unusual to find persons who function nonsymptomatically under resting conditions but have debilitating symptoms under exercise conditions. When an exercise respiratory test is combined with metabolic measures, such as oxygen consumption and carbon dioxide production, it is a very effective, inexpensive, and noninvasive method for diagnosing exercise intolerance.[35]

The purpose of the Exercise Respiratory Test is to examine the influence of exercise upon such dynamic parameters as (a) ventilation, (b) breathing frequency, (c) tidal volume, (d) ventilatory equivalent, and (e) ventilatory threshold. A secondary purpose is to relate a static measurement at rest—maximal voluntary ventilation—to exercise ventilation.

Physiological Rationale

There are measurable differences in exercise respiratory parameters between aerobically fit and nonfit people.[38] In brief, fit people are expected to have lower ventilations, breathing frequencies, and ventilatory equivalents at any given exercise intensity (power). The dynamics of the various respiratory parameters for both fit and nonfit subjects are the following: (a) a positive linear relationship between ventilation versus power level except for the change in linearity at the ventilatory threshold, (b) a positive curvilinear relationship between both breathing frequency and tidal volume versus power level, and (c) a horizontal (nonchanging) relationship between ventilatory equivalent and power levels below the ventilatory threshold. The kinetics of these respiratory variables are similar to those of oxygen consumption, heart rate, and blood pressure. Thus, the time required to achieve steady state usually occurs within 2–6 min, depending primarily upon the intensity of the power level.

Ventilation ($\dot{V}_E$ or $\dot{V}_I$)

The amount of air inspired (I) or expired (E) in one minute is termed ventilation ($L \cdot min^{-1}$). Typical ventilations at rest range from 5 to 10 $L \cdot min^{-1}$, and at exhaustive exercise from 70 to 125 $L \cdot min^{-1}$ with the lower values found in females. Ventilation increases linearly with increased exercise intensity in order to rid the body of carbon dioxide. The increase changes exponentially at a point usually between 50% to 75% of maximal oxygen consumption[31] with less fit persons closer to the 50% value.

Breathing Frequency (f)

The number of breaths taken each minute is referred to as **breathing frequency** or **respiratory rate.** At rest, typical frequencies range from 10 to 20 breaths per minute ($br \cdot min^{-1}$), whereas at maximal exercise they typically range from 40 to 55 $br \cdot min^{-1}$. The curvilinear rise in breathing frequency with increased power levels is gradual at low and moderate powers but rapid at high powers.

Tidal Volume (TV or V_T)

The volume of air inspired or expired with each breath is called the tidal volume. It may be expressed either in milliliters or liters and sometimes as a percentage of the vital capacity. At rest typical tidal volumes are about 350–500 ml (about 10% VC), whereas at maximal aerobic exercise they may reach about 1600 ml and 2400 ml for the typical female and male, respectively (about 50%–60% of VC). The curvilinear rise in tidal volume with increased power levels is opposite that of breathing frequency; there is a rapid increase in TV when progressing from low to moderate powers and smaller increases from moderate to high power levels. The larger tidal volume is due to both greater inspirations and expirations, thus encroaching upon the resting inspiratory and expiratory reserve volumes.[28]

Ventilatory Equivalent (VE)

The ratio of ventilation to oxygen consumption is referred to as the ventilatory (or ventilation) equivalent. The ventilatory equivalent is expressed in formula form in Equation 1.

$$VE = (\dot{V}_E \text{ or } \dot{V}_I) \div \dot{V}O_2 \qquad \text{Eq. 1}$$

Typical ventilatory equivalents at rest are about 20 to 25 L of air for each liter of oxygen consumed, thus 20:1 to 25:1 ratios. Although VE remains relatively constant during subventilatory threshold (ventilatory breakpoint) exercise, it may increase to 30 or more (30^+:1) at oxygen costs exceeding the threshold.

Ventilatory Threshold (Tvent)

The Tvent is an important index of the capacity for prolonged exercise.[3] Originally, the ventilatory threshold was termed the anaerobic threshold (T_{an}), which was used as an indirect, or noninvasive, estimate of the lactate threshold. It was named this because it was thought to represent the start of anaerobic metabolism during exercise. Various researchers and reviewers have quarreled with both the term—T_{an}—and the physiological rationale.[5,7] Other terms often used, and confused, are: (1) *onset of blood lactate accumulation* (OBLA); (2) *lactate threshold;* (3) *ventilatory inflection point—or breakpoint—or threshold;* and (4) *critical lactate clearance point*. The newer terms recognize the nonlinear, or disproportionate, increase in blood lactate or ventilation compared to $\dot{V}O_2$ increase, but do not attribute these to the *beginning* of anaerobiosis.[27,37] Operationally, the lactate threshold, or inflection point, occurs at the oxygen consumption that is associated with at least one millimole (mM)[14] to 2 mM[8] increase in lactate. Although the terms lactate threshold, critical lactate clearance point, and OBLA are similar, the OBLA is usually not designated until lactate levels reach 4.0 mM·L^{-1} of blood.[28] Although the OBLA value of 4 mM is often associated with the critical lactate clearance point (CLCP), this value is not the cause of the CLCP, which reflects the power output beyond the performer's ability to clear lactate and prevent it from continuously rising.[8] Thus, the lactate threshold occurs at a lower oxygen consumption than OBLA and CLCP.

The *ventilatory threshold (Tvent)* or *breakpoint,* controversially referred to as the anaerobic threshold, is associated with the lactate threshold, which, as previously mentioned, occurs at a lower exercise intensity and lactate level than either OBLA[28] or CLCP.[8] A nonlinear increase, or exponential rise, in ventilation (hyperventilation) is thought to be caused by the increase in expired carbon dioxide, which results from the buffering by bicarbonate of the hydrogen ions from lactic acid.[16,37] Usually the Tvent occurs at about 50% to 60% of maximal oxygen consumption in the typical person,[8,9,18] but may vary from 40% to 85% of $\dot{V}O_2$max.[23] An increase in breathing frequency is usually responsible for the increase in ventilation when the exercise level is above the ventilatory threshold; whereas, an increase in tidal volume is mainly responsible for increased ventilation when the exercise level is below the ventilatory threshold. The Tvent has practical implications because fatigue occurs sooner at power levels above the Tvent than below it,[34] and this is even more evident for the critical lactate clearance point.[7]

Maximal Voluntary Ventilation

The maximal voluntary ventilation test (MVV), or sometimes called the maximal breathing capacity test (MBC), reflects the overall capacity of the lungs and respiratory muscles to pump air. Thus, it is an indicator of maximal ventilation ($\dot{V}_E$max) during exercise. However, $\dot{V}_E$max values are only about 70%[5] up to 80% or 86% of 15-s MVV values. The maximum tolerable steady-state exercise ventilation is only about 64% of the 15-s MVV.[19] This is due to the performer's ability to sustain voluntarily a maximal effort during a 12- or 15-second MVV period[4] versus the longer one-minute period for exercise ventilation. Addi-

tionally, maximal exercise does not involuntarily stimulate short-term maximal ventilations, and performers do not voluntarily force themselves to breathe faster and deeper at maximal exercise.

In respiratory patients at exercise, when the ventilation requirement exceeds 50% of the MVV "the patient almost invariably complains of dyspnea (breathlessness)."[20] The correlation was −.49 between MVV and performance time in trained middle distance runners.[13]

The purpose of the MVV test is to measure the maximal amount of air that can be inspired (or expired) within a brief time period under resting conditions.

Maximal Voluntary Ventilation (MVV) Method

If the performer's MVV is going to be compared to maximal ventilation during treadmill ergometry, then the MVV at rest should be measured with the performer standing. If the performer is compared to cycle ergometry, then the resting MVV can be measured with the performer sitting.

Most spirometers today use small and inexpensive microprocessors with digital computers and associated automation. However, the procedures described here use the basic mechanically driven air meter.

Procedural Steps for MVV

1. In the standing position, the performer breathes from a respiratory valve mouthpiece into a dry spirometer or air meter that is connected via ventilatory tubing to a three-way stopcock. Also, the same setup as for the exercise respiratory test may be used (explained later), which has the option of reversing the direction of air flow.
2. Record the present values on the air meter's gauges, or reset the pointers to zero; the value serves as the baseline value.
3. At the "GO" signal, the performer starts breathing as much air as possible. To maximize the MVV, the performer should approximate a breathing rate of 40–80 br·min^{-1} with tidal volumes about 50% of vital capacity; larger breaths may interfere with frequency of breathing.
4. Immediately after the "GO" signal a technician turns the stopcock to direct air from the spirometer to the performer; air continues to exit out the respiratory valve. As soon as the stopcock is turned, another technician starts a stopwatch.
5. At the 12th s (sometimes 15 s) a technician calls "STOP"; the technician turns the stopcock and the performer breathes normally.
6. A technician reads the gauges on the air meter and subtracts the baseline value from this; then this difference is multiplied by five in order to derive the minute value.

$$L \cdot min^{-1} (ATPS) = (12\text{-s meter reading} - Baseline) \times 5$$

7. Repeat the test and use the best trial for data purposes.
8. Convert the ATPS volume to BTPS with the correction factor corresponding to the air temperature and RH.

$$L \cdot min^{-1} (BTPS) = \text{Correction Factor} \times L \cdot min^{-1} (ATPS)$$

Exercise Respiratory Method

The Exercise Respiratory Test described here demonstrates the effect of exercise upon such respiratory factors as ventilation, breathing frequency, tidal volume, ventilatory equivalent, and ventilatory threshold. The equipment, procedures, and calculations are described here.

Equipment

The instruments used to measure respiration during exercise include dry gas meters, respiratory tubing, noseclips, breathing valves, valve support, recorders (optional), calibrating syringe, and ergometers (cycle and treadmill). As with the MVV test, more modern equipment can be used that interfaces pneumotachs (temperature sensitive) or other flowmeters with microcomputers and associated software.[4]

Dry Gas (Airflow) Meters

These nonwater-filled spirometers contrast with wet gas meters (spirometers). They were a welcome invention in the early nineteenth century by gas companies, whose wet meters would freeze and deteriorate.[1] For demonstration and teaching purposes, the gas meter serves very well as an on-line method. Contamination and durability of the dry gas meter may be minimized by measuring inspired air rather than expired air.

Procedure

In addition to the actual conduction of the Exercise Respiratory Test, the technicians should be familiar with the proper preparations, such as calibration, meteorological data, and the exercise protocol.

The technician should record the **meteorological data** onto Form ER 1. This is especially important for respiratory tests because of the influence of temperature, pressure, and saturation on air volumes.

As with most of the exercise tests described in this manual, the **performer** should abide by the standard guidelines prior to exercise testing. The performer should be fitted comfortably and securely with the noseclip and the respiratory valve.

The **exercise protocols** described in Table 1 are for cycle and treadmill ergometry, although other forms of ergometry may be used. The four-minute exercise bouts at each power level are designed to elicit steady-state conditions, especially for those power levels below the ventilatory threshold.[35] It is not expected to be a maximal test. There are three exercise protocols for **cycle ergometry,** depending upon the low, moderate, or high power level of the performer. For example, those persons with $\dot{V}O_2$max values greater than 2.9 L·min^{-1} will use the high-power protocol, which has 4-min stages starting at 100 W, proceeding to 150 W, and ending at 200 W. The cycle recovery period returns to the initial 100-W stage. This cycle protocol will approach maximal levels for persons who are only slightly above the criterion. The single protocol presented for the **treadmill** should be able to be completed by persons with maximal MET capacities near or above 14 METs (about 50 ml·kg^{-1}·min^{-1}) based upon a resting MET equivalent of 3.5 ml·kg^{-1}·min^{-1}.[3]

Conduction of the Test

For cycle ergometry, a technician starts the timer as soon as the performer reaches the appropriate pedal revolutions (50 or 60 rpm in most cases) at the prescribed exercise level. For treadmill ergometry, the time starts when the performer is at the prescribed speed and slope and then releases the hands from the treadmill railings. If a ventilation recorder is used, it can be started simultaneously with the timer. However, only the minute ventilation between the third and fourth minutes of each power level needs to be calculated. If an electronic recorder is not being used, a technician should record the position of the pointers on the dial of the airflow meter at the start of the test and at every minute until the end of recovery. Another technician should count breathing frequency by observing the movements of

Table 1 Exercise Protocols for Respiration During Exercise and Recovery

		Cycle Exercise			
Power History		Low-Power	Moderate-Power	High-Power	
$\dot{V}O_2$max (L·min^{-1})		<2.1	2.1–2.9	>2.9	
Time			Power Prescription (W)		
0:00–4:00		50	75	100	
4:00–8:00		100	125	150	
8:00–12:00		150	175	200	
			Cycle Recovery		
12:00–16:00		50	75	100	
			Treadmill Exercise[a]		
Time	mph	km·h^{-1}	Slope %	$\dot{V}O_2$ ml·kg^{-1}·min^{-1}	MET
0:00–4:00	3	4.8	0	11.55	3.3
4:00–8:00	5	8.0	0	30.1	8.6
8:00–12:00	7	11.2	2.5	45.15	12.9
			Treadmill Recovery		
12:00–16:00	3	4.8	0	11.55	3.3

[a]From *Guidelines for Exercise Testing and Prescription,* Treadmill MET values from Table D-2 and D-3b, pp. 171–172, 1986. Copyright © 1986, Lea & Febiger Publishers, Malvern, PA. Reprinted by permission.

the dial's pointers or the movement of the performer's chest. As with the ventilation measurements, only the third to fourth minute of each power level is needed for the frequency measures unless the kinetics (the approach to steady state) of ventilation are being monitored.

Calculations

As mentioned before, the parameters of concern are ventilation, frequency, tidal volume, ventilatory threshold, and ventilatory equivalent. If the air meter recorder is used, the ventilation, frequency, and tidal volume can be determined directly from the recording paper. If no recorder is used, these parameters may be calculated by simple arithmetic from the technicians' observations. As with the lung volumes measured under resting conditions, the exercise respiratory volumes must be expressed in BTPS form.

BTPS Correction

Because the observed volumes are ATPS liters, they must be converted to BTPS. This means that the inspired or the expired volume is less than a converted BTPS volume because the ATPS volume is at a lower humidity (less water vapor) and at a lower temperature. At least two approaches to this conversion are possible—one that is best for inspired air volumes, and another that is best for expired volumes.

The **inspired-volume approach** uses two tables in conjunction with two equations. First, use Table 2 to find what the water vapor pressure of the ATPS volume at the observed temperature would be if it were at 100% RH. Secondly, use Equation 2 to find the water vapor pressure (P_AH_2O; torr) for the ambient relative humidity.

$$P_AH_2O = RH_A\% \times 100\% \ P\text{-}H_2O \qquad \text{Eq. 2}$$

Then this water vapor pressure is inserted into the temperature (T) ratio times pressure (P) ratio (Eq. 3) as follows:

Table 2 Water Vapor Pressure (P-H$_2$O) at 100% Saturation at Given Temperatures (T)

°C	T °K	P-H$_2$O torr	°C	T °K	P-H$_2$O torr
20	293	18	31	304	34
21	294	19	32	305	36
22	295	20	33	306	38
23	296	21	34	307	40
24	297	22	35	308	42
25	298	24	36	309	45
26	299	25	37	310	47
27	300	27	38	311	50
28	301	28	39	312	52
29	302	30	40	313	55
30	303	32			

$$\text{BTPS CF} = \frac{273 \ °K + T_b \ °C}{273 \ °K + T_A \ °C} \times \frac{P_B - P\text{-}H_2O_A}{P_B - P\text{-}H_2O_b} \quad \text{Eq. 3}$$

where: T_b = body temperature; assumed 37 °C
P_b = water vapor pressure at body T; assumed 47 torr

Lastly, the BTPS volume is found by multiplying the ATPS volume by the BTPS correction factor as in Equation 4.

$$V_I \text{ BTPS (L·min}^{-1}) = \text{BTPS CF} \times V_I \text{ ATPS} \quad \text{Eq. 4}$$

The **expired-volume approach** works well because Table 3 is based upon 100% RH, the same RH in expired air. In Table 3 find the correction factor (CF) for converting ATPS volumes (100% RH) to BTPS volumes by noting the CF in the row of the observed ambient temperature. The ambient temperature may vary depending upon the thermometer's placement in the expiratory system and the amount of time elapsing before sampling the air temperature. Although air temperatures are about 33 °C at the

Table 3 Correction Factors (CF) for Converting ATPS Volumes (100% RH) to BTPS Volumes

T_A (°C)	CF	T_A (°C)	CF
20	1.102	29	1.051
21	1.096	30	1.045
22	1.091	31	1.039
23	1.085	32	1.032
24	1.080	33	1.026
25	1.075	34	1.020
26	1.068	35	1.014
27	1.063	36	1.007
28	1.057	37	1.000

mouth they can decrease rapidly as they circulate past an air meter downstream. Also, if the air is collected in Douglas bags (or meteorological balloons) and not sampled until after the test, the air may be the same as the laboratory's air temperature.

The BTPS volume is then found simply by multiplying the V_E ATPS by the CF as in Equation 5.

$$V_E \text{ BTPS } (L \cdot min^{-1}) = CF \times V_I \text{ ATPS} \qquad \text{Eq. 5}$$

An example of the entire calculation is presented here, given the following conditions observed for the third to fourth minute of the exercise test:

Given Conditions
Ambient: T = 25 °C; RH = 50%; P_B = 758 torr
Ventilation: V_I ATPS = 20.0 L · min⁻¹

The first step in finding the BTPS correction factor is to account for the difference in water vapor pressure in the V_I ATPS at 50% RH versus that from the body at 100% RH. This is done by referring to Table 2, which gives vapor pressures only at 100% RH. By using Equation 2, the water pressure (torr) at 50% RH can be found by simply multiplying the ambient relative humidity (RH_A%) by the pressure listed for the given temperature at 100% RH:

$$P\text{-}H_2O_A = 50\% \text{ RH} \times 24 \text{ torr} = 12 \text{ torr}$$

Then this water vapor pressure is inserted into Equation 3 as follows:

$$\begin{aligned}
\text{BTPS CF} &= \frac{273 \text{ °K} + 37 \text{ °C}}{273 \text{ °K} + 25 \text{ °C}} \times \frac{758 - 12}{758 - 47} \\
&= (310 \text{ °K} / 298 \text{ °K}) \times (746 \text{ torr} / 711 \text{ torr}) \\
&= 1.04 \times 1.05 \\
&= 1.09
\end{aligned}$$

Then the BTPS volume is found by multiplying the ATPS volume by the BTPS correction factor as in Equation 4:

$$\begin{aligned}
V_I \text{ BTPS } (L \cdot min^{-1}) &= \text{BTPS CF} \times V_I \text{ ATPS} \\
&= 1.09 \times 20.0 \text{ L} \cdot min^{-1} \\
&= 21.8 \text{ L} \cdot min^{-1}
\end{aligned}$$

Tidal Volume (TV; V_T)

The average tidal volume could be determined by two methods if using an electronic recorder during the test. It would be possible to measure each tidal volume during the minute's interval and then get the average; however, even without the recorder it is much simpler to derive V_T from Equation 6, which when transposed becomes Equation 7.

$$\dot{V}_E \text{ or } \dot{V}_I \text{ BTPS} = f \times V_T \qquad \text{Eq. 6}$$

$$V_T (L \cdot br^{-1}; ml \cdot br^{-1}) = V_E \text{ or } V_I \div f \qquad \text{Eq. 7}$$

where: f = frequency of breathing in breaths per minute ($br \cdot min^{-1}$)
V_T = tidal volume in liters or milliliters per breath ($L \cdot br^{-1}$; $ml \cdot br^{-1}$)
$\dot{V}_E$ or $\dot{V}_I$ = ventilation expired or inspired in $L \cdot min^{-1}$ or $ml \cdot min^{-1}$

For example, if ventilation equals 60 $L \cdot min^{-1}$ for the 12th min, and the frequency of breathing equals 30 $br \cdot min^{-1}$, then the following calculation would provide the tidal volume:

$$\begin{aligned}
V_T (L \cdot br^{-1}; ml \cdot br^{-1}) &= 60 \div 30 \\
&= 2 \text{ L} \cdot br^{-1} \text{ or } 2000 \text{ ml} \cdot br^{-1}
\end{aligned}$$

A meaningful calculation with respect to tidal volume is that which relates it to vital capacity. Equation 8 can be used to calculate the relative size of each breath:

$$\%VC = (V_T / VC) \times 100 \qquad \text{Eq. 8}$$

For example, if tidal volume is 2000 $ml \cdot br^{-1}$ and vital capacity is 5000 ml, then the following calculation shows that the size of the tidal volume as a percentage of the vital capacity is 40%:

$$\begin{aligned}
\%VC &= (2000/5000) \times 100 \\
&= 0.40 \times 100 \\
&= 40\%
\end{aligned}$$

Ventilatory Equivalent (VE)

The VE is determined by first equating the exercise power levels to oxygen consumption, then dividing these values into the minute ventilation for each exercise level. To equate the power level of cycle ergometry with oxygen consumption, Table 4 or Equation 9, which was first presented in Chapter UN, may be used.

$$\dot{V}O_2 (ml \cdot min^{-1}) =$$

[P (in N·m·min⁻¹) × 0.2] + 300	Eq. 9a
[P (in kgm·min⁻¹) × 2] + 300	Eq. 9b
[P (in W) × 12] + 300	Eq. 9c

Once the estimated oxygen consumption for the given power level is known, the ventilatory equivalent may be calculated from Equation 10.

$$VE = (\dot{V}_I \text{ or } \dot{V}_E) / \dot{V}O_2 \qquad \text{Eq. 10}$$

For example, Table 4 shows that the expected oxygen consumption for cycle ergometry at a power of 150 W is

Table 4 Expected Ranges for Ventilatory Equivalent (VE), Frequency (f), Tidal Volume (TV), and Ventilation ($\dot{V}_E$ or $\dot{V}_I$) During the Exercise Respiratory Test

Power kg·m·min⁻¹	W	$\dot{V}O_2$ L·min⁻¹	$\dot{V}_E$ or $\dot{V}_I$ L·min⁻¹	f br·min⁻¹	TV ml·br⁻¹	VC %	VE ratio
150	25	0.60	12–15	12–19	900–1400	20–35	20–25
300	50	0.90	15–23	13–20	1000–1500	20–40	20–25
450	75	1.20	24–32	15–21	1300–1700	25–45	20–25
600	100	1.50	32–39	17–23	1500–1900	30–50	21–26
750	125	1.80	40–49	20–25	1600–2000	35–55	22–27
900	150	2.10	48–59	23–30	1700–2100	35–55	23–28
1050	175	2.40	58–70	26–35	1800–2200	40–60	24–29
1200	200	2.80	70–84	30–40	1900–2300	40–60	25–30
Recovery (1st min) 300	50	0.90	35–50	20–28	1400–2000	25–40	40–50

Source: Derived from unpublished data from Adams, 1988 and partly from Origenes et al., 1993. Note: It is possible to have values outside these ranges.

2.1 L·min⁻¹. If the ventilation during the twelfth minute is 52.0 L·min⁻¹ BTPS, then the following calculation would provide a ventilatory equivalent of 24.8.

$$\text{VE (ratio)} = 52.0 \text{ L·min}^{-1} / 2.1 \text{ L·min}^{-1}$$
$$= 24.8$$

Thus, 24.8 L of air per minute was breathed by the performer for each liter of oxygen consumed while exercising at a steady-state power level of 150 W.

For the treadmill protocol, oxygen consumption in liters per minute or milliliters per minute may be estimated from the given MET values or ml·kg⁻¹·min⁻¹ values in Table 1 when used in conjunction with Equation 11.

$$\dot{V}O_2 \left(L \cdot min^{-1} \right) = \frac{MET \times 3.5 \text{ ml} \cdot kg^{-1} \cdot min^{-1} \times wt \text{ in kg}}{1000} \quad \text{Eq. 11}$$

For example, what would be the oxygen consumption (L·min⁻¹) if the MET value at the 12th minute of the treadmill protocol (7 mph; 2.5% slope) was 12.9 in a 70 kg person? By multiplying 12.9 by 3.5 ml·kg⁻¹·min⁻¹, the relative value is produced—45.15 ml·kg⁻¹·min⁻¹. When this is multiplied by the weight of the performer, 70 kg, the product is the amount of oxygen consumed expressed in milliliters per minute—3160. This is converted to liters by dividing it by 1000, resulting in an oxygen consumption of 3.16 L·min⁻¹.

Ventilation or oxygen consumption may be approximated if either of these two variables is known. This is because the expected range of ratios for the ventilatory equivalent is between 20 and 25 for submaximal exercise below the ventilatory threshold (Fig. 1). For instance, if only oxygen consumption is measured, then ventilation may be estimated from Equation 12, which is a transposed form of Equation 1.

$$\dot{V}_E \text{ or } \dot{V}_I = \dot{V}O_2 \text{ (L·min}^{-1}) \times 20\text{–}25 \quad \text{Eq. 12}$$

For example, if the oxygen consumption is 3.0 L·min⁻¹, then the ventilation can be estimated as:

$$\dot{V}_E \text{ or } \dot{V}_I = 20\text{–}25 \times 3.0 \text{ L·min}^{-1}$$
$$= 60\text{–}75 \text{ L·min}^{-1}$$

Oxygen consumption may be calculated by using Equation 13,[15] which is also a transposition of Equation 1, or by using Equation 14.

$$\dot{V}O_2 \text{ (L·min}^{-1}) = \dot{V}_E \text{ or } \dot{V}_I \times 0.04 \quad \text{Eq. 13}$$

$$\dot{V}O_2 \text{ (L·min}^{-1}) = (\dot{V}_E \text{ or } \dot{V}_I) / 25 \quad \text{Eq. 14}$$

For example, if the ventilation is 60 L·min⁻¹, then the oxygen consumption can be estimated as follows:

$$\dot{V}O_2 \text{ (L·min}^{-1}) = 60 \text{ L·min}^{-1} \times 0.04$$
$$= 2.40 \text{ L·min}^{-1}$$

or
$$= 60 \text{ L·min}^{-1} / 25$$
$$= 2.40 \text{ L·min}^{-1}$$

Ventilatory Threshold (Tvent; VT)

The Tvent is at the point where ventilatory equivalent increases without a similar increase in the ventilation-to-carbon dioxide ratio when oxygen consumption is plotted on the horizontal axis.[17] Ideally, examination of the $\dot{V}_E/CO_2$ relationship, and more data points for the $\dot{V}_E$ vs. $\dot{V}O_2$ relationship than the three produced by this exercise protocol, are recommended[36] for estimating the ventilatory threshold. Also, ideally, 30-s data points, not just 1-min points, should be plotted in order to determine the change in slope or linearity between $\dot{V}CO_2$ and $\dot{V}O_2$.[33] Despite these limitations, Tvent can be approximated by using the graph developed from Form ER 3 (also see Fig. 1). This is done by connecting the data points for ventilation at the three given exercise intensities and the three corresponding assumed oxygen consumptions of the protocol. The point where there is an obvious change of linearity (change in slope) would represent the approximate ventilatory threshold.[32]

Summary

It becomes apparent from the equations that there is a very close relationship between metabolism (oxygen consump-

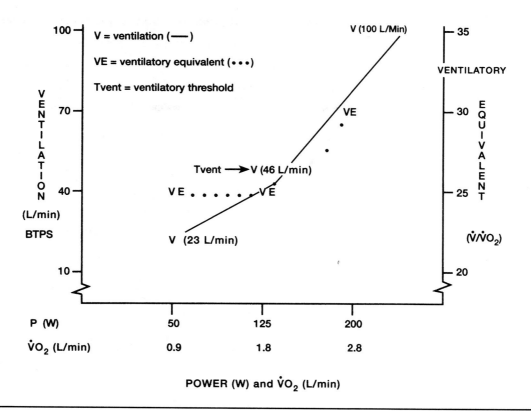

V = ventilation (——)
VE = ventilatory equivalent (•••)
$Tvent$ = ventilatory threshold

V (100 L/Min)

$Tvent \rightarrow$ V (46 L/min)

V (23 L/min)

VENTILATION (L/min) BTPS

VENTILATORY EQUIVALENT ($\dot{V}/\dot{V}O_2$)

| P (W) | 50 | 125 | 200 |
| $\dot{V}O_2$ (L/min) | 0.9 | 1.8 | 2.8 |

POWER (W) and $\dot{V}O_2$ (L/min)

Figure 1 An example of the graph format for estimating ventilatory threshold from ventilation at exercise.

tion) and respiration (ventilation). Only ventilation and breathing frequency are directly measured when not using a ventilation recorder and not measuring oxygen consumption. Thus, tidal volume is a derivation of ventilation and frequency, while ventilatory equivalent is calculated from ventilation and the estimated oxygen consumption for a given exercise intensity.

Results and Discussion

Maximal voluntary ventilation may be indicated by measuring the **resting (static)** maximal voluntary ventilation. One investigator reported an average MVV of 189 L·min^{-1} with the highest being 252 L·min^{-1} in trained middle-distance runners.[13] Some norms use body surface area (m^2) as a basis for categorizing subjects.[6] High school boys average 146 L·min^{-1} (SD = 21).[25] MVV decreases by about 25% from ages in the 20s to the 60s.[10] Various methods of determining normal values are presented as follows:

1. Use a nomogram[24] to predict the expected (normal) MVV based upon age, gender, and height, or use the Kory prediction equation for men only:

Men: MVV (L·min^{-1}) =
$$(1.34 \times Ht \text{ in cm}) - (1.26 \times Age) \qquad \text{Eq. 15}$$

2. A prediction equation (Eq. 16) for MVV in women may be used by multiplying the forced expiratory volume (FEV$_1$) by 35.[19]

$$FEV_1 \times 35 = MVV. \qquad \text{Eq. 16}$$

3. Tables are available that provide norms for adult men and women based upon body surface areas (BSA) between 1.40 and 2.10 square meters (m^2).[6] The regression equations for men (Eq. 17) and women (Eq. 18) are based on their data.

Men: MVV (L·min^{-1}) = $(86.5 - 0.522 \text{ Age}) \times m^2$ Eq. 17

Women: MVV (L·min^{-1}) = $(71.3 - 0.474 \text{ Age}) \times m^2$ Eq. 18

4. Women's MVV may be predicted from age alone in Equation 19.[29]

Women: MVV (L·min^{-1}) = $113 - 0.7 \text{ Age}$ Eq. 19

Exercise respiration may be evaluated by observing the kinetics of ventilation and the steady-state aspects of ventilation. The kinetics of ventilation refers to the non-steady-state condition, whereby the ventilatory parameters are ascending to their plateaus at each exercise power level; kinetics may also refer to the ventilatory parameters descent to baseline during recovery from exercise.

Kinetics of Ventilation

The rise in ventilation at the onset of exercise is similar to the rise in heart rate and oxygen consumption; there is a sudden rise during the first minute, which is followed by a more gradual rise to steady state during the next couple of minutes. Thus, the rise is curvilinear and can be graphed as such from the Exercise Respiratory Test if the first four minutes of ventilation at each exercise stage are recorded.

During recovery, or cool-down, ventilation decreases curvilinearly with time. It is unlikely, however, to return to the steady-state value typical for the given exercise levels within the fourth minute of recovery for the cycle or treadmill (3.3 METs) protocols. Thus, both the ventilation and the ventilatory equivalent are higher during early recovery of the cool-down period than during an equivalent exercise level in the progressive exercise protocol.

Steady-State Ventilatory Values at Submaximal Exercise

Aerobically fit persons have lower ventilations, respiratory frequencies, and ventilatory equivalents for any given level of submaximal exercise. With exercise training, persons with chronic airway obstruction reduce their ventilations and frequencies.[2] The expected ranges for ventilation, breathing frequency, tidal volume, and ventilatory equivalent at given powers and oxygen consumptions are presented in Table 4.

Ventilation

At the higher power levels, or at some point between 50% and 75% maximal oxygen consumption, the ventilation would be expected to increase at an accelerated rate;[7] thus the higher end of the ranges presented in Table 4 would be more appropriate for persons exercising at power levels above their ventilatory threshold. As mentioned previously, low-aerobic-power persons tend toward higher ventilations, frequencies, and ventilatory equivalents, especially at submaximal exercise below their ventilatory threshold.

Tidal Volume and Breathing Frequency

The approximated tidal volumes in Table 4 are based upon typical vital capacities of 4.8 L and 3.2 L for men and women, respectively. Also, a somewhat linear relationship between tidal volume and oxygen consumption (or power) is assumed at the low and moderate exercise intensities (about 25 W to 150 W). As exercise intensity increases beyond the moderate levels, however, the greater ventilation requirement tends to be met by increased frequency, while the tidal volume tends to reach an asymptote (plateau). The change in frequency of breathing is in contrast to its relatively slow increase at low and moderate levels of exercise.

Ventilatory Threshold

The Tvent may be closely related to a perceived exercise intensity of 12 to 15 on the 6–20 RPE scale. Semantically, this would equate to exercise intensities described as "somewhat heavy" (12–14 RPE) to "heavy" (15 RPE).[26] The intensity of exercise at the Tvent (or lactate threshold) coincides roughly with the oxygen consumption maintained by marathoners or 3-h cyclists.[14] Thus, the higher along the

oxygen consumption continuum that Tvent occurs, the faster will be the sustained exercise pace.

Maximal Exercise

Although the final stage of the exercise protocol used for the Exercise Respiratory Test may not stimulate maximal exercise ventilatory values in most performers, the discussion presented here can help interpret the ventilatory values produced by a maximal oxygen consumption test.

Maximal Ventilation

Respiratory parameters are not limiting factors for maximal exercise capacity in the average healthy person. However, they do limit the maximal aerobic capacity of elite endurance athletes.[37] Neither the average person nor the athlete is expected to have a maximal exercise ventilation that equals the 12-s maximal voluntary ventilation (MVV). The breathing reserve may be expressed as the difference between the stationary MVV and the maximal exercise ventilation.[35] If a performer's $\dot{V}_E$ max is within 15 L·min^{-1} of the MVV, then that person may have a clinically significant ventilatory problem.[12] Thus, a normal person should have a ventilatory reserve of at least 15 L·min^{-1}. The ventilatory reserve (Vres) may be calculated from Equation 20.

$$Vres = MVV - \dot{V}_E \text{ or } \dot{V}_I \text{ max} \qquad \text{Eq. 20}$$

Maximal Tidal Volume

In general, the maximal tidal volume at exercise can be expressed by Equation 21 as:[22]

$$V_T \text{ max} = 0.74 \text{ VC} - 1.11 \qquad \text{Eq. 21}$$

Thus, the typical adult male with a vital capacity of 4.8 L would be expected to have a maximal tidal volume of about 2.44 L (2440 mL) or about 50% of the vital capacity; the typical female with a vital capacity of 3.2 would be expected to have a maximal tidal volume of about 1.26 L (1260 mL) or 40% of the vital capacity. Probably, highly motivated exercisers would be able to achieve tidal volumes up to 60% of their vital capacities at their exhaustive point of exercise.

References

1. Adams, A. P., Vickers, M. D. A., Munroe, J. P., & Parker, C. W. (1967). Dry displacement gas meters. *British Journal of Anaesthesia, 39,* 174–183.
2. Alison, J. A., Samios, R., & Anderson, S. D. (1981). Evaluation of exercise training in patients with chronic airway obstruction. *Journal of Physical Therapy, 61,* 1273–1277.
3. American College of Sports Medicine. (1986, 1991). *Guidelines for exercise testing and exercise prescription.* Philadelphia: Lea & Febiger.
4. American Thoracic Society. (1987). Standardization of spirometry—1987 update. *American Review of Respiratory Disease, 136,* 1285–1298.

5. Astrand, P. O., & Rodahl, K. (1986). *Textbook of work physiology.* New York: McGraw-Hill.

6. Baldwin, E. D., Cournand, A., & Richards, D. W. (1948). Pulmonary insufficiency I, Physiologic classification, Clinical methods of analysis, Standard values in normal subjects. *Medicine, 27,* 243.

7. Brooks, G. A., & Fahey, T. D. (1984). *Exercise physiology: Human bioenergetics and its application.* New York: John Wiley & Sons.

8. Brooks, G. A., Fahey, T. D., & White, T. P. (1996). *Exercise physiology: Human bioenergetics and its application.* Mountain View, CA: Mayfield.

9. Casaburi, R., Storer, T. W., Sullivan, C. S., & Wasserman, K. (1995). Evaluation of blood lactate elevation as an intensity criterion for exercise training. *Medicine and Science in Sports and Exercise, 27,* 852–862.

10. Chebotarev, D. F., Korkushka, D. V., & Ivanov, L. A. (1974). Mechanisms of hypoxemia in the elderly. *Journal of Gerontology, 29,* 393–400.

11. Collins, W. E. (1988). *Warren E. Collins Catalog.* Braintree, MA: Author.

12. Cooper, C. B. (1995). Determining the role of exercise in patients with chronic pulmonary disease. *Medicine and Science in Sports and Exercise, 27,* 147–157.

13. Costill, D. L. (1971). Endurance running. In ACSM (Ed.), *Encyclopedia of sport science & medicine* (p. 338). New York: Macmillan.

14. Coyle, E. F. (1995). Integration of the physiological factors determining endurance performance ability. In J. O. Holloszy (Ed.), *Exercise and Sport Sciences Reviews, 23* (pp. 25–63), Baltimore: Williams & Wilkins.

15. Datta, S. R., & Ramanathan, N. L. (1969). Energy expenditure in work predicted from heart rate and pulmonary ventilation. *Journal of Applied Physiology, 26,* 297–302.

16. Davis, J. A. (1985). Anaerobic threshold: Review of the concept and directions for future research. *Medicine and Science in Sports and Exercise, 17,* 6–18.

17. Davis, J. A., Frank, M. H., Whipp, B. J., & Wasserman, K. (1979). Anaerobic threshold alterations caused by endurance training in middle aged men. *Journal of Applied Physiology, 46,* 1039–1045.

18. deVries, H. A. (1986). *Physiology of exercise in physical education and athletics.* Dubuque, IA: Wm. C. Brown.

19. Freedman, S. (1970). Sustained maximum voluntary ventilation. *Respiratory Physiology, 3,* 230–244.

20. Gaensler, E. A., & Wright, G. W. (1966). Evaluation of respiratory impairment. *Archives of Environmental Health, 12,* 146–189.

21. Jones, N. L. (1975). Exercise testing in pulmonary evaluation: Rationale, methods, and the normal respiratory response to exercise. *New England Journal of Medicine, 293,* 541–544.

22. Jones, N. L. (1984). Dyspnea in exercise. *Medicine and Science in Sports and Exercise, 16,* 14–19.

23. Jones, N. L., & Ehrsam, R. E. (1982). The anaerobic threshold. In R. Terjung (Ed.), *Exercise and sport sciences review* (pp. 49–83). New York: Franklin Institute Press.

24. Kory, R. C., Callahan, R., Boren, H. G., & Syner, J. C. (1961). The Veterans Administration—Army cooperative study of pulmonary function. *American Journal of Medicine, 30,* 243–258.

25. Pease, G. F. (1961). *Maximum breathing capacity in high school boys.* Unpublished master's thesis, San Diego State University, California.

26. Prusacyzk, W. K., Cureton, K. J., Graham, R. E., & Ray, C. A. (1992). Differential effects of dietary carbohydrate on RPE at the lactate and ventilatory thresholds. *Medicine and Science in Sports and Exercise, 24,* 568–575.

27. McArdle, W. D., Katch, F., & Katch, V. (1986). *Exercise physiology.* Philadelphia: Lea & Febiger.

28. McArdle, W. D., Katch, F., & Katch, V. (1996). *Exercise physiology. Energy, nutrition, and human performance.* Philadelphia: Williams & Wilkins.

29. Needham, C. D., Rogan, M. C., & McDonald, J. (1954). Normal standards for lung volumes, intrapulmonary gas-mixing and maximum breathing capacity. *Thorax, 9,* 313.

30. Origenes, M. M., Blank, S. E., & Schoene, R. B. (1993). Exercise ventilatory response to upright and aero-posture cycling. *Medicine and Science in Sports and Exercise, 25,* 608–612.

31. Powers, S. K., & Beadle, R. E. (1985). Onset of hyperventilation during incremental exercise: A brief review. *Research Quarterly for Exercise and Sport, 56,* 352–360.

32. Powers, S. K., & Howley, E. T. (1990). *Exercise physiology.* Dubuque, IA: Wm. C. Brown.

33. Schneider, D. A., Phillips, S. E., & Stoffolano, S. (1993). The simplified V-slope method of detecting the gas exchange threshold. *Medicine and Science in Sports and Exercise, 25,* 1180–1184.

34. Wasserman, K. (1986). Anaerobiasis, lactate and gas exchange during exercise: The issues. *Federation Proceedings, 45,* 2904–2909.

35. Wasserman, K., Hansen, J. E., Sue, D. Y., Whipp, B. J., & Casaburi, R. (1994). *Principles of exercise testing and interpretation.* Philadelphia: Lea & Febiger.

36. Wasserman, K., Whipp, B. J., Koyal, S. N., & Beaver, W. L. (1973). Anaerobic threshold and respiratory gas exchange during exercise. *Journal of Applied Physiology, 35,* 236–243.

37. Wilmore, J. H., & Costill, D. L. (1994). *Physiology of sport and exercise.* Champagne, IL: Human Kinetics.

38. Wilmore, J. H., & Norton, A. C. (1974). *The heart and lungs at work.* Schiller Park, IL: Beckman Instruments.

Form ER 1

Individual Data for the Exercise Respiratory Test

Name _____ Date _____ Time _____ a.m. _____ p.m.

Age _____ y   Gender (M or F) _____   Ht _____ cm   Wt _____ kg   BSA _____ m²

Temperature (T_A) _____ °C P_B _____ torr RH_A (dry spirometer) _____ % (if $\dot{V}_I$)

P-H_2O at 100% RH (Table 2) _____ torr × RH_A _____ = P-H_2O_A _____ torr

VC BTPS _____ L   MVV _____ L·min⁻¹ $\dot{V}O_2$max _____ L·min⁻¹

BTPS Correction Factors (CF): If inspiratory volume _____   If expiratory _____

$$\text{BTPS} \atop \text{CF} = \left[\frac{273\ °K + T_b \ \underline{37^+}\ °C}{273\ °K + T_A \ \underline{\quad}\ °C} \right] \times \left[\frac{P_B \underline{\quad} \text{torr} - \text{P-}H_2O_A \underline{\quad} \text{torr}}{P_B \underline{\quad} \text{torr} - \text{P-}H_2O_b \ \underline{47}\ \text{torr}} \right]$$

= (___310___ °K / _____ °K) × (_____ torr/ _____ torr)

= _____   × _____ = _____ CF

Ergometry Mode (check one): Cycle _____   Treadmill _____   Step _____   Other _____

Time min	P W	MET	AIR METER	$\dot{V}$ATPS L·min⁻¹	$\dot{V}$BTPS L·min⁻¹	f br/min	TV mL/br;	BTPS %VC	$\dot{V}O_2$ L·min⁻¹	VE ratio
3:00			_____							
4:00			_____							
7:00			_____							
8:00			_____							
11:00			_____							
12:00			_____							
15:00	POST		_____							
16:00			_____							

Form ER 2

Graphic Analysis of Tidal Volume and Frequency

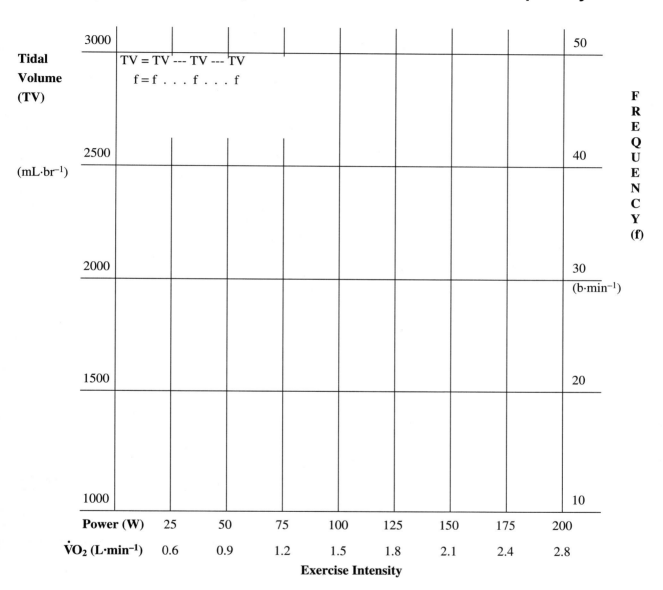

Tidal Volume (TV)

$(mL \cdot br^{-1})$

FREQUENCY (f)

$(b \cdot min^{-1})$

TV = TV --- TV --- TV

f = f . . . f . . . f

Power (W)	25	50	75	100	125	150	175	200
$\dot{V}O_2$ $(L \cdot min^{-1})$	0.6	0.9	1.2	1.5	1.8	2.1	2.4	2.8

Exercise Intensity

Form ER 3

Graphic Analysis of Ventilation and Ventilatory Equivalent

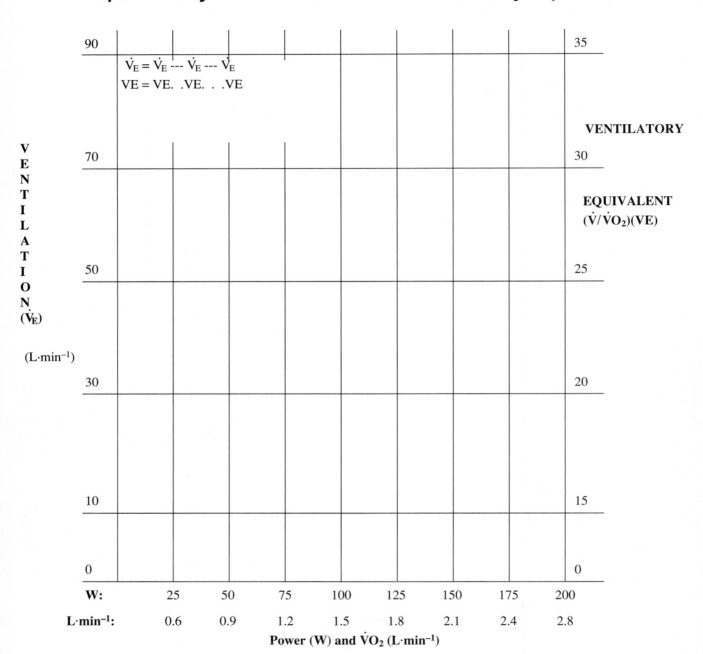

$\dot{V}_E = \dot{V}_E$ --- $\dot{V}_E$ --- $\dot{V}_E$
VE = VE. .VE. . .VE

VENTILATION ($\dot{V}_E$) (L·min⁻¹)

VENTILATORY EQUIVALENT ($\dot{V}/\dot{V}O_2$)(VE)

W: 25 50 75 100 125 150 175 200
L·min⁻¹: 0.6 0.9 1.2 1.5 1.8 2.1 2.4 2.8

Power (W) and $\dot{V}O_2$ (L·min⁻¹)

Chapter FL

Lower Trunk Flexibility

Although the term *flexibility* is a popular one, it may be a misnomer because it implies that flexibility is only concerned with flexion. However, flexibility also consists of extension, abduction, adduction, and circumduction. Furthermore, flexion implies bending or folding of the tissue when, in fact, it is really a stretching or elongation of the tissue. The extensibility of the muscles and tendons allows them to stretch; their elasticity permits them to return from stretch to their original length.[16]

Flexibility may be defined and then subdefined in various ways. One meaningful definition of flexibility is the optimal range of motion (ROM) permitted by connective and muscle tissue. This definition not only lends itself to quantifying flexibility in terms of distance or degree of ROM, but also includes the two main tissues influencing flexibility.

Indirectly, the fitness component of flexibility was responsible for the formation of the President's Council on Physical Fitness and Sports (PCPFS). This organization was formed in the mid-1950s by President Eisenhower after his disenchantment with the fitness of our youth. He was stirred to action when two investigators[28] reported that American children from 6–16 y old compared poorly with Europeans. More than half of the American children had failed a fitness battery composed of six tests; this compared to less than one-tenth of the European children (Fig. 1). Most of the American failures were due to poor flexibility, specifically the "floor-touch" (Kraus-Weber) test, which caused 44% of the American children to fail.

Sit-and-Reach (SR) Test

Most Americans will suffer from low back pain at least once in their lifetime. Because poor flexibility of low-back extensors and hamstrings may cause, or be associated with, muscular low-back pain,[5,29] tests for these two muscle groups have received the most attention. For example, the Sit-and-Reach Test has been incorporated as a health-related physical fitness item in such national fitness batteries as *AAHPERD Physical Best,*[4] the President's Council on Physical Fitness and Sports,[36] the Fitnessgram,[24] the AAHPERD Functional Fitness Assessment for Adults over 60 years,[7,35] and the American Alliance for Health, Physical Education, Recreation and Dance Health-Related Test.[2] In addition, poor hamstring flexibility may predispose injury to hamstrings.[40,44]

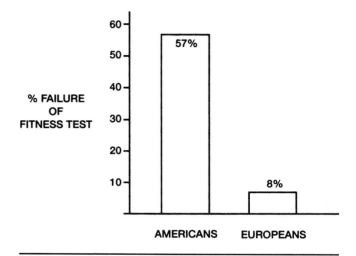

Figure 1 Fitness of American and European children in the 1950s based on a six-item fitness test.

Method

Four methods to perform the Sit-and-Reach (SR) Flexibility Test include modifications of the traditional one prescribed by the American Alliance for Health, Physical Education, Recreation, and Dance.[2,3,4] The three modifications are the YMCA,[13] Canadian,[11] and Wall[17–20] SR tests (Table 1).

Equipment

Table 1 presents the equipment for the four SR tests. The test apparatus for the Traditional SR Test is a wooden, box-like structure with a measuring scale on its upper surface labeled in 1-cm gradations. The 23rd-cm (9-in.) line is exactly in line with the vertical plane of the participant's soles and heels, which are against the front edge of the box (Figures 2 and 3).

Procedures Common to All SR Tests

Certain procedures are the same for all four tests. Because flexion places strain on spinal ligaments, especially when performed ballistically,[1] and raises intradiscal pressures,[32,38] the participant should be "warm and loose" and perform the movement slowly. Although only the Canadian test prescribes a standard preparatory regimen, it seems that

Accuracy of the Sit-and-Reach (SR) Test

Validity

Scientifically significant evidence to support the association between low-back pain and inflexibility is not clearly apparent.[34] Although the SR Test is presumed to measure both lower back and hamstring flexibility, investigators conclude that the test, or its modification, is more valid for hamstring than for back flexibility.[9,25,26,30] It is, secondarily, a test for the lower back, buttocks, and calf muscles. Specifically, these muscles are the biceps femoris, semitendinosus, semimembranosus, erector spinae, gluteus maximus and medius, and gastrocnemius.

Many investigators agree that there is no such phenomenon as general flexibility.[15,21,22,23,31,39] In other words, one joint's range of motion cannot predict the range of motion of another joint. Few correlations between one body part and another exceed .40. Some exceptions are cited in a review of flexibility,[8] but a factor analytic study was quite convincing toward a specificity characteristic for flexibility.[15] It is reasonable that the relationship between the SR Test and the Standing Toe-Toucher Test is high ($r = .90$)[43] because these tests, essentially, are measuring the same muscle groups.

Not only is flexibility specific from one type of joint in the body to another type of joint in the body (e.g., legs vs. shoulders) but it is specific with respect to the same joint but on different sides of the body. For example, one shoulder is usually more flexible than the other shoulder.

Reliability

The test-retest reliability of the SR Test can be as high as .98[30] and is usually greater than .70, based upon the testing of over 12,000 boys and girls 6–18 y of age; the test-retest correlation over an 8-month period in older persons (45–75 y) was .83.[39] The test-retest reliability of the modified Wall-SR Test for males and females tested on the same day ranges from .91 to .97.[20]

Table 1 Types of Sit-and-Reach Tests and Their Basic Characteristics

Type	Equipment	Heel-Line (Index)	Hold (s)	Trials
Traditional	Box: 12.75 in. high	23 cm; 9 in.	1–2	1st 3 unofficial 4th = recorded
Canadian	Meter-stick and adjustable box—toe level	26 cm; ~10 in.	2	2
YMCA	Yard-stick; tape; floor level	15 in.; 38 cm	~2	3
Wall SR	Traditional box with m/yd-stick or Acuflex 1™	0 cm; 0 in.	≥2	2 (3-phase stretch for each trial)

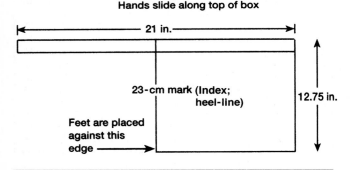

Figure 2 The sit-and-reach test apparatus.

a standard prior exercise regimen of slow stretching and walking/jogging-in-place for five minutes would enhance the reliability and validity of the other three tests.

The shoeless participants fully extend their legs, meaning that the back of the knees are against the floor, table, or bench. The hands are placed with palms down and one palm on top of the backhand of the other. The performer holds the final reach trial for at least a second or two.

Specific Procedures for the SR Tests

Traditional SR Test

Figure 3 illustrates the proper technique to perform the Sit-and-Reach Test. The procedural steps are as follows:

Participant
1. Perform a short bout of prior exercise (e.g., 5 min).
2. Remove shoes.
3. Sit on the floor, bench, or table with feet against the testing apparatus (index; heel-line); the apparatus is against a wall to prevent it from sliding.
4. Fully extend the legs, with the feet about shoulder width (about 8–12 in. or 20–30 cm) apart.

Technician
5. Hold one hand lightly against the performer's knees to ensure full leg extension.

Participant
6. Extend arms forward with the hands placed on top of each other, palms down.
7. Slowly bend forward along the measuring scale, not necessarily to the maximal.

254 Lower Trunk Flexibility **FL-2**

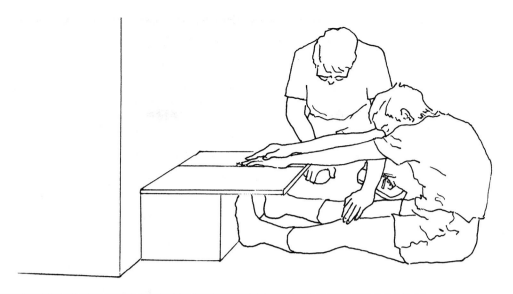

Figure 3 A subject performing the Sit-and-Reach flexibility test.

8. Repeat this forward stretch two more times.
9. Repeat the same stretch a fourth time, but now hold both hands at the maximal position for 1–2 s.

Technician

10. Observe and record the cm value to the nearest centimeter. For example, if the performer extends beyond the index line (heels), then the value will be greater than 23 cm (9 in.).
11. Interpret SR value from Table 2.

Canadian SR Test[10,11]

Except for the prior exercise regimen, the beginning steps of the Canadian test are similar to those of the traditional test. The later steps include minor differences related to the height of the meter stick, separation of the performer's feet, and the number of trials.

1. Participant performs the modified hurdle stretch (bent leg's sole of foot against inside of other leg), holding for 20 s, and repeated twice for each leg.
2. Performer removes shoes, sits on floor, table, or bench, and extends legs.
3. Technician places a meter stick at the performer's toe-level height; or uses a height-adjustable box with meter stick attached.
4. The meter stick crosses the heel-line (index) at the 26-cm (~10 in.) mark.
5. Performer's heels are about 5 cm (~2 in.) apart.
6. Performer places hands on top of each other, and slowly bends forward running hands along meter stick, keeping head down.
7. Performer holds for 2 s.
8. Technician notes the distance of the reach. For example, if the performer reaches exactly to the index line at toe level, the cm score is recorded as 26.
9. Participant performs a second trial.

Table 2 Percentile (%ile) Norms for the Traditional Sit-and-Reach Test for Men and Women 18–21 y of Age

%ile	Sit and Reach (cm)[a]							
	M e n				W o m e n			
AGE	18	19	20	21	18	19	20	21
99	50	49	49	50	52	52	51	50
95	45	45	46	45	47	47	46	46
90	42	43	43	42	46	45	45	44
85	41	42	41	41	44	43	43	43
80	40	40	41	40	43	42	42	42
75	39	39	40	39	42	41	41	42
70	38	38	39	38	41	40	39	40
65	37	37	38	36	40	40	38	39
60	36	36	37	35	39	38	38	38
55	35	35	36	35	38	38	37	37
50	34	34	35	33	38	37	37	36
45	34	33	34	32	37	36	36	36
40	32	32	33	31	36	36	35	35
35	31	31	32	31	35	34	34	34
30	30	29	31	30	34	33	33	33
25	29	28	30	28	33	32	32	32
20	27	27	27	27	32	31	31	31
15	25	26	25	25	30	29	30	29
10	23	23	22	24	29	27	28	27
5	19	19	18	20	26	23	24	25

Note: [a]Index (heel-line) is at 23 cm.
Reprinted from "Norms for College Students" with permission of the American Alliance for Health, Physical Education, Recreation and Dance, 1900 Association Dr., Reston, VA.

10. Technician records and interprets the best of the two trials using Form FL 1 and Table 3, respectively.

YMCA SR Test[13]

Except for the placement of the yardstick, its index line, and the number of trials, most of the Y's procedures are the same as the traditional SR test.

FL-3   Lower Trunk Flexibility   **255**

Table 3 Sit-and-Reach Flexibility Norms and Percentiles (%ile) in Canadian Men (M) and Women (W) Ages 15–69

Age (y)		15–19		20–29		30–39 Sit and Reach (cm)a		40–49		50–59		60–69	
	%ile	M	W	M	W	M	W	M	W	M	W	M	W
High	81–100	38	42	39	40	37	40	34	37	34	38	32	34
>Ave	61–80	34–38	38–42	34–39	37–40	33–37	36–40	29–34	34–37	28–34	33–38	25–32	31–34
Ave	41–60	29–33	34–37	30–33	33–36	28–32	32–35	24–28	30–33	24–27	30–32	20–24	27–30
<Ave	21–40	24–28	29–33	25–29	28–32	23–27	27–31	18–23	25–29	16–23	25–29	15–19	23–26
Low	1–20	24	29	25	28	23	27	18	25	16	25	15	23

Note: aIndex line (heel-line) is at 26 cm.
From Fitness and Lifestyle in Canada, Fitness and Lifestyle Research Institute, 1983. Fitness and Amateur Sport, Ottawa, Canada.

Table 4 YMCA Sit-and-Reach Norms for Men (M) and Women (W) Ages 20 to 60+a

Category		20–29		30–39		Age(y) 40–49		50–59		60+	
		M	W	M	W	M	W	M	W	M	W
High	in.	>21	>23	>20	>22	>19	>21	>18	>20	>17	>19
	cm	>53	>58	>51	>56	>48	>53	>46	>51	>43	>48
>Ave.	in.	19–21	22–23	18–20	21–22	17–19	20–21	16–18	19–20	15–17	18–19
	cm	48–53	56–58	46–51	53–56	43–48	51–53	41–46	48–51	38–43	46–48
Ave.	in.	13–18	16–21	12–17	15–20	11–16	14–19	10–15	13–18	9–14	12–17
	cm	33–46	41–53	30–43	38–51	28–41	36–48	25–38	33–46	23–36	30–43
<Ave.	in.	10–12	13–15	9–11	12–14	8–10	11–13	7–9	10–12	6–8	9–11
	cm	25–30	33–38	23–28	30–36	20–25	28–46	18–23	25–30	15–20	23–28
Low	in.	<10	<13	<9	<12	<8	<11	<7	<10	<6	<9
	cm	<25	<33	<23	<30	<20	<28	<18	<25	<15	<23

Note: aIndex line (heel-line) is at 15 in. (38 cm).
Adapted from Golding, L. A., Myers, C. R., & Sinning, W. E. (Eds.). *The Y's Way to Physical Fitness,* National Board of YMCA (1982).

The technician places a yard/meter stick on the floor, table, or bench. Because the yardstick is at a lower level than when it is on top of a 12 in. box, the reach scores may be about 1 in. or 2.5 cm lower than the reaches measured on the traditional box.[27]

1. Technician intersects the index line by placing tape across the yardstick at 15 in. (38 cm).
2. Performer removes shoes, sits on floor, table, or bench, and extends legs, straddling yard/meter stick or measuring tape.
3. Performer separates legs by 10–12 in. (25–30 cm), and places heels perpendicular to and at the index tape mark.
4. Performer places hands on top of each other, and slowly bends forward, running hands along the top of the meter/yard stick.
5. Performer holds for about 2 s.
6. Technician notes the distance of the reach to the closest one-fourth in. For example, if the performer reaches exactly to the index line at toe level, the score is recorded as 15 in. (38 cm).
7. Participant performs a second and third trial.
8. Technician records and interprets the best of the three trials using Form FL 1 and Table 4, respectively.

Wall SR Test[17-20]

This test has an added preliminary phase to the other three SR tests. This phase is performed against a wall in order to correct for any inter-individual differences in appendage proportions.[6,18,19,41]

1. The participant performs a short bout of prior exercise.
2. Performer removes shoes.
3. Performer sits on the floor, (or bench, or table) with the back, hips, and head against a wall.
4. The performer places soles and heels of feet against the testing apparatus, which can be a commercial box (Acuflex 1™) or the traditional box. The apparatus should be braced against the technician's feet or some object in order to prevent it from sliding away from the performer's feet.
5. The performer fully extends the legs, with the feet about shoulder width (about 8–12 in. or 20–30 cm) apart. The technician does not need to hold the knees of the performer but legs remain straight.
6. The performer places one hand on top of the other as in the other tests.
7. The **starting (zero) position** is found by:
   a. the **performer** reaching forward as far as possible along the measuring device without having the

Table 5 Percentiles (%ile) for the Wall Sit-and-Reach Test

Age (y) %ile	<35		36–49		>50	
			Flexibility Score (in.)^a			
	Men	Women	Men	Women	Men	Women
99	24.7	19.8	18.9	19.8	16.2	17.2
95	19.5	18.7	18.2	19.2	15.8	15.7
90	17.9	17.9	16.1	17.4	15.0	15.0
80	17.0	16.7	14.6	16.2	13.3	14.2
70	15.8	16.2	13.9	15.2	12.3	13.6
60	15.0	15.8	13.4	14.5	11.5	12.3
50	14.4	14.8	12.6	13.5	10.2	11.1
40	13.5	14.5	11.6	12.8	9.7	10.1
30	13.0	13.7	10.8	12.2	9.3	9.2
20	11.6	12.6	9.9	11.0	8.8	8.3
10	9.2	10.1	8.3	9.7	7.8	7.5
5	7.9	8.1	7.0	8.5	7.2	3.7
1	7.0	2.6	5.1	2.0	4.0	1.5

Note: ^{a}The index (heel-line) is at zero in.
From *Principles and Laboratories for Physical Fitness and Wellness* (1991). Englewood, CO: Morton Publishing. Reprinted with permission.

Table 6 Idealized Sit-and-Reach Standards for All Ages^a

Percentile	Flexibility^b			
	Males		Females	
	in.	cm	in.	cm
99	10	25	10.5	27
90	7.5	19	8.5	22
80	6	15	7.5	19
75	5.5	14	7	18
70	5	13	6.5	17
60	4	10	6	15
50	3	8	5.5	14
40	2.5	6	5	13
30	1.5	4	4	10
25	1	3	3.5	9
20	−0.5	1	3	8
10	−2	−5	1	3

Note: ^{a}Based on persons 18 years of age.
^{b}Index line (heel-line) converted from the original 12-in. mark to a zero index.
Adapted from Ross, J. G., Dotson, C. O., & Gilbert, G. G. (1985, January). New standards for fitness measurement: The National Children and Youth Fitness Study. *JOPERD*, pp. 62–66 (20-NCYFS-24-NCYFS). © 1985 AAHPERD; 1900 Association Dr; Reston, VA 22091.

head and back leave the wall; however, the shoulders are permitted to hunch forward into a rounded position.

   b. the **technician** observing and recording the inch-mark to the closest 0.5 in. onto Form FL 1, or if using the Acuflex 1 simply sliding the reach indicator to the person's finger tips.

8. After the recording or adjustment is made, the performer slowly reaches forward three times along the device, with the third reach being held for 2 s or more.
9. The technician records the third reach.
10. The technician records the actual back/hamstring flexibility value by subtracting the starting value from the end-reach value.
11. The participant performs another three-phase reach trial.
12. The technician records the second trial, then calculates and records the average flexibility value of the two trials.
13. The technician interprets the flexibility value by referring to Table 5.

Results and Discussion

Unlike two of the other major fitness components—aerobic and anaerobic—*maximal* flexibility may not be best. For that reason, a better term might be *optimal* flexibility. Optimal implies that "too much" or "too little" flexibility may exist. For example, the optimal flexibility of a football player is different from that of a gymnast. In fact, too much flexibility (laxity) may increase the susceptibility to dislocations, subluxations, or sprains. On the other hand, too little flexibility (tightness) may increase the player's susceptibility to strains.[12,33] In the gymnast, high flexibility is important for success, but too much laxity in the spine may cause lordotic vertebral problems; too much tightness in the swimmer may cause "swimmer's shoulder" (impingement

syndrome).[14] For these reasons high flexibility scores are not classified as "excellent." A nonqualitative classification system ranging from low to high is used instead.

A remedial flexibility program is advised by AAHPERD if anyone falls below the 25th percentile (Table 2) in their traditional SR test. The 50th percentile is the average score. Standard scores (i.e., scores that are recommended) may be found in AAHPERD's *Physical Best* pamphlet.[4]

Anthropometric factors may cause normal boys and girls between the ages of 10 and 14 to be unable to reach the 23-cm index mark in the traditional test.[2] This may be due to the preadolescent and adolescent growth spurt, which makes the legs disproportionately longer than the trunk. Three of the Sit-and-Reach Tests may favor persons with longer arms and/or trunk and disproportionately shorter legs.[18] This might be one of the reasons leading to higher scores in women than men—lower average leg length compared to their height.[42] Despite the bias attributed to disproportionate lengths, it appears that the non-wall SR tests would be independent of total height.[6,39,41]

Norms for the Canadian SR Test in Table 3[11] are for a wider age range than those for the traditional test in Table 2. The absolute values (cm) of the two tests cannot be compared directly because the index point is different. One way to compare the scores of all four tests is to standardize the scores by making the index lines (heel-lines) of all the tests start at zero. As a general guide to interpreting such scores, the National Children and Youth Fitness Study (NCYFS 1) norms in Table 6[37] have been idealized by assuming that flexibility should not change with age after a mature age of 18 y. Thus, the NCYFS flexibility values and percentiles for the typical 18-y-old male and female represent an idealistic view of flexibility and age.

Norms for the YMCA SR Test are presented in Table 4.[13] The original American inches have been converted to include the metric centimeters.

The norms for the Wall SR Test are presented in Table 5.[17,20] The flexibility categories are based on the same percentile (%ile) categories as those for the Canadian SR Test. Thus, >81st %ile is equivalent to the High category; 61–80 = >Ave.; 41–60 = Ave.; 21–40 = <Ave.; and <20th %ile = Low.

References

1. Adams, M. A., & Hutton, W. C. (1983). The mechanical function of the lumbar apophyseal joints. *Spine, 8,* 327–330.

2. American Alliance for Health, Physical Education, Recreation, and Dance. (1980). *AAHPERD health related physical fitness test.* Reston, VA: AAHPERD.

3. American Alliance for Health, Physical Education, Recreation, and Dance. (1985). *Norms for college students—The health related physical fitness test.* Reston, VA: AAHPERD.

4. American Alliance for Health, Physical Education, Recreation, and Dance. (1988). *Physical best.* Reston, VA: AAHPERD.

5. American College of Sports Medicine. (1991). *Guidelines for exercise testing and prescription.* Philadelphia: Lea & Febiger.

6. Broer, M. R., & Galles, N. R. G. (1958). Importance of relationship between various body measurements in performance of toe touch test. *Research Quarterly, 29,* 253–263.

7. Clark, B., Osness, W., Adrian, M., Hoeger, W. W. K., Raab, D., & Wiswell, R. (1989). Tests for fitness in older adults: AAHPERD Fitness Task Force. *Journal of Physical Education, Recreation, and Dance, 60,* 66–71.

8. Clarke, H. H. (1975). Joint and body range of movement. *Physical Fitness Research Digest, 5,* 1–22.

9. Corbin, C. B., & Pangrazi, R. P. (1992). Are American children and youth fit? *Research Quarterly for Exercise and Sport, 63,* 96–106.

10. Fitness and Amateur Sport Canada. (1987). *Canadian Standardized Test of Fitness (CSTF) operations manual.* 3d ed. Ottawa, Ontario: Canadian Association of Sport Sciences.

11. Fitness and Lifestyle Research Institute. (1983). *Fitness and lifestyle in Canada.* Ottawa, Canada: Fitness and Amateur Sport.

12. Gerber, S., & Marshall, J. (1974, October). Searching for loose and tight joints. *The Physician and Sportsmedicine,* pp. 50; 81–83.

13. Golding, L. A., Myers, C. R., & Sinning, W. E. (1982). *The Y's way to physical fitness: The complete guide to fitness testing and instruction.* Rosemont, IL: YMCA.

14. Greipp, J. F. (1985, August). Swimmer's shoulder: The influence of flexibility and weight training. *The Physician and Sportsmedicine,* pp. 92–98; 101–105.

15. Harris, M. L. (1969). A factor analytic study of flexibility. *Research Quarterly, 40,* 62–70.

16. Hinson, M. M. (1977). *Kinesiology.* Dubuque, IA: Wm. C. Brown.

17. Hoeger, W. W. K. (1989). *Lifetime physical fitness and wellness.* Englewood, CO: Morton Publishing.

18. Hoeger, W. W. K, & Hopkins, D. R. (1992). A comparison of the sit and reach and the modified sit and reach in the measurement of flexibility in women. *Research Quarterly for Exercise and Sport, 63,* 191–195.

19. Hoeger, W. W. K., Hopkins, D. R., Button, S., & Palmer, T. A. (1990). Comparing the sit and reach with the modified sit and reach in measuring flexibility in adolescents. *Pediatric Exercise Science, 2,* 156–162.

20. Hoeger, W. W. K., Hopkins, D. R., & Johnson, L. C. (1993). *The assessment of muscular flexibility.* Rockton, IL: Authors/Novel Products, Inc.

21. Holland, G. J. (1968). The physiology of flexibility. *Kinesiology Review, 49.* Cited by Clarke (1975).

22. Hubley, C. (1982). Testing flexibility. In D. McDougall, H. Wenger, & H. Green (Eds.), *Physiological testing of the elite athlete,* 117–132. Ottawa, Canada: Canadian Association of Sport Sciences.

23. Hupperich, F. L., & Sigerseth, P. O. (1950). The specificity of flexibility in girls. *Research Quarterly, 21,* 25–33.

24. Institute for Aerobics Research. (1988). *The Fitnessgram.* Dallas: Institute.

25. Jackson, A. W., & Baker, A. A. (1986). The relationship of the sit and reach test to criterion measures of hamstring and back flexibility in young females. *Research Quarterly for Exercise and Sport, 57,* 183–186.

26. Jackson, A. W., & Langford, N. J. (1989). The criterion-related validity of the sit and reach test: Replication and extension of previous findings. *Research Quarterly for Exercise and Sport, 60,* 384–387.

27. Jones, G. R., Boyce, R. W., Coolidge, W. A., & Hiatt, A. R. (1989). Comparison of two methods of sit and reach trunk flexion assessment. *Medicine and Science in Sports and Exercise, 21,* (Suppl.), Abstract #691, S116.

28. Kraus, H., & Hirschland, R. P. (1954). Minimum muscular fitness tests in school children. *Research Quarterly, 125,* 178–188.

29. Kraus, H., & Raab, W. (1961). Hypokinetic disease. Springfield, IL: Charles C Thomas.

30. Liemohn, W., Sharpe, G. L., & Wasserman, J. F. (1994). Criterion related validity of the sit-and-reach

test. *Journal of Strength and Conditioning Research, 8,* 91–94.

31. Munroe, R. A., & Romance, T. J. (1975). Use of the Leighton flexometer in the development of a short flexibility test battery. *American Corrective Therapy Journal, 29,* 22–29.

32. Nachemson, A. (1975). Towards a better understanding of low back pain: A review of the mechanics of the lumbar disc. *Rheumatic Rehabilitation, 14,* 129–143.

33. Nicholas, J. A. (1970). Injuries to knee ligaments: Relationship to tightness and looseness in football players. *JAMA, 212,* 2236–2239.

34. O'Connor, J. S., Hines, K., & Warner, C. A. (1996). Flexibility and injury incidence. *Medicine and Science in Sports and Exercise, 28*(5), Abstract #376, S63.

35. Osness, W. H, Adrian, M., Clark, B., Hoeger, W., Raab, D., & Wiswell, R. (1990). *Functional fitness assessment for adults over 60 years: A field-bond assessment.* Reston, VA: AAHPERD.

36. President's Council on Physical Fitness and Sports. (1990). *PCPFS President's challenge physical fitness program test manual.* Washington, D.C.: PCPFS.

37. Ross, J. G., Dotson, C. O., & Gilbert, G. G. (1985, January). New standards for fitness measurement: The National Children and Youth Fitness Study. *JOPERD,* pp. 62–66 (20-NCYFS-24-NCYFS).

38. Schultz, A., Andersson, G., Ortengren, R., Haderspeck, K., & Nachemson, A. (1982). Loads on the lumbar spine: Validation of a biomechanical analysis by measurement of intradiscal pressures and myoelectric signals. *Journal of Bone and Joint Surgery, 64A,* 713–720.

39. Shephard, R. J., Berridge, M., & Montelpare, W. (1990). On the generality of the "Sit and Reach" test: An analysis of flexibility data for an aging population. *Research Quarterly for Exercise and Sport, 61,* 326–330.

40. Sullivan, M. K., Dejulia, J. J., & Worrell, T. W. (1992). Effect of pelvic position and stretching method on hamstring muscle flexibility. *Medicine and Science in Sports and Exercise, 24,* 1383–1389.

41. Wear, C. L. (1963). Relationships of flexibility measurements to length of body segments. *Research Quarterly, 23,* 115–118.

42. Wells, C. L. (1985). *Women, sport, and performance: A physiological perspective.* Champaign, IL: Human Kinetics.

43. Wells, K. F., & Dillon, E. K. (1952). The sit and reach test: A test of back and leg flexibility. *Research Quarterly, 34,* 234–238.

44. Worrell, T., Perrin, D., Gansneder, B., & Gieck, J. (1991). Comparison of isokinetic strength and flexibility measures between injured and noninjured athletes. *Journal of Orthopodic Sports Physical Therapy, 13,* 118–125.

Form FL 1

Individual Data for Sit-and-Reach Flexibility Tests

Name _____ Date _____ Time ____ a.m. ____ p.m. ____

Age ____ y   Gender (M or F) ____   Ht ____ cm   Wt ____ kg

Temperature (T_A) ____ °C

Trials	1st	2nd	3rd	4th		Index
AAHPERD	____	____	____	____	cm (circle best)	23 cm; 9 in.
YMCA	____	____	____		in. (circle best)	38 cm; 15 in.
CANADA	____	____			cm (circle best)	26 cm; 10 in.
WALL	____	____			in. (Average = ____ in.)	0 cm; 0 in.

Sit and Reach Score:

____ in.   ____ cm (AAHPERD method fourth trial; held 1–2 s)   ____ %ile

____ in.   ____ cm (YMCA; best of 3 trials)   ____ category

____ in.   ____ cm (Canadian; best of 2 trials; held 2 s)   ____ category; %ile

____ in.   ____ cm (Wall; average of 2 trials)   ____ %ile

Form *FL 2*

Group Data for Sit-and-Reach Flexibility

MEN					**WOMEN**				
Initials	**AAHPERD**	**YMCA**	**CANADA**	**WALL**	**Initials**	**AAHPERD**	**YMCA**	**CANADA**	**WALL**
1.					1.				
2.					2.				
3.					3.				
4.					4.				
5.					5.				
6.					6.				
7.					7.				
8.					8.				
9.					9.				
10.					10.				
11.					11.				
12.					12.				
13.					13.				
14.					14.				
15.					15.				
16.					16.				
17.					17.				
18.					18.				
19.					19.				
20.					20.				
M					*M*				

Chapter BM Body Mass Index

The Body Mass Index (BMI), the term proposed by Keys and his colleagues[13] in 1972,[25] also has been referred to as Quetelet's Index,[15] named after its 1869 originator, who is sometimes considered the Father of Anthropometry.[12] The most popular stature-weight index, the Body Mass Index (BMI), has been used to categorize persons with respect to their health fitness[1] and their degree of obesity.[8,9] High BMI is associated with higher death rates in men, either from all-causes or coronary heart disease.[10]

Method

Body weight can be assessed from various stature/weight indexes, thus indicating the degree of obesity. Stature-weight indexes for assessing body weight are probably the simplest and least expensive methods of all, requiring only the measurement of weight and stature (height).

Procedure

The first two steps in obtaining the BMI are to measure weight (mass) and height. Both of these were described in Chapter UN. The third and final step in getting the BMI requires a simple calculation or the use of a nomogram (Fig. 1).[23]

Calculation of BMI

As presented in Equation 1, BMI is a ratio of the person's weight (kg) to the height squared (m^2). In other words, BMI (kg/m^2 or $kg \cdot m^{-2}$) is the result of dividing a person's weight by the square of that person's height.

$$BMI = Wt\ (kg) \div Ht^2\ (m) \qquad Eq.\ 1$$

where: m = meters; 100 cm = 1 m

For example, if a person weighs 68.0 kg and is 174.0 cm tall (1.740 m), then Equation 1 is used to calculate the BMI as follows:

$$BMI = 68.0\ kg \div 1.74\ m^2$$
$$= 68\ kg \div 3.03$$
$$= 22.44\ (22.4\ to\ closest\ tenth)$$

Calculation of Percent Body Fat from BMI

Percent body fat (%BF) can be estimated in adults up to 83 years of age by using Equation 2.[8]

Accuracy of BMI

BMI has a "somewhat higher" association with body fat than the popular height-weight tables.[18] BMI has moderate correlations (r) between .70 and .80 with the percent fat predicted from hydrostatic weighing[13] and .64 to .69 for skinfold predictions.[19] These represent a slight improvement of the correlation (r = .6) between percent fat and weight alone, hence giving a standard error of predicting percent fat from BMI of about 5%–6%.[20]

The prediction of percent body fat by using BMI, age, and gender in a group of over 1,000 males and females was comparable to the prediction error obtained with such measurements as skinfolds and bioelectrical impedance.[8] The *SEE* was 4.1% body fat when compared to densitometrically-determined (underwater weighing) body fat percentage. When obese persons were evaluated the BMI was "not much less accurate" than the average body fat from hydrodensitometry, body water, and body potassium.[12] Although the BMI may be acceptable for predicting percent fat in a typical group of persons, and for predicting obesity,[12] it is prone to error in persons exceptionally lean, such as bodybuilders or power athletes[19] and in older persons,[12] unless the latter group's ages are factored.[8] For example, about 12% of male athletes were deemed obese (>27.2 kg · m^{-2}) by BMI; however, only 2% of the female athletes were falsely positive for obesity.[19] BMI ignores the nebulous factor of body-frame size, a factor that may be both ill defined and unnecessary in anthropometry.[21]

$$\%BF = 1.20 \times BMI + (0.23 \times Age) - (10.8 \times sex) - 5.4 \qquad Eq.\ 2$$

where: sex = 0 for women; 1 for men

For example, if a 30-y-old woman's BMI is 20 kg·m^{-2}, then the following calculation predicts her hydrodensitometry (underwater weight) percent fat as 25.5%.

$$\%BF = 1.20 \times 20\ kg\cdot m^{-2} + (0.23 \times 30\ y) - (10.8 \times 0) - 5.4$$
$$= 24 + 6.9 - 0 - 5.4$$
$$= 25.5\%$$

If a 30-y-old man's BMI was also 20 kg·m^{-2}, then his predicted underwater-determined percent body fat would be 14.7%.

$$\%BF = 1.20 \times 20\ kg\cdot m^{-2} + (0.23 \times 30\ y) - (10.8 \times 1) - 5.4$$
$$= 24 + 6.9 - 10.8 - 5.4$$
$$= 14.7\%$$

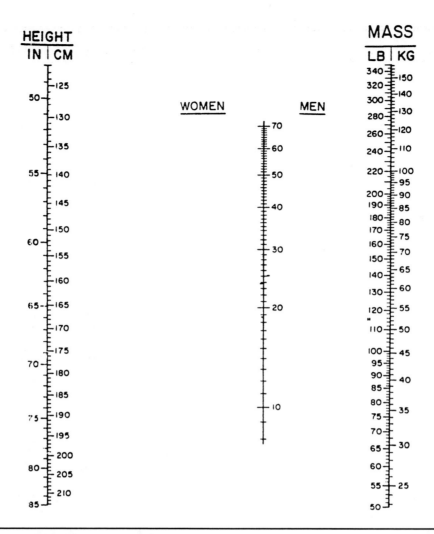

Figure 1 A nomogram for assessing body weight. Adapted from Thomas, A. E., McKay, D. A., & Cutlip, M. B. (1976). A nomograph method for assessing body weight. *The American Journal of Clinical Nutrition, 29,* 302–304. Reprinted with permission of American Society for Clinical Nutrition.

Results and Discussion

Cautious interpretation should be made of the BMI value as a direct measurement of the degree of fatness. Norms for BMI may imply that the higher the BMI value, the greater the fat percentage; this would not be the case in "athletic" persons with high amounts of lean mass. AAHPERD established health fitness standards for 18-y-old males and females as 18–26 $kg \cdot m^{-2}$.[1] The Canadian Standardization Test of Fitness (CSTF) provides percentiles for men and women ages 20–69 years (Table 1).[11] The CSTF places percentiles greater than the 84th (low BMI) into the *excellent* category, and percentiles less than the 25th (high BMI) into the *poor* category. Consistent with the *poor* criterion, some researchers define obesity as an index higher than 85% of the population between 18 and 24 years old (or below the 15th %ile in Table 1).

Overweight has been defined as a BMI between 24.0 (women), or 25.0 (men), and 30.0 $kg \cdot m^{-2}$, whereas obesity's criterion is a BMI greater than 30.0.[5] Using a BMI of 30 as the criterion for obesity, about 9–12% of North Americans are obese.[7] Obviously, a typical non-obese adult, who has about 25 billion fat cells, will weigh less at a given height, than the obese person, who has about 75 billion fat cells.[22] Classifications in Table 2 relate to the degree of obesity, normality, and starvation for men and women.[4,9,24] Authors[18] cited reports revealing that 26% of the U.S. population was overweight based on the body mass index. More African Americans and Hispanics were overweight than Whites, with Hispanic men and African American women having the highest prevalence of overweight. As of 1980 the average White woman 25 to 34 years of age had a BMI of 23.8, whereas the average African American woman averaged 26.2. The mean BMI for a large group of 43-year-old men was 25.4 (*SD* = 3.1), ranging from an extremely lean BMI of 16.96 to a morbidly obese BMI of 46.63 $kg \cdot m^{-2}$.[16]

BMI in men is directly related to mortality, indicating a greater risk of death the higher the BMI.[14] A body-mass index of 21.4 $kg \cdot m^{-2}$ in males between 20 and 29 years of

Table 1 Percentiles for Body Mass Index (BMI) in Men (M) and Women (W) Ages 20–69

%ile	20–29		30–39		40–49		50–59		60–69	
	M	W	M	W	M	W	M	W	M	W
95	19	18	20	19	21	19	21	20	21	20
90	20	18	21	19	22	20	22	21	22	21
85	21	19	22	20	23	20	23	22	23	22
80	21	19	22	20	23	21	24	22	24	22
75	22	20	23	21	24	21	24	23	25	23
70	22	20	23	21	24	22	24	23	25	23
65	22	20	24	22	25	22	25	23	25	24
60	23	21	24	22	25	23	25	24	26	24
55	23	21	24	22	25	23	25	24	26	25
50	23	21	25	23	26	24	26	25	27	25
45	24	22	25	23	26	24	26	25	27	26
40	24	22	26	23	27	25	27	26	27	26
35	25	22	26	24	27	25	27	26	28	27
30	25	23	27	24	28	26	28	27	28	28
25	26	23	28	25	28	27	28	28	28	28
20	27	24	28	26	29	28	29	29	29	29
15	27	25	29	27	30	29	30	30	30	30
10	28	26	30	29	31	31	31	31	31	32
5	30	28	32	31	32	34	32	34	33	34

Source: Data from Fitness and Amateur Sport Canada, Canadian Standardized Test of Fitness (CSTF) Operations Manual, 3d edition, Appendix I: Table 1, p. 30, 1987 by Canadian Association of Sport Sciences, Ottawa, Ontario.

Table 2 Body Mass Index (BMI) and Its Categories

Category	BMI ($kg \cdot m^{-2}$)[a]		BMI ($kg \cdot m^{-2}$)[b]	
	Men	Women	Men	Women
Starved[c]				≤15
Non-obese	<25	<27	<28	<27
Obese				
Moderate	25–30	27–30	28–31	27–32
Massive		30–40		
Severely			>31	>32
Morbid		>40		

Source: Adapted from (a) M. DiGirolamo, March, 1986, "Body Composition-Roundtable", in The Physician and Sportsmedicine, 144–152; 157; 161–2 table depicting body mass index (BMI) and degree of obesity; (b) US Surgeon General; (c) Blackburn & Kanders (1987)

age, and 26.6 $kg \cdot m^{-2}$ in both sexes between 60–69 years of age was associated with a minimum mortality.[3] Thus, the BMI value that is related to the least risk of mortality within age groups increases with age in both sexes.[6] The American College of Sports Medicine reports that BMI values at or above 27.8 $kg \cdot m^{-2}$ and 27.3 $kg \cdot m^{-2}$ for men and women, respectively are associated with significant increases in mortality risk.[2] For women, BMI values over 29 represent a doubling of mortality risk.[17] The BMI for 27% of American women is greater than 27. Although fatter women may have fewer problems associated with menopause, they are at greater risk of cancer mortality.[26]

References

1. American Alliance for Health, Physical Education, Recreation, and Dance. (1988). *Physical best.* Reston, VA: AAHPERD.

2. American College of Sports Medicine. (1991). *Guidelines for exercise testing and prescription.* Philadelphia: Lea & Febiger.

3. Andres, R. (1984). *Principles of geriatric medicine.* New York: McGraw-Hill.

4. Blackburn, G., & Kanders, B. (1987). Evaluation and treatment of the medically obese patient with cardiovascular disease. *American Journal of Cardiology, 60,* 11.

5. Bray, G. A. (1978). Definition, measurement, and classification of the syndromes of obesity. *International Journal of Obesity, 2,* 99–112.

6. Bray, G. A. (1985). General discussion of adipose tissue. In A. F. Roche (Ed.), *Body-composition assessments in youth and adults,* (pp. 20–21). Columbus, OH: Ross Laboratories.

7. Bray, G. A., & Gray, D. S. (1988). Obesity: Part 1— Pathogenesis. *Western Journal of Medicine, 149,* 429–441.

8. Deurenberg, P., Weststrate, J. A., & Seidell, J. C. (1991). Body mass index as a measure of body fatness: age- and sex-specific prediction formulas. *Journal of Nutrition, 65,* 105–114.

9. DiGirolamo, M. (1986, March). Body composition— Roundtable. *The Physician and Sportsmedicine,* pp. 144–152, 157, 161, 162.

10. Dorn, J. P., Trevisan, M., & Winkelstein, W. (1996). The long-term relationship between body mass index, coronary heart disease and all-cause mortality. *Medicine and Science in Sports and Exercise, 28* (Suppl.), Abstract #662, p. S111.

11. Fitness and Amateur Sport Canada. (1987). *Canadian Standardized Test of Fitness (CSTF) operations manual.* Ottawa, Ontario: Canadian Association of Sport Sciences.

12. Garrow, J. S., & Webster, J. (1985). Quetelet's Index (W/H^2) as a measure of fatness. *International Journal of Obesity, 9,* 147–153.

13. Keys, A., Fidanza, F., Karvonen, M. J., Kimura, N., & Taylor, H. L. (1972). Indices of relative weight and obesity. *Journal of Chronic Diseases, 25,* 329–343.

14. Lee, I-M, Manson, J. A., Hennekens, C. H., & Paffenbarger, R. S. (1993). Body weight and mortality: A 27-year follow-up of middle-aged men. *JAMA, 270,* 2823–2828.

15. Lee, J., Kolonel, L. N., & Hinds, M. W. (1981). Relative merits of the weight-corrected-for-height indices[1-3]. *The American Journal of Clinical Nutrition, 34,* 2521–2529.

16. Macera, C. A., Jackson, K. L., Hagenmaier, G. W., Kronenfeld, J. J., Kohl, H. W., & Blair, S. N. (1989). Age, physical activity, physical fitness, body composition, and incidence of orthopedic problems. *Research Quarterly for Exercise and Sport, 60,* 225–233.

17. Manson, J. E., Willett, W. C., Stampfer, M. J., Colditz, G. A., Hunter, D. J., Hankinson, S. E., Hennekens, C. H., & Speizer, F. E. (1995). Body weight and mortality among women. *New England Journal of Medicine, 333,* 677–685.

18. McArdle, W. D., Katch, F. I., & Katch, V. L. (1996). *Exercise physiology: Energy, nutrition, and human performance.* Baltimore: Williams & Wilkins.

19. Mullins, N. M., Sinning, W. E. (1996). Diagnostic utility of the body mass index as a measure of obesity in athletes and non-athletes. *Medicine and Science in Sports and Exercise, 28,* Abstract #1148, S193.

20. Pollock, M. (1985). General discussion of sports medicine. In A. F. Roche (Ed.), *Body-composition assessments in youth and adults* (p. 83). Columbus, OH: Ross Laboratories.

21. Roche, A. F. (1984). Research progress in the field of body composition. *Medicine and Science in Sports and Exercise, 16,* 579–583.

22. Stern, J. S. (1973, May). Adipose cellularity: Metabolic and chemical significances. Symposium conducted at American College of Sports Medicine Convention, Seattle, WA.

23. Thomas, A. E., McKay, D. A., & Cutlip, M. B. (1976). A nomograph method for assessing body weight. *The American Journal of Clinical Nutrition, 29,* 302–304.

24. U.S. Department of Health and Human Services. (1988). The Surgeon General's report on nutrition and health (DHHS (PHS) Publication No. 88-50210). Washington, D.C.: U.S. Government Printing Office.

25. Weigley, E. S. (1989). Adolphe Quetelet (1796–1874): Pioneer anthropometrist. *Nutrition Today, 24,* 12–16.

26. Wells, C. (1993, November). Megatrends in women's health. Symposium conducted at Southwest American College of Sports Medicine Convention, San Diego, CA.

Form BM 1

Individual Data for BMI

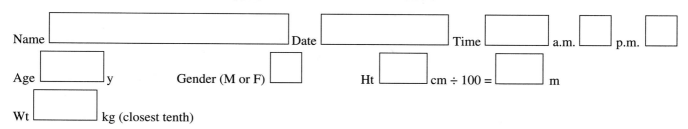

Name [ ] Date [ ] Time [ ] a.m. [ ] p.m. [ ]

Age [ ] y   Gender (M or F) [ ]   Ht [ ] cm ÷ 100 = [ ] m

Wt [ ] kg (closest tenth)

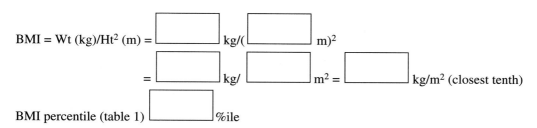

$BMI = Wt (kg)/Ht^2 (m) =$ [ ] $kg/($ [ ] $m)^2$

$=$ [ ] $kg/$ [ ] $m^2 =$ [ ] kg/m^2 (closest tenth)

BMI percentile (table 1) [ ] %ile

BMI %ile vs. BMI Category (Table 1):

%ile	BMI Category (circle one)
≥85	Low BMI (Very thin)
65–84	<Ave. (Thinner than average)
45–64	Average
25–44	>Ave. (Fatter than average)[a]
<25	High BMI (Very fat)[a]

[a]Exceptions: Highly muscular persons.

Form BM 2

Group Data for BMI

MEN				WOMEN			
Initials (or ID#)	Height m	Mass kg	BMI kg·m^{-2}	Initials (or ID#)	Height m	Mass kg	BMI kg·m^{-2}
1.				1.			
2.				2.			
3.				3.			
4.				4.			
5.				5.			
6.				6.			
7.				7.			
8.				8.			
9.				9.			
10.				10.			
11.				11.			
12.				12.			
13.				13.			
14.				14.			
15.				15.			
16.				16.			
17.				17.			
18.				18.			
M				M			
Range				Range			

Chapter GR Girth

A strong case could be made for classifying many anthropometric tests as either field tests or field/lab tests. They could be classified as field tests because they are simple, portable, and inexpensive. For example, some linear tests simply require the measurement of height and/or weight on a platform scale or anthropometer; others measure girths, skinfolds, or diameters with such hand-held instruments as tape measures and calipers. However, some of these tests may be classified as field/lab tests because they may require expert anatomical knowledge and instrument handling by the technician in addition to computerized calculations.

A girth measure is simply a circumference measure that results in a linear dimension such as inches or millimeters. Waist/hip girth ratios, indicating both fat distribution and fat percentage, are important factors in cardiovascular disease.[4,5,6,16,28,29,49] Persons with a high ratio of waist-to-hip girth are twice as susceptible to heart attack, stroke, hypertension, diabetes, gall bladder disease, and death.[11] This fat patterning is thought to cause a negative effect on liver metabolism due to the release of fat directly into the portal (liver) circulation by the close-proximity abdominal fat cells.[11,12]

Various equations, tables, or nomograms are available for predicting percent fat from girth data.[24] Prediction of percent fat can be made from equations derived from a single girth (waist) and body weight of men, or a single girth (hip) and body stature (height) of women.[51,52] This simple method may be referred to as the **1-Girth Method.** A slightly more complex prediction of percent fat uses stature and two or three circumference measures to predict body density in men or women, respectively; then percent fat is calculated from the body density value.[21,22] This more complex method may be referred to as the **2–3-Girth Method** or the Naval Health Research Center (NHRC) method.

Physiological Rationale

Relationship Between Girth and Percent Fat

Compartmentalization of the body into fat and fat-free divisions may be estimated from such measures as body girths, diameters, skinfolds, and/or hydrostatic weight (hydrodensitometry).[9] Because hydrodensitometric measures are so valid, researchers commonly correlate body density measures from hydrostatic weighing tests with the measures from such linear anthropometric measures as skinfolds, diameters, and girths. Regression equations formed from the linear and densitometric relationship are then used to predict the body composition from only the linear measures. Thus, the linear measures can be used to predict the percent fat that would have been determined from hydrodensitometric methods.

In the 1-Girth method for the women, the hip girth at a given height is positively related to percent fat. Thus, higher percent fats occur in persons of the same height but with higher hip girths, or vice versa—in shorter persons but with the same hip girth. For men, according to the 1-Girth method, the lower the mid-abdominal girth is for any given weight, the lower is the percent fat. Also, the more a man weighs for any given mid-abdominal girth, the lower is his percent fat. In the 2–3-Girth method, the neck and hip girth is less important than the abdominal girth for the fat factor. Height weighs heavily for the lean factor.

Relationship Between Girth and Fat Distribution

Fat deposits around the upper abdominal area deserve more serious attention with respect to health than fat deposits elsewhere. A greater deposit of fat at this abdominal "waist" area than at the hip area is more common in adult men than adult women, hence it is often referred to as the android characteristic or the "apple" shape. Women tend to deposit fat in the hip, lower abdominal, gluteal, and appendage areas more than the upper abdominal waist area, hence this girth is often referred to as the gynoid characteristic or the "pear" shape. Coincidentally, the acronym for the girth ratio is A:G, regardless of using the initials for abdomen to gluteal or android to gynoid ratio.

Method

The equipment for measuring girth is very simple. Ideally, a measuring tape made of reinforced fiberglass or metal should be used. Some anthropometric tapes have a calibrated spring at the tip. The purported advantage of anthropometric spring tapes is that the proper tape pressure can be applied repeatedly, although not everyone recommends these.[41] It is helpful to make a "handle" or "tab" from masking or adhesive tape to be attached at the tip of a regular tape. This prevents the technician's thumb and finger from obscuring the zero/index line when reading the circumference. A tape labeled with an inch scale on one side and a metric scale on the other is preferred.

Accuracy of Girth Measurements

All measures of fat in living bodies are merely estimates. The first anthropometric prediction of body fat was published in 1951.[13] Since then, over 100 predictive equations have been developed.

Traditionally, hydrostatic weighing has been the criterion by which other predictive methods are evaluated. The error of estimate (SEE) is about 3.5% for most linear (not hydrostatic) anthropometric predictive tests.[31,33] For example, if an individual was predicted to be 20% fat by girth, skinfold, and/or diameter measures, then an assumed error of 3.5% would mean that there is a 67% chance that the "true" value as predicted by hydrostatic weighing is between 16.5 and 23.5% (20% ± 3.5%).

The 2–3-Girth Method, which was developed from data on large samples of Navy women and men, has moderate to high correlations (r = .85 and .90, respectively) and reasonable standard errors (SEE = 3.7% and 2.7% body fat units, respectively) when compared with hydrostatic weighing. In general, the Navy equation tends to overpredict body fat in lean persons and underestimate it in fat persons.[21,22]

Investigators evaluating the accuracy of three different military equations (Army, Marine, and Navy) concluded that only the Navy equation was not significantly different from hydrostatic weight for group estimations of percent fat in 50-y-old women, but none were a substitute for underwater weighing for individual estimations for the middle-aged women.[48]

Test-retest reliabilities of girth measures are .97 or higher.[10]

Because both girth methods for the women and the 2-3-Girth Method for the men requires a stature measurement, familiarity with anthropometers or stadiometers is essential. The same is true for weight scales, because the weight is measured in men for the 1-Girth Method. These instruments and the proper procedures for stature and weight are described in Chapter UN.

Nomograms are provided in the manual for deriving the percent fat for the men's and women's 1-Girth method. To make the calculations for the 2–3-Girth method, a good pocket calculator (or computer-calculator) with a "log" function is necessary.

Procedures for Measuring Girth

1. Technician measures the weight of the man and records it to the closest pound or 0.5 kg onto Form GR 1.
2. Technician measures the height of the man or woman and records it to the closest one-fourth in. or 0.5 cm onto Form GR 1.
3. The subject stands while the technician determines the exact anatomical sites of the girth measurements as shown in Figure 1. The measurement sites for the 1-Girth[51] and 2–3-Girth Methods[21,22] are explained in Table 1.

4. The technician measures the girths, careful to avoid any air space between the skin and the tape. On the other hand, the tape should not be pulled so tightly that it indents the skin.[23]
5. The technician holds the tape horizontally, except for neck girth, and reads the tape to the closest one-fourth in. and 0.5 cm. Metric measures are used for the 2–3-Girth equations and the Canadian Fitness Test (CSTF); however, either system provides the same ratio value.
6. Technician reads-off the values as another technician records them onto the form.

Calculation of Waist (Android; Abdominal) to Hip (Gynoid; Gluteal) Ratio (W:H; A:G)

Although a W:H (A:G) nomogram is available from various sources,[11] the ratio is so simple to calculate that the nomogram is actually less convenient than a pocket calculator. The girth sites and the calculation of the W:H (A:G) ratio are the same for men and women. The ratio is found simply by dividing the waist (upper abdominal) girth by the hip (gluteal) girth (Eq. 1).

W:H (A:G) = Upper abdominal girth ÷ Gluteal girth   Eq. 1

For example, if a woman's upper waist (upper abdominal) girth is 30 in. (~76 cm) and her hip (gluteal) girth is 40 in. (~101.5 cm), then her W:H (A:G) ratio is calculated as follows:

$$W:H (A:G) = \frac{30 \text{ in.}}{40 \text{ in.}} \quad \text{or} \quad \frac{76 \text{ cm}}{101.5 \text{ cm}}$$
$$= 0.75$$

Calculation of Percent Body Fat from Girth

The 1-Girth Method uses the appropriate nomogram for men (Fig. 2) or women (Fig. 3). Thus, for the men, a straightedge is placed on the weight on the left vertical axis and then pivoted to the mid-abdominal girth on the right vertical axis; percent fat is then read where the straightedge intersects the diagonal axis. For the women, the percent fat is found by placing the straightedge on the hip girth on the left vertical axis and then pivoted to the height on the right vertical axis. As much as possible, the placements should be at the closest pound or 0.5 kg, and at the closest one-fourth in. or 0.5 cm.

The 2–3-Girth Method uses tables[1,21,22] or multiple regression equations—Equation 2 (men)[21] and Equation 3 (women)[22]—to predict body density from circumferences (cm) and stature (cm). The extensive tables also require calculations, but are not quite so intimidating as the multiple regression equations presented here. The advantage of the multiple regression equations is that they can be programmed into a calculator or computer quite easily, thus avoiding the search through the tables. The Siri[45] equation (Eq. 4) for converting body density to percent fat can also be programmed into the calculator or computer. Thus, there is an ultimate savings in time and convenience by using the

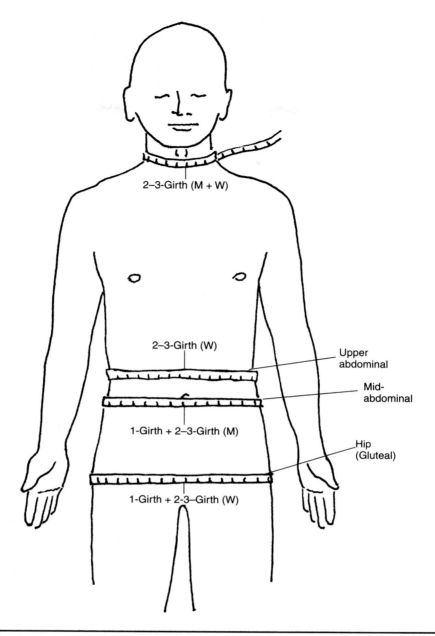

2–3-Girth (M + W)

2–3-Girth (W)

Upper abdominal

Mid-abdominal

1-Girth + 2–3-Girth (M)

Hip (Gluteal)

1-Girth + 2-3–Girth (W)

Figure 1 Girth sites for the 1-Girth-Method (men: mid-abdominal; women: hip/gluteal) and 2–3-Girth-Method (men: neck and mid-abdominal; women: neck, upper abdominal/waist, hip/gluteal).

Table 1 Measurement Sites for the 1-Girth and the 2–3-Girth Methods

Men (M)	Women (W)
1-Girth Method Weight (closest lb; 0.5 kg)	**1-Girth Method** Height (closest one-fourth in.; 0.5 cm)
Mid-abdominal girth—level of umbilicus (navel)	Hip girth—widest point
2–3-Girth Method	**2–3-Girth Method**
Height (closest one-fourth in.; 0.5 cm)	
Neck girth—just inferior to the larynx (Adam's apple) with the tape sloping slightly downward to the front	
Mid-abdominal girth—level of umbilicus (navel)	Upper abdominal girth (waist)—at the narrowest point above navel; often midway between xiphoid process and navel
	Hip (gluteal)—at the level of symphysis pubis and greatest protrusion of the gluteal muscles
Men's A:G Sites Same as upper abdominal (waist) and hip (gluteal) of women's 2–3-Girth Method	**Women's A:G Sites** Same as abdominal and gluteal for 2–3-Girth Method

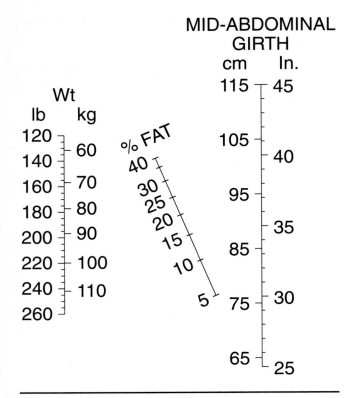

Figure 2 Men's nomogram for determination of percent body fat (%fat) from weight and mid-abdominal girth. From J. H. Wilmore, *Sensible Fitness,* Fig. 13, p. 30, 1988. Copyright © 1988.

regression equation instead of the tables, especially if testing many people.

Men:
$$D_b = 1.0324 + [0.15456 \times Log_{10}(Ht)]$$
$$- [0.19077 \times Log_{10}(Ab - N)] \qquad \text{Eq. 2}$$

where:

D_b = body density
$Log_{10}(Ht)$ = expressed in cm[a]; enter ht, then press "log" on calculator
Ab = mid-abdominal girth (cm)
N = neck girth (cm)

Women:
$$D_b = 1.29579 + [0.22100 \times Log_{10}(Ht)]$$
$$- [0.35004 \times Log_{10}(Ab + Hip - N)] \qquad \text{Eq. 3}$$

For example, if a man, who is 174.0 cm tall, has a mid-abdominal girth of 80.0 cm and a neck girth of 41.9 cm, then the following process would calculate his body density:

---

[a]Logarithm—the exponent expressing the power to which a fixed number (the base) must be raised in order to produce a given number (the antilogarithm): logs are normally computed to the base of 10 and are used for shortening math calculations.

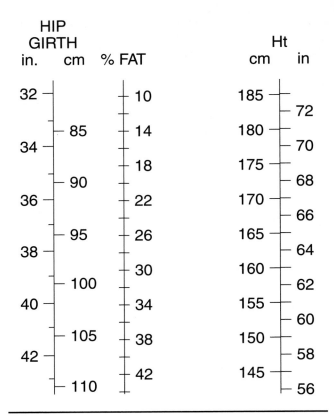

Figure 3 Women's nomogram for determination of percent body fat (%fat) from height and hip girth. From J. H. Wilmore, *Sensible Fitness,* Fig. 14, p. 31, 1988. Copyright © 1988 Human Kinetics Publishers, Champaign, IL.

$$D_b = 1.0324 + [0.15456 \times Log_{10}(174)]$$
$$- [0.19077 \times Log_{10}(80 - 41.9)]$$
$$= 1.0324 + (0.15456 \times 2.2405) - [0.19077 \times Log_{10}(38.1)]$$
$$= 1.0324 + 0.3463 - (0.19077 \times 1.5809)$$
$$= 1.3787 - 0.3016$$
$$= 1.0771$$

$$\%Fat = 100 \times [(4.95 \div D_b) - 4.50] \qquad \text{Eq. 4}$$

Using the same man as in our prior example, his body density of 1.0771 converts to a percent body fat of 9.6%:

$$\%Fat = 100 \times [(4.95 \div 1.0771) - 4.50]$$
$$= 100 \times (4.596 - 4.50)$$
$$= 100 \times 0.096$$
$$= 9.6\%$$

Calculation of Ideal Weight

After the percent fat is known, a person usually wishes to know how much fat should be lost (occasionally, gained) in order to be ideal or perfect. The criterion for what is perfect is open to speculation and is based on health, aesthetics, and performance, or, simply, on the eye of the beholder. A formerly proposed value of 14% for men and 20% for women[26] may be used as an example for demonstrating the calculation of ideal or desired weight. A range of ideal values, rather than a single ideal percent fat value, for each gender is suitable, and its selection should be left up to the discretion of the counselor and/or investigator and the subject.

The calculation of ideal weight may be performed by using various equations. Equation 5 may be referred to as the **approximate equation** because of its approximation of ideal weight, whereas Equations 6 and 7 may be referred to as **exact equations** because of their more exact and logical approach. Although both the approximated and the exact equations use 14% as the constant ideal fat percentage for men, and 20% as the constant ideal fat percentage for women, other desired values (or ranges) for percent body fat may be chosen and inserted in their place.

The approximate equation is based upon a very simple concept and often can be calculated in one's head. It basically calls for the subtraction of the unwanted fat from the initial body weight (B wt) of the man (M) or woman (W).

Approximate Equation: Eq. 5
$$\text{Ideal Wt} = \text{B wt} - [(F - 0.14_M \text{ or } 0.20_W) \times \text{B wt}]$$

where: F = observed percent fat in decimal form

For example, if a man weighing 70 kg (154 lb) was estimated to be 20% body fat, then the following calculation would approximate his ideal weight:

$$\text{Ideal Wt (kg)} = 70 \text{ kg} - [(0.20 - 0.14) \times 70 \text{ kg}]$$
$$= 70 \text{ kg} - (0.06 \times 70 \text{ kg})$$
$$= 70 \text{ kg} - 4.2 \text{ kg}$$
$$= 65.8 \text{ kg}$$

The exact equations (Eq. 6 and 7) for calculating ideal body weight are based upon the lean body weight (LBW) of the individual.[8,40] These equations emphasize the importance of maintaining or gaining lean weight while losing fat weight when dieting and/or exercising. Both equations use the ideal (I-%Fat) criteria of 14% and 20% fat for men and women, respectively.

Exact Equation (A): Eq. 6
$$\text{Ideal Wt} = \left[\frac{100 - \text{Pre \%Fat}}{100 - \text{I-\%Fat}}\right] \times \text{Pre B wt}$$

where: Pre %Fat and Pre B wt = the measured %Fat and body wt
I-%Fat = the ideal %Fat (e.g., 14% in men; 20% in women)

Exact Equation (B): Eq. 7
$$\text{Ideal Wt} = \frac{\text{LBW}}{\text{Ideal LBW Fraction of B wt}}$$
$$= \frac{\text{B wt} - \text{Fat wt}}{0.86 \text{ (men) or } 0.80 \text{ (women)}}$$

If the exact equation (Eq. 6) is used to calculate the ideal or desired weight of the same male in the previous example, then the following calculations would be made:

Table 2 Health and Fitness Standards for Percent Body Fat

Classification	Men	Women
Essential fat	5%	8%
Optimal fitness	12–18%	16–25%
Optimal health	10–25%	18–30%
Overfat	>25%	>30%

Source: From M. DiGirolamo, "Body Composition: A Roundtable" in The Physician and Sportsmedicine, 14, 144–162, March 1986.

$$\text{Ideal Wt} = \left[\frac{100 - 20\%\text{Fat}}{100 - 14\%\text{Fat}}\right] \times 70 \text{ kg}$$
$$= (80/86) \times 70$$
$$= 0.93 \times 70$$
$$= 65.1 \text{ kg}$$

As can be observed by the two examples, the exact method produces a greater amount of weight (fat) that must be lost (4.9 kg) than the approximate method (4.2 kg).

Results and Discussion

Percent Fat Interpretation. Authorities differ as to the recommended body composition for the average person. Average values may not always be recommended values. For example, we do not know if the 16% body fat of babies born in the United States[20] is healthy even though infant mortality is very low. Also, some may feel that elderly persons should carry slightly extra fat in case of severe prolonged illness.

The recommended body composition for athletes also varies; usually, it is dependent upon the sport and/or gender. For example, successful male marathoners are about 7.5% fat,[15] whereas female marathoners usually are less than 20% fat; however, some investigators[14] caution that there may be a critical set point of percent body fat for each female amenorrheic (absence of menstruation) runner, although this has not been confirmed by most studies.[43] Successful middistance and distance swimmers tend to carry more fat than successful sprint swimmers.[38] If high school wrestlers drop below 5% fat, they are either banned from competition in some conferences,[30] or are advised to obtain medical clearance.[3] One authority[47] advises a minimum of 7% fat for wrestlers under 16 years of age. Thus, it appears that the ideal percent fat is dependent upon the goal of the individual. It may be inappropriate to use a single value as a standard for specific-sport athletes, using, instead, a suitable range of values.[51] Also, if an indirect method is used, then a person's predicted percent fat should be presented as a value within the range of the standard error; thus a percent fat of 20% should be presented as 14%–26% if the standard error is 6%. Some of the fat categories suggested by various investigators are presented in Tables 2 and 3.

Table 3 Percent Fat Categories in College-Aged People

Category	Percent Fat (%)	
	Men	Women
Very Lean[18]	8	14
Underweight[35]		$<17^a$
Lean[18]	11	20
Average	10.5 ± 5	23 ± 6
	$12–16^{50}$	$22–26^{50}$
	15^{18}	25^{18}
	15	27
	$10–15^{17}$	$15–20^{17}$
Suitable	$10–22^{32}$	$20–32^{32}$
Optimal Health	$10–25^{42}$	$18–30^{42}$
Recommended (Goal-Dependent)	$15–20^{25}$	$22–28^{25}$
	$8–10^{37}$	
	$10–14^{27}$	
Optimal Fitness	$12–18^{42}$	$16–25^{42}$
Adult Fitness	$15–22^8$	$23–28^8$
Navy Standard		$<30^{48}$
Overfat	$>20^{35}$	$>30^{35}$
Moderately Overfat	$>20^{18}$	$>31^{18}$
Obese	$>25^{34}$	$>34^{34}$
	$>25^{42}$	$>30^{42}$
	$>25^{48}$	$>35^{48}$
		$>38^{44}$
	$>30^{18}$	$>44^{18}$
Massively Obese	$>55^{36}$	$>55^{36}$

Note: ^{a}Accompanied by <20th %ile in body mass by stature.

Although some investigators have reported percent fat values of less than 3%, these are "generally considered to be underestimates of the true relative body fat."[51] For example, one study of a group of professional football players found one player at 0% body fat and eight players at less than 0%![2] Olga Korbut, the girl who helped popularize gymnastics, was found to be 1.5% body fat.[39] The lowest value I have ever measured was 4% in a Black wrestler trying out for the U.S. Olympic team. Underfat males and females of less than 5% and 15% fat,[42] respectively, may not be healthy. A 70% body fat is the highest value I have ever seen reported.[46]

Waist:Hip (Abdominal:Gluteal) Ratio Interpretation. W:H (A:G) ratios are presented in Table 4.[19] Percentiles above the 84th are in the excellent category; those between the 65th and 84th are better than average; the average includes persons between the 45th and 64th percentiles, and the below average are between the 25th and 44th; the poorest category includes those lower than the 25th percentile. *Playboy* centerfolds and Miss Americas over several decades have had a waist–hip ratio of 0.67 to 0.72.[7]

A waist–hip ratio below 0.80^{28} or 0.86^5 for women and 0.95^{28} or 1.0^6 for men are the criteria ratios to avoid a greater risk for several diseases.

Table 4 Percentiles for Waist–Hip Ratios for Men (M) and Women (W) Ages 15 to 69 y

%ile	15–19		20–29		30–39		40–49		50–59		60–69	
	M	W	M	W	M	W	M	W	M	W	M	W
95	0.73	.65	.76	.65	.80	.66	.81	.66	.82	.67	.84	.71
90	.75	.67	.80	.67	.81	.68	.83	.69	.85	.71	.88	.73
85	.76	.68	.81	.68	.82	.69	.84	.71	.87	.72	.89	.74
80	.77	.69	.81	.69	.83	.71	.86	.72	.89	.73	.90	.75
75	.79	.71	.82	.71	.84	.72	.87	.73	.89	.74	.90	.76
70	.80	.72	.83	.72	.84	.73	.88	.74	.90	.75	.91	.77
65	.81	.73	.83	.73	.85	.74	.89	.75	.91	.76	.92	.78
60	.81	.73	.84	.73	.86	.75	.90	.76	.92	.77	.93	.79
55	.82	.74	.85	.74	.87	.75	.91	.76	.92	.77	.94	.80
50	.83	.75	.85	.75	.88	.76	.92	.77	.93	.78	.94	.81
45	.83	.75	.86	.76	.89	.77	.92	.78	.94	.79	.95	.82
40	.84	.76	.87	.76	.90	.78	.93	.79	.95	.80	.96	.83
35	.85	.77	.87	.77	.91	.78	.94	.79	.95	.81	.97	.84
30	.85	.78	.88	.78	.92	.79	.95	.80	.96	.82	.98	.85
25	.86	.78	.89	.78	.93	.80	.95	.82	.98	.84	.99	.86
20	.87	.79	.91	.79	.94	.81	.97	.84	.99	.85	1.00	.87
15	.87	.80	.93	.80	.95	.83	.99	.86	1.01	.86	1.02	.88
10	.88	.82	.94	.82	.96	.85	1.01	.87	1.02	.88	1.03	.91
5	.92	.86	.96	.85	1.01	.87	1.03	.92	1.04	.92	1.04	.94

Source: Data from Canadian Standardized Test of Fitness (CSTF) Operations Manual, pp. 30–31, 1987. Fitness and Amateur Sport Canada, Ottawa, Ontario, Canada.

References

1. Adams, G. M. (1994). *Exercise physiology laboratory manual.* Dubuque, IA: Brown & Benchmark.
2. Adams, J., Mottola, M., Bagnall, K. M., & McFadden, K. D. (1982). Total body fat content in a group of professional football players. *Canadian Journal of Applied Sport Science, 7,* 36–40.
3. American College of Sports Medicine. (1979). Position statement on weight loss in wrestlers. *Sports Medicine Bulletin, 22,* 2–3.
4. American College of Sports Medicine. (1991). *Guidelines for exercise testing and prescription.* Philadelphia: Lea & Febiger.
5. American College of Sports Medicine. (1995). *ACSM's guidelines for exercise testing and prescription.* Philadelphia: Williams & Wilkins.
6. American Heart Association. (1991). *1992 heart and stroke facts.* Dallas: American Heart Association.
7. Anonymous. (1994, January/February). Vital statistics. *Health,* p. 12.
8. Baumgartner, T. A., & Jackson, A. S. (1987). *Measurement for evaluation in physical education and exercise science.* Dubuque, IA: Wm. C. Brown.
9. Behnke, A. R., & Wilmore, J. H. (1974). *Evaluation and regulation of body build and composition.* Englewood Cliffs, NJ: Prentice-Hall.
10. Bemben, M. G., Massey, B. H., Bemben, D. A., Boileau, R. A., & Misner, J. E. (1995). Age-related patterns in body composition for men aged 20–79 y. *Medicine and Science in Sports and Exercise, 27,* 264–269.
11. Bray, G. A., & Gray, D. S. (1988). Obesity: Part 1—Pathogenesis. *Western Journal of Medicine, 149,* 429–441.
12. Brooks, G. A., Fahey, T. D., & White, T. P. (1996). *Exercise physiology: Human bioenergetics and its application.* Mountain View, CA: Mayfield Publishing Company, pp. 26–27.
13. Brozek, J., & Keys, A. (1951). The evaluation of leanness-fatness in man: Norms and intercorrelations. *British Journal of Nutrition, 5,* 194–205.
14. Carlberg, K. A., Buckman, M. T., Peake, G. T., & Riedesel, M. L. (1983). Body composition of oligo/amenorrheic athletes. *Medicine and Science in Sports and Exercise, 15,* 215–217.
15. Costill, D. L., Bowers, R., & Kammer, W. F. (1970). Skinfold estimates of body fat among marathon runners. *Medicine and Science in Sports, 2,* 93–95.
16. Despres, J.-P., Moorjani, S., Lupien, P. J., Tremblay, A., Nadeau, A., & Bouchard, C. (1990). Regional distribution of body fat, plasma lipoproteins, and cardiovascular disease. *Arteriosclerosis, 10,* 497–511.
17. deVries, H. A. (1986). *Physiology of exercise for physical education and athletics.* Dubuque, IA: Wm. C. Brown.
18. Falls, H. B., Baylor, A. M., & Dishman, R. K. (1980). *Essentials of fitness.* Philadelphia: Saunders College Publishing.
19. Fitness and Amateur Sport Canada. (1987). *Canadian Standardized Test of Fitness operations manual.* 3d ed. Ottawa, Ontario: Minister of Supply and Services Canada.
20. Hager, A., et al. (1977). Body fat and adipose tissue cellularity in infants: A longitudinal study. *Metabolism, 26,* 607–614.
21. Hodgdon, J. A., & Beckett, M. B. (1984). *Prediction of percent body fat for U.S. Navy men from body circumferences and height.* Report No. 84-11. San Diego, CA: Naval Health Research Center.
22. Hodgdon, J. A., & Beckett, M. B. (1984). *Prediction of percent body fat for U.S. Navy women from body circumferences and height.* Report No. 84-29. San Diego, CA: Naval Health Research Center.
23. Hodgdon, J. A., & Beckett, M. B. (1984). *Technique for measuring body circumferences and skinfold thicknesses.* Report No. 84-39. San Diego, CA: Naval Health Research Center.
24. Jackson, A. S. (1984). Research design and analysis of data procedures for predicting body density. *Medicine and Science in Sports and Exercise, 16,* 616–620.
25. Jackson, A. S., & Pollock, M. L. (1985, May). Practical assessment of body composition. *The Physician and Sportsmedicine,* pp. 76–80, 82–90.
26. Johnson, P. B. (1968, Nov.–Dec.). Metabolism and weight control. *JOHPER,* pp. 39–40.
27. Johnson, P. B., Updyke, W. F., Schaefer, M., & Stolberg, D. C. (1975). *Sport, exercise, and you.* San Francisco: Holt, Rinehart, & Winston.
28. Joint Dietary Guidelines Advisory Committee of the United States, Department of Agriculture, Health, and Human Services. (1990). U.S. Dept of Agriculture.
29. Larsson, B., Svardsudd, K., Welin, L., Wilhelmsen, L., Bjorntorp, P., & Tibblin, G. (1984). Abdominal adipose tissue distribution, obesity, and risk of cardiovascular disease and death: 13-year follow-up of participants in the study of men born in 1913. *British Medical Journal, 288,* 1401–1404.
30. Legwold, G. (1984, March). When sports medicine groups speak, who listens? *The Physician and Sportsmedicine,* 162–166.
31. Lohman, T. G. (1981). Skinfolds and body density and their relation to body fatness: A review. *Human Biology, 53,* 181–225.
32. Lohman, T. G. (1982, Dec.). Body composition methodology in sportsmedicine. *The Physician and Sportsmedicine,* 46–58.
33. Lohman, T. G. (1986, March). Body composition—A round table. *The Physician and Sportsmedicine,* pp. 157, 161, 162.
34. Mayer, J. (1968). *Overweight.* Englewood Cliffs, NJ: Prentice-Hall.

35. McArdle, W. D., Katch, F. I., & Katch, V. L. (1991, 1996). *Exercise physiology: Energy, nutrition, and human performance.* Philadelphia: Lea & Febiger.

36. McArdle, W. D., Katch, F. I., & Katch, V. L. (1994). *Essentials of exercise physiology.* Philadelphia: Lea & Febiger.

37. Myers, C. R., Golding, L. A., & Sinning, W. E. (1973). *The Y's Way to Fitness.* Rodale Press.

38. Noble, B. J. (1986). *Physiology of exercise and sport.* St. Louis: Times/Mirror College Publishers.

39. Parizkova, J. (1977, January). Nutritional practices in athletics abroad. *The Physician and Sportsmedicine,* pp. 32–36, 39–40, 42–44.

40. Pate, R. R., McClenaghan, B., & Rotella, R. (1984). *Foundation of Coaching.* Philadelphia: Saunders College Publishing.

41. Ross, W. D., & Marfell-Jones, M. J. (1991). Kinanthopometry. In J. D. MacDougall, H. A. Wenger, & H. J. Green (Eds.), *Physiological testing of the high performance athlete* (pp. 223–308). Champaign, IL: Human Kinetics.

42. Roundtable. (1986, March). Body composition methodology in sportsmedicine. *The Physician and Sportsmedicine,* pp. 46–58.

43. Sanborn, C. F., Albrecht, B. H., & Wagner, W. W. (1987). Athletic amenorrhea: Lack of association with body fat. *Medicine and Science in Sports and Exercise, 19,* 207–212.

44. Sharkey, B. J. (1975). *Physiology and physical activity.* San Francisco: Harper & Row.

45. Siri, W. E. (1961). *Body composition from fluid spaces and density: Analysis of methods in techniques for measuring body composition.* Washington, D.C.: National Academy of Science, National Research Council.

46. Stern, J. S. (1973, May). Adipose cellularity: Metabolic and chemical significances. Symposium at ACSM 20th Annual Convention, Seattle, WA.

47. Tipton, C. M. (1987, January). Commentary: Physicians should advise wrestlers about weight loss. *The Physician and Sportsmedicine,* pp. 160, 163.

48. U.S. Department of the Navy, Navy Military Personnel Command, Code 6H. (1986, August). Office of the Chief of Naval Operations Instruction 6110.1C. Physical Readiness Program.

49. Van Itallie, T. B. (1988). Topography of body fat: Relationship to risk of cardiovascular and other diseases. In T. G. Lohman, A. F. Roche, & R. Martorell (Eds.), *Anthropometric standardization reference manual* (pp. 143–149). Champaign, IL: Human Kinetics.

50. Wells, C. L., & Plowman, S. A. (1983, August). Sexual differences in athletic performance: Biological or behavioral? *The Physician and Sportsmedicine,* pp. 52–56, 59–63.

51. Wilmore, J. H. (1986). *Sensible fitness.* Champaign, IL: Human Kinetics.

52. Wilmore, J. H., & Behnke, A. R. (1969). An anthropometric estimation of body density and lean body weight in young men. *Journal of Applied Physiology, 27,* 25–31.

Form GR 1

Individual Data for Girth Prediction of %Fat and W:H Ratio

Name [＿＿＿＿＿＿＿＿＿] Date [＿＿＿＿＿＿] Time [＿＿＿＿] a.m. [＿＿] p.m. [＿＿]

Age [＿＿＿] y   Gender (M or W) [＿＿]   Ht [＿＿] in. = [＿＿] cm   Wt [＿＿] kg = [＿＿] lb

Girths (in.)

Upper Abdominal Waist [＿＿＿]   Mid-Abdominal [＿＿＿]   Hip (gluteal) [＿＿＿]   Neck [＿＿＿]

Girths (cm) [＿＿＿]   [＿＿＿]   [＿＿＿]   [＿＿＿]

% Fat

1-Girth Method (Nomograms)

Men (Fig. 2): Wt and Mid-Abdomen Girth = [＿＿＿] % Fat

Women (Fig. 3): Ht and Hip Girth = [＿＿＿] % Fat

2–3-Girth Method (Equations)

Men:

$D_b = 1.0324 + [0.15456 \times \text{Log}_{10}$ [＿＿＿] Ht (cm)$] - [0.19077 \times \text{Log}_{10} ($ [＿＿＿] $-$ [＿＿＿] $)]$

$= 1.0324 + (0.15456 \times$ [＿＿＿] $) - (0.19077 \times \text{Log}_{10}$ [＿＿＿] $)$

$= 1.0324 +$ [＿＿＿] $- (0.19077 \times$ [＿＿＿] $) =$

Women:

$D_b = 1.29579 + [0.22100 \times \text{Log}_{10}$ [＿＿＿] Ht (cm)$] - [0.35004 \times \text{Log}_{10} ($ [＿＿＿] $+$ [＿＿＿] $-$ [＿＿＿] $)]$

$= 1.29579 + (0.22100 \times$ [＿＿＿] $) - (0.35004 \times \text{Log}_{10}$ [＿＿＿] $)$

$= 1.29579 +$ [＿＿＿] $- (0.35004 \times$ [＿＿＿] $) =$

Ideal Wt (Equations)

Approximate (Eq. 5): Ideal Wt = B wt [＿＿＿] kg $-$ [(F [＿＿＿] $- 0.14_M$ or 0.20_W [＿＿＿]) $\times$ B wt [＿＿＿] kg]

Ideal Wt = B wt [＿＿＿] kg $-$ ([＿＿＿] $\times$ B wt [＿＿＿] kg)

= B wt [＿＿＿] kg $-$ [＿＿＿] kg = [＿＿＿] kg

Exact (Eq. 6):

Ideal wt = [(100% $-$ F [＿＿＿] %)/(100 $- 14_M$ or 20_W [＿＿＿] %)] $\times$ B wt [＿＿＿] kg

= ([＿＿＿] %/ [＿＿＿] %) $\times$ B wt [＿＿＿] kg

= [＿＿＿] $\times$ B wt [＿＿＿] kg = [＿＿＿] kg

Waist-Hip (A:G) Ratio

Waist (Upper abdominal) Girth [＿＿＿] in./Hip (Gluteal) Girth [＿＿＿] in. = [＿＿＿] ratio = [＿＿＿] Percentile

Percentile Category[19] (check one)

Excellent   (>84th)   [＿＿＿]

>Average   (65th–84th)   [＿＿＿]

Average   (45th–64th)   [＿＿＿]

<Average   (25th–44th)   [＿＿＿]

Poor   (<25th)   [＿＿＿]

Form GR 2

Group Data for Girth-Prediction of % Fat and W:H Ratio

Initials (or ID#)	MEN 1-Girth %	2–3 Girth %	W:H (A:G) ratio	Initials (or ID#)	WOMEN 1-Girth %	2–3-Girth %	W:H (A:G) ratio
1.				1.			
2.				2.			
3.				3.			
4.				4.			
5.				5.			
6.				6.			
7.				7.			
8.				8.			
9.				9.			
10.				10.			
11.				11.			
12.				12.			
13.				13.			
14.				14.			
15.				15.			
16.				16.			
17.				17.			
18.				18.			
M				M			
Range				Range			

Chapter SF Skinfolds

Within the field of kinanthropometry (kin = movement; anthropo = human; metry = measure) there is a subarea called body composition. Body composition is a term referring to the components of the human body. In exercise physiology it often means dividing the body into a two-component model of a fat-free mass and a fat mass.

The purpose of numerous body composition methods is to determine the desirable weight of a person. Some of these methods (e.g., height-weight-age charts) do not indicate the body composition per se but do make an assumption that too much weight for a certain height and age is an indicator of excess fat. Desirable weight can be more validly assessed by examining body composition than by examining standard height-weight-age charts. For example, the body weights of lean, muscular athletes may be 30% greater than the average body weight for stature (height) listed in standard height-weight-age tables.[30] Obviously these muscular athletes should not be classified as overweight. Thus, a body weight that is above average has a much different meaning if it is due to a preponderance of lean weight (e.g., muscle) rather than fat. Another example can be made of typical major-league baseball coaches who were found to weigh approximately the same as the average major-league baseball player; however, body composition assessments revealed that the coaches averaged 6.4 kg less lean weight than the players. This resulted in a body fat percentage of 20% in the baseball coach versus 12.6% in the major league baseball player.[13] Thus, the measurement of body composition is a more valid method of determining desirable weight than is body weight alone.

When studying the various methods of determining body composition, it should be remembered that there is no direct measure of all the fat in the body in living persons—all methods make assumptions.[17] The only sure method is to "blenderize" the body and then make a chemical analysis of the constituents, obviously a very traumatic and complicated procedure. Very few human cadavers have been analyzed by chemical extraction of lipids for direct assessment of body composition. All of the body composition methods on living organisms are indirect estimates, ranging greatly in sophistication and expense. A list of many of the indirect methods of determining body composition are presented in Table 1.[18,22]

The use of calipers to measure subcutaneous skinfolds for the prediction of percent body fat has become popular in health and fitness clinics. Although traditionally the skinfold caliper has been thought of as a laboratory instrument, its portability and recent modification to an inexpensive plastic caliper would qualify it also as a field instrument. In addition, the recommendation of AAHPERD to incorporate skinfold measures in physical education classes,[2,3] characterizes skinfold testing as a field test. Because the location of fat (regional distribution) may be as important clinically and aesthetically as the total amount of fat, skinfolds have an advantage over some other body composition measures.

Physiological Rationale

Fat is not bad. In fact, it is a very economical way to store energy. For instance, one gram of fat contains slightly more than twice the amount of kilocalories as do either carbohydrates or proteins. In addition to its economical storage of fuel, fat also provides a storage place for vitamins. Also, fat is important because it serves as an insulator. Because of these important roles, fat is often subdivided into two compartments—storage fat and essential fat.

The **essential** fat necessary to sustain life in the theoretical reference male (ht = 170–174 cm; 70 kg) represents about 2%–5% of total body weight,[37] and that of the reference female (ht = 163.8 cm; 56.7 kg) up to 12% of total body weight (Table 2).[7,37] Essential fat may be stored in the bone marrow, heart, intestines, kidneys, liver, spleen, central nervous system (myelination), muscles, and other organs and tissues. In women an additional gender-related site for essential fat is the breast area, and possibly the pelvis, buttocks, and thighs.[37]

Storage fat is stored subcutaneously between the skin and muscles; it is also between muscles (intermuscularly) and surrounding various organs. The subcutaneous fat represents about half of the fat in the body of a young adult,[42] whereas the other half is internalized. In older adults the visceral (internal) fat becomes proportionally greater.[37]

Regression equations for predicting percent body fat from body density estimations are based upon correlations between anthropometric measures and hydrostatic measures of body density. Numerous sites may be measured originally, with the combination of sites best predicting body density and/or body fat being chosen for the regression equation. In some cases the regression equation is transformed into a table or nomogram based upon two or more skinfolds (or their sum), which is then used to find the corresponding percent body fat.

Table 1 Some Indirect Methods of Determining Body Composition

Linear-Anthropometry	Densitometry	Spectrometry	Radiology
Stature-Weight	Hydrostatic weighing	Potassium	Computer Axial-
		Deuterium	Tomography (CAT)
Body Mass Index	Buoyancy	Tritiium	X-ray
Ponderal Index	Volume Displacement	Electrical Conductivity	Neutron Activation Analysis (NAA)
Body Surface Area	Water	Total Body (TOBEC)	Nitrogen
	Air plethysmograph	Bioimpedance	Potassium (^{40}K)
		Bioresistance	Magnetic Resonance Imaging (MR)
Diameters	Ultrasonic	Metabolic	Nuclear (NMRI)
Girths	A-mode	Urinary creatine	Photon Absorptiometry (^{125})
Skinfolds	B-mode[24]	Plasma creatine	Dual photon
Somatotype	Portable	Urinary 3-methylhistidine	Dual energy X-ray absorptiometry
Somatogram	Hydrometry	N_2 balance	Light Wave
Visual Inspection	Total body water:	Gas Absorption	Infrared
	D_2O-Deuterium & tritium oxide	xenon; cyclopropane;	Near infrared
	Antipyrine-ethanol	radiokrypton; O_2-labeled water	

Accuracy of the Skinfold-Prediction of Body Fat

Of the over 100 equations for the prediction of body density (with subsequent conversion to percent body fat), the ones from skinfold measurements are considered the most accurate.[27] The relationship between body density and skinfold fat is nonlinear. Thus, when using a linear equation, accurate predictions would be made for those in the middle values but not at the extremes where the obese person would be underestimated and the lean person overestimated. On the other hand, quadratic equations eliminate this bias.[27]

Validity

Correlation coefficients between skinfolds and hydrostatically determined body fatness have consistently ranged from .70 to .90.[1] In general, the inclusion of three skinfold sites in the regression equation produces a better prediction (lower standard error of estimate; *SEE*) of body density than fewer sites. However, neither the feasibility nor accuracy is improved by using more than three sites.[41] The standard error of the estimate for skinfold prediction of hydrodensitometrically determined body fat is about 3.5% body fat units with the acceptable *SEE* of 1%–1.5% probably impossible to attain via skinfold methods.[8,25,28,45,49] For example, using the sum of three skinfolds, described as the J-P method in this chapter, resulted in an *SEE* of 2.7% fat in young adult men.[47] The skinfold *SEE* should be added to the error of hydrodensitometry, making the error of determining true body fat from skinfolds about 4.6%.[15] The sum of the skinfolds itself may be a more valid indicator of adiposity and progressive monitoring of fatness than the prediction of percent fat derived from the skinfolds.

Reliability

The reliability of skinfold measurements is high. The test-retest correlation was .96 in 28 subjects after a one-day waiting period.[a] This is consistent with test-retest reliabilities (r = .94–.98) of other researchers.[9,31]

As with girth estimations, skinfold predictions of body fat are not without controversy. One investigator said that using skinfolds to predict body fat mass "is like trying to find the weight of the peel of an orange by measuring the thickness of the peel, but ignoring the size of the orange."[17] Nevertheless, for the determination of desirable weights, it is logical to conclude that skinfolds are superior to the height-weight-age tables, girths, and diameters.

[a]Adams, G. M. (1970). Unpublished raw data.

Method

A detailed description of skinfold techniques is found in Chapter 5 of *Anthropometric Standardization Reference Manual*.[21] The technique of measuring skinfolds accurately requires considerable practice—the technician must learn to sense (feel) the subcutaneous fold. This feel, however, is not consistent from one subject to another or from one site to another. The ease with which the skinfold, or fatfold, can be separated from the underlying muscle varies between persons and at different sites within the same person. There are also variations in the compressibility of the skin or adipose tissue, which may affect the feel and the measurement. For example, the skinfold is more likely to change its dimension while being grasped in younger subjects due to their greater tissue hydration.[21]

Table 2 Body Composition of the Reference Man and Woman Aged 20–30 y

	Reference Man[a]			Reference Woman[a]		
	kg	lb	%[b]	kg	lb	%[b]
Total Fat Wt	11	23	15	16	35	27
Essential fat	2	5	3	7	15	12
Stored fat	9	19	12	9	20	15
Total Lean Wt	59	131	85	41	91	73
Muscle	31	69	45	20	45	36
Bone	10	23	15	7	15	12
Remainder	18	39	25	14	31	25
Total Body Wt	70	154.0	100	57	126	100

[a]Rounded values
[b]Percent of total body weight
Source: Data from A. R. Behnke & J. H. Wilmore, p. 61, 1974.

Equipment

The basic instrument for skinfold measurement is the caliper. It simplifies and improves the crude use of a ruler to measure the pinch of skinfold held by the technician's fingers. Thus, calipers apply a standard pinch pressure and provide an easily read measure of the width (mm) of the pinch. High quality calipers, such as the Harpenden® and the Lange®, have scales that can be read to a precision of 0.2 mm and 1.0 mm, respectively, whereas lesser quality calipers, such as McGaw®, Ross®, Fat-O-Meter®, and Skin-Guide®, can usually be read to the nearest 2 mm.[23] These cheaper calipers are apparently acceptable for non-research purposes.[34]

A tape measure is used to locate the precise site of some skinfolds (e.g., triceps). It is best to use a metric tape because the midpoint of any measure is often simpler to find using a metric dimension than an inches dimension (e.g., the halfway point of 13.75 in. vs. 34.2 cm). A felt marker (or body marker) or ballpoint pen may be used to mark the site of the skinfolds on the subject.

Subject Preparation

The subjects should wear loose-fitting shirts and shorts. The male subjects are encouraged to go shirtless, while the female subjects are encouraged to wear a bathing-suit top. Leotards should not be worn. The skinfold should not be measured while the subject is overheated, due to the increased fluid volume in the skinfold from cutaneous capillary blood flow. On the other hand, the skinfold will be reduced up to 15% if the subject is dehydrated.[10]

General Procedures for Measuring Skinfolds

Subject Position

All skinfold sites are measured with the subject standing, except for the calf, which can be measured at either the sitting or standing position. Although some authorities state that there is little practical difference as to which side of the body to use for girth measures,[36] it appears that most skinfold equations, including those in this manual, are based on right-side measurements. The description of the skinfold sites corresponds mainly with those methods described by AAHPERD,[1,2] Jackson and Pollock (J-P),[26,29] and the *Anthropometric Standardization Reference Manual*.[21,35]

Skinfold Technique

The caliper should be handled very carefully. While holding it in the right hand, the technician uses the thumb and index finger of the left hand to pinch the skinfold at a distance of about 1 cm proximal (towards the trunk of the body) to the skinfold site (or mark). This fold represents two layers of skin and fat. The long axis of the fold is a natural one, which is smooth and untwisted. This may be referred to as the natural cleavage of the skin. The axis direction of the cleavage may be different in obese persons than in those of normal weight. The points of the caliper should be placed across the long axis of the skinfold at the designated skinfold site (mark). The 1-cm separation between the technician's fingers and the calipers should prevent the skinfold dimension from being affected by the pressure of the fingers. The depth of caliper placement is about half the distance between the base of the normal skin perimeter and the crest (top) of the skinfold. Because of the compressibility of the skinfold,[6] the jaws of the caliper should not press longer than 2 to 4 s at the skinfold site so they do not force fluid from the tissues and reduce the measurement.[32,42] Technicians should be consistent in the timing of the reading, not relying on the end of the rapid decrease in the measurement.[21] For example, all technicians should agree that they will record the reading observed at the first, second, third, or fourth second. While still holding the skinfold, the technician reads the gauge (dial) of the skinfold caliper to the closest 0.5 or 1 mm (e.g., Lange® caliper) to 0.1 or 0.2 mm (Harpenden® caliper), depending on what type of caliper is used.

Number of Measurements

Although most investigators repeat three measurements at one site before moving on to another skinfold site, one authority on anthropometric measures, suggests that the technician make a complete circuit of the measurement sites, then repeat the circuit.[b] In the case of the AAHPERD skinfold test, this would mean that one of the skinfolds (e.g., triceps) would be measured once and not repeated until the other skinfold (e.g., subscapular) is measured. The measurements should be repeated three times (three circuits) or more if the skinfold thicknesses differ by more than 10%.[51] In nonobese persons, the skinfolds at any given site should not differ by more than 1 or 2 mm. Either the median (middle) or mean value of the three trials is used for evaluation.

---

[b]Personal communication, Dr. J. L. Carter, SWACSM Convention, Las Vegas, 1983.

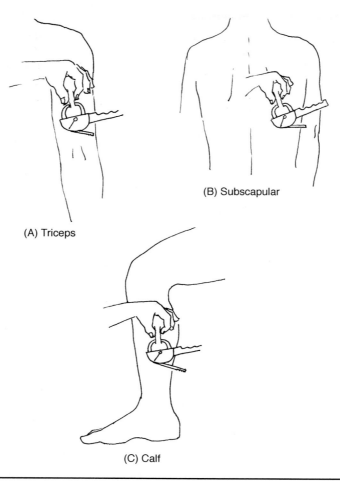

(A) Triceps

(B) Subscapular

(C) Calf

Figure 1 The skinfold sites for the AAHPERD method. The sites for college-aged population are: (a) Triceps and (b) Subscapular; for students younger than college age: (a) Triceps and (c) Calf.

Summary of General Procedures

1. The technician marks the sites to be measured on the right side of the subject's body.
2. The technician pinches the skinfold, at about 1 cm proximal to the marked site, using the thumb and index finger.
3. The jaw points of the caliper are placed on the marked site at a depth of about half the distance between the base of the normal skin perimeter and the crest of the fold.
4. While the technician maintains a firm grip on the skinfold, the gauge of the skinfold caliper is read within 4 s to the closest 0.5 to 1 mm (e.g., Lange®) or closest 0.1 to 0.2 mm (e.g., Harpenden®).
5. The circuit of skinfold measurements is made three times and recorded for each site during each circuit.
6. Either the median or mean value is used for analytical purposes.

Specific Procedures for the AAHPERD and the J-P Methods

Two popular methods of predicting percent fat from skinfold measurements are those using the tables provided by the American Alliance for Health, Physical Education, Recreation and Dance (AAHPERD) and those using the Jackson and Pollock (J-P) multiple-skinfold equations or nomogram for a generalized population of men[26] and women.[29]

AAHPERD Skinfold Measurements

The AAHPERD method derives percent fat from the sum of only two skinfolds—the triceps and subscapular or calf. The subscapular fold is used with the triceps in order to derive percent body fat and percentiles for the college-aged population.[2] The calf measurement was substituted later for the subscapular site in younger students partly to circumvent the sensitive situation of lifting the shirt of the subject.[3] The calf value is added to the triceps skinfold, and this sum is compared to accepted standards for students under college age.[3] The procedures for measuring triceps, subscapular, and calf skinfolds are as follows:

Triceps (Fig. 1a)

1. The subject bends the right arm at a right angle, keeping the elbow close to the side.

Table 3 Percent Fat (%Fat), Sum of Skinfolds (SSF), and Percentiles (%ile) in College-Aged Persons for the AAHPERD Test

%ile	Men SSF (mm) (Triceps + Subscapular)	%Fat	Women SSF (mm) (Triceps + Subscapular)	%Fat
95	12	3.9	17	13.7
75	16	6.6	24	19.0
50	21	9.4	30	22.8
25	26	13.1	37	27.1
5	40	20.4	51	33.7

Reprinted by permission of the American Association for Health, Physical Education, Recreation and Dance, 1900 Association Dr., Reston, VA 22091.

2. The technician, standing behind the subject, places the start of the measuring tape at the top lateral portion of the shoulder (acromion process of the scapula) and runs it down the arm (straightest line possible) to the tip of the bent elbow (inferior portion of the olecrenon process of the ulna).
3. The technician marks the arm at the midpoint between the acromion and olecrenon.
4. The subject allows the arm to fall to a hanging position.
5. With the thumb and index finger pointed downward, the technician grasps a vertical skinfold at the back of the arm, 1 cm above the mark.
6. The technician applies the points of the calipers to the back of the arm at the marked level.
7. The median value of the three measurements is recorded onto Form SF 1.
8. This value is added to the subscapular value in order to obtain percent fat from Table 3.

Subscapular (Fig. 1b)

1. The technician locates by inspection or palpation the inferior angle of the scapula (lowest point). It helps if the subject places the arm behind the back in an arm-lock position.
2. The technician marks the skin of the subject just inferior (about 1 cm; 0.5 in.) to the lower tip of the scapula.
3. The technician grasps the skinfold on a diagonal (about 45°) plane directed from the upper medial position to the lower lateral position. This typically follows the natural cleavage of the skin.
4. The technician applies the jaw points of the caliper at the mark about 1 cm distal from the grasp.
5. The median value of the three measurements is recorded onto Form SF 1.
6. To estimate percent body fat for the college-aged population, first sum the median values of the triceps and subscapular skinfolds.
7. Secondly, refer the sum to Table 3, where the associated percent body fat is found. For example, a

man with a sum of skinfolds equal to 26 mm has 13.1% fat; a woman with a sum of 24 mm has 19.0% fat. Interpolate values between the given table values by noting the gaps between the table skinfold values and the associated %Fat values.

Calf (Fig. 1c) (not necessary for ages 18–35 y)

1. The subject may sit or stand with the right knee bent about 90° and the right foot resting comfortably at a right angle.
2. The technician marks the caliper site at the level of the medial side of the maximum calf circumference.
3. The technician grasps the fold parallel to the long axis of the calf on its medial aspect.
4. The technician applies the jaw points of the caliper at the mark about 1 cm distal from the grasp.
5. The median value of the three measurements is recorded onto Form SF 1.
6. Sum the median values for the tricep and calf skinfolds.
7. Refer the sum to the AAHPERD Standard box.[3]

J-P Skinfold Measurements

The Jackson/Pollock (J-P) Method utilizes a nomogram, equations, or tables in order to determine the percent body fat from the sum of *three* skinfolds for each sex. The three sites for the men are (1) thigh, (2) chest, and (3) abdomen, whereas those for women are (1) thigh, (2) triceps, and (3) suprailium.

Thigh (male and female) (Fig. 2a)

1. The subject flexes the right hip in order to help the technician visualize the location of the inguinal crease at the junction of the hip and the right leg.
2. The technician places the top of the measuring tape at the anterior groin area of the hip (the midpoint of the inguinal ligament, which is halfway between the anterior superior iliac spine and the symphysis pubis).
3. The technician extends the tape to the top (proximal or superior) border of the patella.
4. The technician marks the midpoint on the anterior-most aspect of the thigh.
5. The subject relaxes the thigh muscles of the right leg by standing mainly on the left leg.
6. The technician grasps a vertical skinfold about 1 cm above the mark and then places the caliper's jaw points across the axis of the skinfold at the mark.
7. The technician records the median value onto Form SF 1.

Chest (male) (Fig. 2b)

1. After visual inspection, the technician makes a mark at half the distance from the anterior axillary fold (the front of the armpit) and the nipple.
2. The technician grasps the chest skinfold about 1 cm diagonally above the mark, that is, with the long axis of the fold towards the nipple.

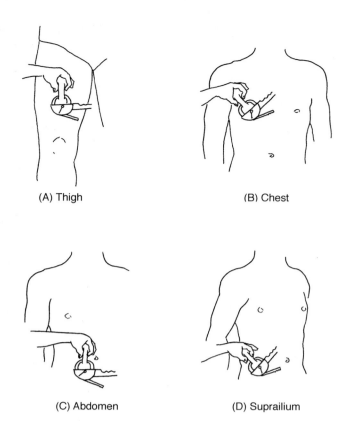

(A) Thigh

(B) Chest

(C) Abdomen

(D) Suprailium

Figure 2 Skinfold sites for the J-P method. Men: (a) Thigh, (b) Chest, and (c) Abdomen. Women: (a) Thigh, (d) Suprailium and Triceps (Fig. 1a).

3. The technician applies the caliper's jaw points across the fold 1 cm inferior to the grasp.
4. The technician records the median value of the three chest measurements onto Form SF 1.

Abdomen (male) (Fig. 2c)

1. The technician marks the site about 2 cm (slightly less than 1 in.) to the right of the umbilicus. (A tape measure is not always necessary for experienced technicians.)
2. The technician grasps a vertical skinfold at a point about 1 cm above the marked site.[c]
3. The technician places the points of the caliper at the marked site across the long axis of the skinfold.
4. The technician records the median value onto Form SF 1.

Triceps (female) (Fig. 1a)

The technician follows the same procedures as for the AAHPERD method.

Suprailium (female) (Fig. 2d)

1. The technician marks the site just above the right iliac crest in the anterior axillary line.[d]

2. The technician grasps the skinfold posterior and superior to the marked site; the natural cleavage of the skinfold normally runs diagonally from the crest toward the umbilicus.
3. The technician places the points of the caliper across the long axis of the typically diagonal fold.
4. The technician records the median value onto Form SF 1.
5. The technician uses any of the three ways to derive the percent body fat from the three skinfold measures of the J-P method:
   a. The sum of the skinfold measures, which can be inserted into appropriate equations for men and women. Because the skinfolds from Lange® calipers are about 10% greater than those from Harpenden® calipers, the 10% difference in the sum should be added.[40]
   b. Refer the sum to a special nomogram[5] derived from the equations (Fig. 3).
   c. Use tables that are available for the J-P method but are not presented in this manual.[16,42,52]

The J-P Equation for Predicting %Fat

The J-P nomogram was derived from the following gender-specific regression equations (Eq. 1 and 2) for body density (D_b) in combination with the equation (Eq. 3) for percent body fat.[46]

[c]Some recommend taking horizontal fold, 3 cm to right, and 1 cm inferior, to the center of the umbilical.[21]
[d]Some recommend taking the measurement 3 cm above the crest[19] or at the midaxillary line.[21]

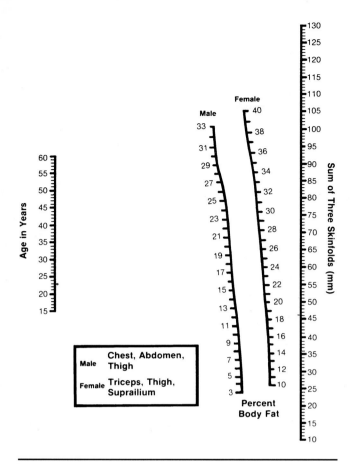

Figure 3 The J-P nomogram for the estimate of percent body fat. From W. B. Baun et al., "A nomogram for the estimate of percent body fat from generalized equations," from Research Quarterly for Exercise & Sport, 52, 380–384. Permission of Tenneco Health & Fitness Dept., PO Box 2511, Houston, TX 77001; and Copyright © 1981, AAHPERD.

Male:

$D_b = 1.1093800 - (0.0008267 \times SSF) + (0.0000016 \times SSF^2) - (0.0002574 \times Age)$ 　　　Eq. 1

Female:

$D_b = 1.0994921 - (0.0009929 \times SSF) + (0.0000023 \times SSF^2) - (0.0001392 \times Age)$ 　　　Eq. 2

where: 　D_b = body density in g·ml^{-1}
　SSF (male) = sum of chest, abdomen, and thigh skinfolds (mm)
SSF (female) = sum of triceps, thigh, and suprailium (mm)

$$\% \text{ Body Fat} = \left[\frac{495}{D_b}\right] - 450 \qquad \text{Eq. 3}$$

The Siri equation has been modified by eliminating the decimals, except for body density, and the need to multiply by 100. Obviously, the calculations can be quite cumbersome when done without the aid of a computer.[4] Nevertheless, the equations can be done, somewhat tediously (about 5 min), using a pocket calculator. For example, if a 48-y-old man's skinfold sum is 43 mm, then the following calculations reveal his percent body fat as 15%.

$$\begin{aligned} D_b &= 1.1093800 - (0.0008267 \times 43) + [0.0000016 \times (43^2)] \\ &\quad - (0.0002574 \times 48) \\ &= 1.1093800 - 0.0355481 + (0.0000016 \times 1849) \\ &\quad - 0.0123552 \\ &= 1.0738319 + 0.0029584 - 0.0123552 \\ &= 1.064 \text{ (rounded off to nearest thousandths)} \end{aligned}$$

$$\begin{aligned} \%\text{Fat} &= \left[\frac{495}{1.064}\right] - 450 \\ &= 465 - 450 \\ &= 15\% \end{aligned}$$

Some authorities recommend that the higher body density of African Americans justifies a different percent-fat equation (Eq. 4).[12,43,48]

$$\% \text{ Body Fat} = \left[\frac{437.4}{D_b}\right] - 392.8 \times 100 \qquad \text{Eq. 4}$$

The J-P Nomogram for Predicting %Fat

The nomogram in Figure 3 is nearly self-explanatory.[5] The percent body fat is found by placing a straightedge (e.g., ruler) at the point on the left vertical line that is closest to the subject's age; then the other end of the straightedge is pivoted to the appropriate value on the far right vertical line (sum of the three skinfolds). The percent body fat is read to the closest 0.5% on the wavy vertical line for the appropriate sex. When using the same example as for the J-P equation, the nomogram also gives a value of 15% for a 48-y-old man with a skinfold sum of 43 mm.

Resting Daily Energy Expenditure (RDEE)

An approximate estimate of the RDEE may be made from the fat-free mass (FFM) by a simple regression equation.[14] First, the fat mass is found by multiplying the total body mass (TBM) by the percent fat (Eq. 5).

$$\text{FM (kg)} = \%\text{F} \times \text{TBM (kg)} \qquad \text{Eq. 5}$$

The fat-free mass (FFM) is calculated by subtracting the fat mass (FM) from the total body mass (TBM) as in Equation 6.

$$\text{FFM (kg)} = \text{TBM} - \text{FM} \qquad \text{Eq. 6}$$

The resting daily energy expenditure (RDEE) in kilocalories is calculated from Equation 7.

$$\text{RDEE (kcal)} = 370 + (21.6 \times \text{FFM}) \qquad \text{Eq. 7}$$

For example, if a man weighing 70 kg has a body fat percentage of 15%, then his RDEE is estimated as 1655 kcal, or 6919 kJ, according to the following calculations:

$$\begin{aligned} \text{FM (kg)} &= 0.15 \times 70 \text{ kg} \\ &= 10.5 \text{ kg} \end{aligned}$$

Older Persons' Equations

Because the AAHPERD and J-P procedures mainly apply to college age and persons less than 60 y of age, respectively, the "older person" equations and procedures are more suitable for persons older than 60 y of age, and, perhaps, as young as 35 y.[50,51] These men's and women's equations are derived from a three-component model (fat and two fat-free body components—water and bone) which enhance their validity (SEE = 2.9% and 3.8% for men and women, respectively) compared to the AAHPERD and J-P two-component models (fat and fat-free weight). A fourth skinfold for the men is taken vertically at the midaxillary site at the level of the xiphoid-sternal junction.[21] The regression equation for the prediction of percent fat, density, water, and bone (PFDWB) of men is presented as Equation 8.

Men: $\qquad$ PFDWB = (0.486 × Sum 4 SF) − (0.0015 × Sum 4 SF^2)

$\qquad\qquad\qquad$ + (0.067 × Age) − 3.83 $\qquad\qquad\qquad$ Eq. 8

where: Sum of 4 SF (mm) = Chest + Subscapular + Midaxillary + Thigh

For women, an additional skinfold to the AAHPERD's subscapular, triceps, and calf is the abdomen site. Equation 9 presents the regression for the prediction of percent fat, density of water and bone (PFDWB).

Women: $\qquad$ PFDWB = (0.428 × Sum 4 SF) − (0.0011 × Sum 4 SF^2)

$\qquad\qquad\qquad$ + (0.127 × Age) − 3.01 $\qquad\qquad\qquad$ Eq. 9

$$\begin{aligned} \text{FFM (kg)} &= 70 \text{ kg} - 10.5 \text{ kg} \\ &= 59.5 \text{ kg} \\ \text{RDEE (kcal)} &= 370 + (21.6 \times 59.5) \\ &= 370 + 1285 \\ &= 1655 \text{ kcal} \\ \text{RDEE (kJ)} &= 1655 \text{ kcal} \times 4.18 \\ &= 6919 \text{ kJ} \end{aligned}$$

Results and Discussion

AAHPERD Interpretation

There are two sets of norms presented for the AAHPERD test. One set is for younger students (under 19 years) and is simply the standards for the sum (mm) of skinfolds (triceps + calf) recommended by AAHPERD.[3]

> AAHPERD Health Fitness Standards (Ages 5–18 y)
> Boys: 12–25 mm $\qquad$ Girls: 16–36 mm

The second set of norms is for college-aged students enrolled in physical education classes and includes five percentiles for their percent body fats (Table 3). This table is the same one that was used to derive the percent body fat from the sum of skinfolds. No age categories are presented for it because only small age differences were found among the college-age group.[2] The greater percent body fat in women for any given sum of skinfolds is attributed presumably to a smaller lean body mass and more essential fat.

J-P Interpretation

The J-P generalized method of predicting body density for adult males was based on the data from over 300 men between the ages of 18 and 61 y (M = 33 y) and who ranged from 1% to 33% fat (M = 18%).[26] The J-P method for women was based on about 250 women between the ages

of 18 and 55 y (M = 31 y) and who ranged from 4% to 44% fat (M = 24%).[29]

The J-P nomogram illustrates the fact that age is an independent factor in body composition. Thus, the same skinfold total in an old person and a young adult would predict a higher fat percentage in the older person. Aging is associated with an increase in internal (besides subcutaneous) fat and a decrease in bone density. Unless age is factored into the equation an underestimation of percent fat with skinfolds will occur in the older person.[11]

General Interpretation

Fat varies from 1–2% of body weight in a severely starved person to 50% in a clinically normal, but obese, person.[46] The lowest acceptable percent fat in adult men is about 3–5%, that is, the amount of essential fat found in bone marrow, central nervous system, and internal organs. The lower limit for adult women is about 8–12%, and includes the same amount of essential fat as in the men, but, additionally, the amount of sex-specific fat, such as that in the breasts.

Although various criteria for fatness and leanness are presented in *Exercise Physiology Laboratory Manual*, the criteria presented also in Figures 4 and 5 emphasize the importance of using ranges, rather than one specific value, for the criteria.[33] The figures should not be interpreted rigidly because not all authorities would have the same criteria. For example, Figure 5 shows that a woman with 16% body fat would be categorized as "ideal," whereas other investigators[38] would suggest that any woman under 17% fat meets one of the criteria for being classified as "underweight." Also, caution is advised when using only one skinfold as an indicator of obesity.[39] For example, triceps skinfolds of 20 mm and 29 mm are obesity criteria for 25-y-old men and women, respectively.[44] Based on U.S. surveys in the 1970s, these skinfold criteria place 25 year olds near the 85th percentile.[20]

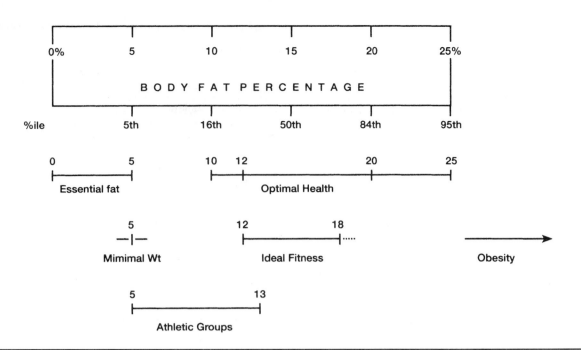

Figure 4 Body fat criteria and percentiles in men. Source: Courtesy of Dr. Timothy Lohman.

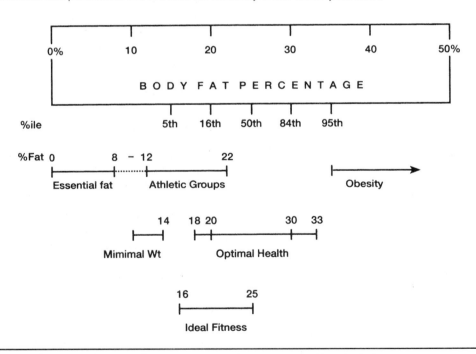

Figure 5 Body fat criteria and percentiles for women. Source: Courtesy of Dr. Timothy Lohman.

References

1. American Alliance for Health, Physical Education, Recreation, and Dance (AAHPERD). (1980). *AAHPERD health-related physical fitness test.* Reston, VA: AAHPERD.

2. American Alliance for Health, Physical Education, Recreation, and Dance (AAHPERD). (1985). *Norms for college students.* Reston, VA: AAHPERD.

3. American Alliance for Health, Physical Education, Recreation, and Dance (AAHPERD). (1988). *Physical best.* Reston, VA: AAHPERD.

4. Baumgartner, T. A., & Jackson, A. S. (1987). *Measurement for evaluation in physical education and exercise science.* Dubuque, IA: Wm. C. Brown.

5. Baun, W. B., Baun, M. R., & Raven, P. B. (1981). A nomogram for the estimate of percent body fat from

generalized equations. *Research Quarterly for Exercise and Sport, 52,* 380–384.

6. Becque, B. D., Katch, V. L., & Moffatt, K. J. (1986). Time course of skin-plus-fat compression in males and females. *Human Biology, 58,* 33–42.

7. Behnke, A. R., & Wilmore, J. H. (1974). *Evaluation and regulation of body build and composition.* Englewood Cliffs, NJ: Prentice-Hall.

8. Bouchard, C. (1985). General discussion of sports medicine. In A. F. Roche (Ed.), *Body-composition assessments in youth and adults,* (p. 95). Columbus, OH: Ross Laboratories.

9. Bouchard, C. (1985). Reproducibility of body-composition and adipose-tissue measurements in humans. In A. F. Roche (Ed.), *Body-composition assessments in youth and adults* (pp. 9–13). Columbus, OH: Ross Laboratories.

10. Brooks, G. A., Fahey, T. D., & White, T. P. (1996). *Exercise physiology: Human bioenergetics and its application.* Mountain View, CA: Mayfield.

11. Bunt, J. C., Lohman, T. G., Slaughter, M. H., Boileau, R. A., Lussier, L., & Van Loan, M. (1983). Bone mineral content as a source of variation in body density in children and youth. [Abstract]. *Medicine and Science in Sports and Exercise, 15,* 172.

12. Clark, R. R., Kuta, J. M., & Sullivan, J. C. (1994). Cross-validation of methods to predict body fat in African-American and Caucasian collegiate football players. *Research Quarterly for Exercise and Sport, 65,* 21–30.

13. Coleman, A. G. (1981). Skinfold estimates of body fat in major league baseball players. *The Physician and Sports Medicine, 9*(10): 77–82.

14. Cunningham, J. J. (1982). Body composition and resting metabolic rate: The myth of feminine metabolism. *American Journal of Clinical Nutrition, 36,* 721.

15. Cureton, K. J. (1984). A reaction to the manuscript of Jackson. *Medicine and Science in Sports and Exercise, 16,* 621–622.

16. deVries, H. A., & Housh, T. J. (1994). *Physiology of exercise for physical education and athletics.* Dubuque, IA: Wm. C. Brown.

17. Dugdale, A. E., & Griffiths, M. (1979). Estimating fat body mass from anthropometric data. *American Journal of Clinical Nutrition, 32,* 2400–2403.

18. Eckerson, J. M., Housh, T. J., & Johnson, G. O. (1992). The validity of visual estimations of percent body fat in lean males. *Medicine and Science in Sports and Exercise, 24,* 615–618.

19. Fitness and Amateur Sport Canada. (1987). *Canadian Standardized Test of Fitness (CSTF) operations manual.* Ottawa, Ontario, Canada: Fitness and Amateur Sport.

20. Frisancho, A. R. (1990). *Anthropometric standards for the assessment of growth and nutritional status.* Ann Arbor, MI: University of Michigan Press.

21. Harrison, G. G., Buskirk, E. R., Carter, J. E. L., Johnston, F. E., Lohman, T. G., Pollock, M. L., Roche, A. F., & Wilmore, J. H. (1988). Skinfold thicknesses and measurement technique. In T. G. Lohman, A. F. Roche, & R. Martorell (Eds.), *Anthropometric standardization reference manual* (pp. 55–70). Champaign, IL: Human Kinetics.

22. Heymsfield, S. B. (1985). Clinical assessment of lean tissues: Future directions. In A. F. Roche (Ed.), *Body-composition assessments in youth and adults.* Columbus, OH: Ross Laboratories.

23. Heyward, V. H. (1991). *Advanced fitness assessment and exercise prescription.* Champaign, IL: Human Kinetics.

24. Ishida, Y., Kanehisa, H., Carroll, J. F., Pollock, M. L., Graves, J. E., & Leggett, S. H. (1995). Body fat and muscle thickness distributions in untrained young females. *Medicine and Science in Sports and Exercise, 27,* 270–274.

25. Israel, R. G., Houmard, J. A., O'Brien, K. F., McCammon, M. R., Zamora, B. S., & Eaton, A. W. (1989). Validity of a near-infrared spectrophotometry device for estimating human body composition. *Research Quarterly for Exercise and Sport, 60,* 379–383.

26. Jackson, A. S., & Pollock, M. L. (1978). Generalized equations for predicting body density of men. *British Journal of Nutrition, 40,* 497–504.

27. Jackson, A. S., & Pollock, M. L. (1985, May). Practical assessment of body composition. *The Physician and Sportsmedicine,* pp. 76–80; 82–90.

28. Jackson, A. S., Pollock, M. L., Graves, J. E., & Mahar, M. T. (1988). Reliability and validity of bioelectrical impedance in determining body composition. *Journal of Applied Physiology, 64,* 529–534.

29. Jackson, A. S., Pollock, M. L., & Ward, A. (1980). Generalized equations for predicting body density of women. *Medicine and Science in Sports and Exercise, 12,* 175–182.

30. Katch, V. L., Katch, F. I., Moffatt, R., & Gittleson, M. (1980). Muscular development and lean body weight in body builders and weight lifters. *Medicine and Science in Sports and Exercise, 12,* 340–344.

31. Kolkhorst, F. W., & Dolgener, F. A. (1994). Nonexercise model fails to predict aerobic capacity in college students with high $\dot{V}O_2$ peak. *Research Quarterly for Exercise and Sport, 65,* 78–83.

32. Lohman, T. G. (1987). *Measuring body fat using skinfolds.* [Video]. Champaign, IL: Human Kinetics.

33. Lohman, T. G. (1989, June). Tutorial on body composition. Presented at ACSM Convention, Baltimore.

34. Lohman, T. G., Pollock, M. L., Slaughter, M. H., Brandon, L. J., & Boileau, R. A. (1984). Methodological factors and the predicting of body fat in female athletes. *Medicine and Science in Sports and Exercise, 16,* 92–96.

35. Lohman, T. G., Roche, A. F., & Martorell, R. (Eds.). (1988). *Anthropometric standardization reference manual.* Champaign, IL: Human Kinetics.

36. Martorell, R., Mendoza, F., Mueller, W. H., & Pawson, I. G. (1988). Which side to measure: Right or left? In A. F. Roche (Ed.), *Body-composition assessments in youth and adults* (pp. 73–78). Columbus, OH: Ross Laboratories.

37. McArdle, W. D., Katch, F. I., & Katch, V. L. (1991). *Exercise physiology: Energy, nutrition, and human performance.* Malvern, PA: Lea & Febiger.

38. McArdle, W. D., Katch, F. I., & Katch, V. L. (1991). *Exercise physiology: Energy, nutrition, and human performance.* Baltimore: Williams & Wilkins.

39. Nieman, D. C. (1995). *Fitness and sports medicine: A health-related approach.* Palo Alto, CA: Bull Publishing.

40. Pollock, M. L., Garzarella, L., & Graves, J. E. (1995). The measurement of body composition. In P. J. Maud/Carl Foster (Eds.), *Physiological assessment of human fitness* (pp. 167–204).

41. Pollock, M. L., Jackson, A. S. (1984). Research progress in validation of clinical methods of assessing body composition. *Medicine and Science in Sports and Exercise, 16,* 606–613.

42. Pollock, M. L., Schmidt, D. H., & Jackson, A. S. (1980). Measurement of cardiorespiratory fitness and body composition in the clinical setting. *Comprehensive Therapy, 6,* 12–27.

43. Schutte, J. E., Townsend, E. J., Hugg, H., Schoup, R. F., Malina, R. M., & Bloomquist, C. G. (1984). Density of lean body mass is greater in blacks than in whites. *Journal of Applied Physiology, 56,* 1647–1649.

44. Selzer, C. C., & Mayer, J. (1965). A simple criterion of obesity. *Postgraduate Medicine, 38*(2), A-101.

45. Sinning, W. E., Dolny, D. G., Little, K. D., Cunningham, L. N., Racaniello, A., Siconolfi, S. F., & Sholes, J. L. (1985). Validity of "generalized" equations for body composition in male athletes. *Medicine and Science in Sports and Exercise, 17,* 124–130.

46. Siri, W. E. (1961). *Body composition from fluid spaces and density: Analysis of methods in techniques for measuring body composition.* Washington, D.C.: National Academy of Science, National Research Council.

47. Stout, J. R., Eckerson, J. M., Housh, T. J., Johnson, G. O., & Betts, N. M. (1994). Validity of percent body fat estimations in males. *Medicine and Science in Sports and Exercise, 26,* 632–636.

48. Thorland, W. G., Johnson, G. O., & Housh, T. J. (1993). Estimation of body composition in black adolescent male athletes. *Pediatric Exercise Science, 5,* 116–124.

49. Thorland, W. G., Johnson, G. O., & Tharp, G. D. (1984). Validity of anthropometric equations for the estimation of body density in adolescent athletes. *Medicine and Science in Sports and Exercise, 16,* 77–81.

50. Williams, D. P., Going, S. B., Lohman, T. G., Hewitt, M. J., & Haber, A. E. (1992). Estimation of body fat from skinfold thickness in middle-aged and older men and women: A multiple component approach. *American Journal of Human Biology, 4,* 595–605.

51. Williams, D. P., Going, S. B., Milliken, L. A., Hall, M. C., & Lohman, T. G. (1995). Practical techniques for assessing body composition in middle-aged and older adults. *Medicine and Science in Sports and Exercise, 27,* 776–783.

52. Wilmore, J. H., & Costill, D. L. (1988). *Training for sport and activity.* Dubuque, IA: Wm. C. Brown.

Form **SF 1**

Individual Data for Skinfolds—Males

Name [ ] Date [ ] Time [ ] a.m. [ ] p.m. [ ]

Age [ ] y   Gender (M or F) [ ]   Ht [ ] in. = [ ] cm

Wt [ ] kg   Temperature (T_A) [ ] °C   Caliper Model [ ]

Skinfolds: (mm) Circle median value of each site

SKINFOLD SITE	METHOD	TRIAL #1	TRIAL #2	TRIAL #3
Triceps	AAHPERD (college age)			
	AAHPERD (<19 y)			
Subscapular	AAHPERD (college age)			
	Older Men (35+ y)			
Calf	AAHPERD (<19 y)			
Chest	J-P (<60 y)			
	Older Men (35+ y)			
Abdomen	J-P (<60 y)			
Thigh	J-P (< 60 y)			
	Older Men (35+ y)			
Mid-Axillary	Older Men (35+ y)			

AAHPERD (Median Values)

College Age

Triceps [ ] mm

+

Subscapular [ ] mm

Sum [ ] mm = [ ] %Fat (Table 3)

= [ ] %ile (Table 3)

5–18 y Age

Triceps [ ] mm

+

Calf [ ] mm

Sum [ ] mm = [ ] %Fat

AAHPERD Standard (12–25 mm) [ ] Yes [ ] No

J-P Nomogram (Median Values; mm)

Chest [ ] + Abdomen [ ] + Thigh [ ] = [ ] mm = [ ] %F (Fig. 3)

D_b = 1.1093800 – (0.0008267 × SSF [ ] mm) + [0.0000016 × (SSF [ ] mm)^2]

  – (0.0002574 × Age [ ] y)

= 1.1093800 – [ ] + (0.0000016 × [ ]) – [ ]

  (0.0008267 × SSF)   (SSF^2)   (0.0002574 × Age)

= [ ] + [ ] – [ ] = [ ] g·ml^{-1}

%Fat = (495/ [ ] g·mL^{-1}) – 450 = [ ] – 450

  (D_b)   (495/D_b)

= [ ] %Fat   = [ ] %ile (from Fig. 4)

Form SF 2

Individual Data for Skinfolds—Females

Name [_____] Date [_____] Time [_____] a.m. [_____] p.m. [_____]

Age [_____] y   Gender (M or F) [_____]   Ht [_____] in. [_____] cm

Wt [_____] kg   Temperature (T_A) [_____] °C   Caliper Model [_____]

Skinfolds: (mm) Circle median value of each site

SKINFOLD SITE	METHOD	TRIAL #1	TRIAL #2	TRIAL #3
Subscapular	AAHPERD (college age)			
	Older Women (35+ y)			
Calf	AAHPERD (<19 y)			
	Older Women (35+ y)			
Triceps	AAHPERD (college age)			
	AAHPERD (<19 y)			
	J-P (<60 y)			
Thigh	J-P (<60 y)			
Suprailium	J-P (<60 y)			
Abdominal	Older Women (35+ y)			

AAHPERD (Median Values)

College Age

Triceps [_____] mm

+

Subscapular [_____] mm

Sum [_____] mm = [_____] %Fat (Table 3)

= [_____] %ile (Table 3)

5–18 y Age

Triceps [_____] mm

+

Calf [_____] mm

Sum [_____] mm = [_____] %Fat

AAHPERD Standard (16–36 mm) [_____] Yes [_____] No

J-P Nomogram (Median Values; mm)

Triceps [_____] + Thigh [_____] + Suprailium [_____] = [_____] mm = [_____] %F (Fig. 3)

$D_b = 1.10994921 - (0.0009929 \times SSF$ [_____] mm$) + [0.0000023 \times (SSF$ [_____] mm$)^2]$

     $- (0.0001392 \times Age$ [_____] y$)$

= 1.0994921 − [_____] + (0.0000023 × [_____]) − [_____]

     (0.0009929 × SSF)   (SSF²)   (0.0001392 × Age)

= [_____] + [_____] − [_____] = [_____] g·ml⁻¹

%Fat = (495/ [_____] g·mL⁻¹) − 450 = [_____] − 450

     (D_b)   (495/D_b)

= [_____] %Fat   = [_____] %ile (from Fig. 5)

Form SF 3

Group Data for Skinfolds

MEN Initials (or ID#)	PERCENT FAT AAHPERD	J-P	OLDER
1.			
2.			
3.			
4.			
5.			
6.			
7.			
8.			
9.			
10.			
11.			
12.			
13.			
14.			
15.			
16.			
17.			
18.			
M			
Range			

WOMEN Initials (or ID#)	PERCENT FAT AAHPERD	J-P	OLDER
1.			
2.			
3.			
4.			
5.			
6.			
7.			
8.			
9.			
10.			
11.			
12.			
13.			
14.			
15.			
16.			
17.			
18.			
M			
Range			

Chapter 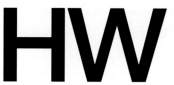 Hydrostatic Weighing

Hydrostatic weighing is sometimes referred to as underwater weighing because the subject's weight is measured while being submerged in water. It also may be referred to as hydrodensitometry because its unit of measure is body density $g \cdot ml^{-1}$. Dual energy x-ray (DXA) and hydrostatic weighing are probably the most valid, or the gold standard, of body composition determinations, meaning that they are the criteria by which other methods are compared. Despite hydrostatic weighing's prominent position among tests of body composition, it can qualify as a simple field test under certain conditions. For example, many hydrostatic weighings can be performed in any body of water such as jacuzzis, swimming pools, or lakes. By indirectly predicting residual volume, rather than measuring it, the hydrostatic technique is greatly simplified. However, when residual volume is measured directly and the underwater weight is measured under controlled conditions, it truly is a laboratory test, not a field test.

Physical and Anatomical Rationales

The rationales for hydrostatic weighing are based on the interaction between physical and anatomical factors. For example, the buoyancy of the human body during hydrostatic weighing is affected by its anatomical compartments, some being more buoyant or less dense than others.

Fat can be disadvantageous, both mechanically and aesthetically, because its density, that is, weight (mass) for any given volume is lower than lean tissue. Thus, 1 g of fat occupies more space than 1 g of protein (Fig. 1). This means that different circumference gains (e.g., thigh) would occur if identical weight gains were made, but one from fat storage and the other from protein growth (e.g., muscle hypertrophy). Thus, if two people of identical height and weight were of different body compositions, the leaner individual would occupy less space than the fatter individual.

Physical Rationale

Specifically, hydrostatic weighing is a method to determine the density of the body. Once the density of the body is known, special equations can be used to convert it to percent body fat. The density (D) of matter is a function of its mass (M) per unit volume (V), and may be calculated from Equation 1:

$$D = M/V \text{ or } M \cdot V^{-1} \qquad \text{Eq. 1}$$

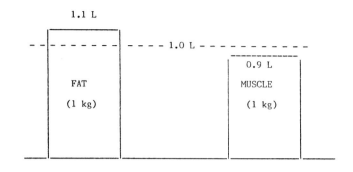

Figure 1 Density of 1 kg of fat and muscle reflecting the volume of each.

Thus, the density ($g \cdot ml^{-1}$) of the body can be determined by knowing the mass (or weight in grams) and volume (milliliters) of the body.[7] The mass of the body is referred to as body mass-in-air and often abbreviated as BM_a. The body volume is determined on the basis of Archimedes's principle, which relates the loss of mass ($BM_a - BM_w$) of an immersed body (BM_w) to the volume of that body. Thus, the principle of deriving body density (D_b) from hydrostatic weighing is conceptualized by Equation 2:

$$\text{Body Density } (D_b) = \frac{BM_a}{BM_a - BM_w} \qquad \text{Eq. 2}$$

In essence, Archimedes's principle states that an immersed body loses mass equivalent to the mass of the displaced fluid, or, as Archimedes stated, "a body immersed in water is buoyed up with a force equal to the weight of the water displaced."[8,13] The mass of the displaced fluid can be converted to a volume measure. An example of this is the entrance of a person into a jacuzzi filled completely to the top. If all of the water that spills over the brim is collected while the subject is completely submerged, then the mass of that collected water would be equal to the mass lost by that person at submersion. Thus, either the mass of the displaced water (volumetric method) or the mass of the submerged body (hydrostatic method) can be inserted into the proper equations to calculate body density. Usually it is easier to measure the mass of the submerged body.[39]

Anatomical Rationale

In general, the estimation of percent body fat is based upon the compartmentalization of total body mass (TBM) into fat

Accuracy of Hydrostatic Weighing

Although hydrostatic weighing has been considered a gold standard of body composition methods, it has not gone without criticism.

Validity

Its validity has been questioned mainly because of the limitations of the cadaver studies that have provided the typical tissue densities. For example, a classic equation for predicting body fat from body density is based upon a sample of only six cadavers.[15] In a study of twelve White cadavers, investigators revealed a much larger variability in muscle and body density than originally supposed.[38] The 1.100 g·ml^{-1} density value for lean tissue used in the equation to predict body fat now is recognized as a varying value within White adults and especially so in various population subgroups. For example, the densities of children (1.085), Blacks (1.113), and the elderly, especially the lower values in postmenopausal women,[25] differ significantly. The greater skeletal densities of Black males[3,59] contribute to their greater lean tissue density. Children have lower densities than adults due to their greater water concentration and lower bone mineral levels in their lean tissue component.[17] Older adults also have a less dense skeleton than younger adults. Thus, unless specific population equations[51,52] are used, the fat percentage in Blacks will be underestimated, and will be overestimated in young and elderly when using such popular equations as the Brozek and the Siri equations.

The variability of the density value is a major problem with hydrostatic weighing; consequently, this problem transfers to all of the other anthropometric methods, such as girths and skinfolds, that predict the hydrostatically determined body density. The problem is not with the density of fat but with that of the highly variable density of the fat-free mass.[45] The fallibility of densitometry was apparent in a study of 29 professional football players, 9 of whom were found to have 0% fat or less.[2] The standard error of the estimate by hydrostatic weighing is about 2.5% body fat,[45] with most of this error attributed to biological variability, not measurement error.[53,54] Ideally, to reduce inherent errors in the two-compartment models or equations (Brozek and Siri), laboratory procedures should measure not only body density, but also body water density and bone mineral density. However, equations using the combination of three or four components are few.[28]

Errors in body density up to 10% may result from estimating residual volume.[32] An average error of 0.7% body fat units occurs for each error of 100 ml in lung volume; the error may accumulate to 3.6% body fat units.[61] Indirectly measuring residual volume by using the standard 24% and 28% vital capacity values for men and women, respectively, may overestimate the residual volume of persons with large vital capacities. Hence, the accuracy of densitometry is greatly improved by directly measuring the residual lung volume (RV) rather than by predicting it from regression equations or from a certain percentage of the vital capacity.[43] The results of various investigators concerning the measurement of residual volume with the subject in air versus in water are conflicting. It appears that it makes little practical difference as long as the subsequent RV method is performed in the same medium (air or water) as the TLC, FRC, or VC,[47] and in the same body position, because RV either decreases or stays the same in water.[11]

Reliability

The reliability of body densitometry is high ($r = .95$).[18] This obviously can vary with the experience of the investigators, the accuracy of the equipment, and the experience and control of the subject. Correlative statistics, however, are not always the best reflector of the repeatability of a test. Statistics may produce high correlations on a heterogeneous group (e.g., widely varied in fat content). Thus, both the correlation values and the standard error values should be used to interpret the accuracy of a test.

---

mass (FM) and fat-free mass (FFM) or lean body mass (LBM). The fat mass is stored mainly in fat cells (adipocytes). However, not even this fat is all fat; it is about 62% pure fat, 31% water, and 7% protein.[53] The fat-free mass is composed of its two largest components—skeletal (20% of FFM)[4] and muscle (about 45% of FFM for a male)—and skin, blood, brain, and organs. The primary constituents of FFM are water, mineral, protein, and glycogen.[6] Although the terms FFM and LBM are often used interchangeably, the LBM is a slightly larger mass because it includes essential fat found in internal organs, bone marrow, and the central nervous system.[19,40,56] For example, essential fat can be found in cell walls and protoplasm of all tissues.[53] The concept of a two-part (FFM and FM) body compartmentalization is presented in Equation 3:

$$TBM = FFM + FM \qquad Eq. 3$$

Thus, fat mass (FM) may be expressed in percentage form as Equation 4:

$$\%Fat = (FM/TBM) \times 100 \qquad Eq. 4$$

Interaction of Compartmentalization and Density

Because fat is less dense than lean body mass, fat weighs less than fat-free tissue when both are placed in water. Thus, greater differences between the person's mass on land (in air) versus the mass in water mean lower densities and, consequently, higher fat percentages.

When the body density is known, that number is inserted into another equation that relates it to the density of lean and fat tissue. Figure 1 schematically depicts the fact that the volume of a less dense tissue, such as fat, occupies more space (volume) than that of a more dense tissue, such as muscle, at any given mass.[12] This concept can be stated another way: the mass of a less dense tissue is less than a more dense tissue for any given volume. Bone is relatively dense and sinkable, having a density of 1.28 g·ml^{-1}[4] compared to 1.100 for lean tissue, ~1.000 for water, and 0.9001 for fat tissue. Fat floats because its density is less than water's density.

Table 1 Relationship Between Water Temperature (Tw) and Water Density (Dw)

	Tw		Dw			Tw		Dw
	°C	°F	g·ml⁻¹			°C	°F	g·ml⁻¹
	0	32	0.999			32	89.5	0.9950
	4	39	1.000	Comfort		33	91	0.9947
	22	72	0.9978			34	93	0.9944
	25	77	0.9971			35	95	0.9941
	26	79	0.9968	Range		36	97	0.9937
	27	81	0.9965			37	98.6	0.9934
	28	82	0.9963			38	100	0.9930
	29	84	0.9960			39	102	0.9926
	30	86	0.9957			40	104	0.9922
	31	88	0.9954					

Source: Data from J. Brozek and A. Keys. Derived from the B-K equation, 1963.

Method

There are at least two methods to determine body density from the submersion of a human in water. One of these methods, the volumetric method, uses a narrow, cylindrical chamber (a volumeter) that facilitates the measurement of the displaced water from the submerged human. The conversion of this volume change to a density measure was first proposed in 1942.[8] The hydrostatic weighing method also measures body density and is the technique that is the focus of this manual.

Equipment

Scales

The traditional scale to weigh a person underwater resembles a supermarket's produce scale (e.g., Chatillon autopsy model) and usually has a maximum range of 9 to 15 kg (Fig. 2). In the 9 kg autopsy scale, there are 1, 2, and 3 kg (1000, 2000, and 3000 g) markers on the main face of the dial; another gauge is on the extension bar from the bottom of the scale, which represents the number of cycles made by the main dial's pointer. For example, if the large-faced dial is at 1500 g (1.5 kg), and the protruding bar is between the 2 and 3, then the actual underwater weight is 7.5 kg or 7500 g [(2 cycles × 3000 g) + 1500].

More sophisticated scales are based upon the strain-gauge, load-cell, or force-transducer principle and can be interfaced with a recorder and/or a computer.[41,48] A regular platform scale may be used to measure the subject's mass in air (BM_a).

Water Tanks

Water tanks vary in style and weight (e.g., redwood, cedar, plexiglass, stainless steel, fiberglass, tile, etc.), but are usually similar in size—just large enough to allow the subject to sit (usually) totally submerged in the water without touching the bottom or sides of the tank. The water tanks include a water filter and heater. The temperature of the water can be monitored with a water thermometer, such as

a basic pool thermometer. The water density may be monitored with a hydrometer or be derived from an appropriate table for water temperature versus density (Table 1).

Tare Weight

The equipment that supports the subject, or attaches to the subject, is called the tare weight equipment. It consists of the supporting device, linkage, and weight belt. The suspension support ("chair") or harness also varies in style and weight (webbing, nylon rope, PVC piping, etc.). Support linkage (chains, rope) is needed to attach the chair to the scale's hook. A weight-belt (e.g., a scuba-type belt) is worn by some subjects to aid in submergence and to minimize the oscillations on the scale's dial. Tare weight will usually vary between 3–6 kg with overfat persons requiring the higher weights.[46]

Lung Volume Equipment

Residual volume (RV) may be measured by nitrogen washout, helium dilution rebreathing, or by the simplified method, requiring only oxygen and carbon dioxide analyzers, not nitrogen or helium ones.[63] RV can be estimated by measuring vital capacity with various spirometers or pneumotachs, and then using either equation 5, 6, 7, or 8.

Subject Preparation

The subject should bring a towel and skimpy bathing suit (preferably nylon; two-piece for females) to the laboratory if these are not provided. Some subjects might bring their own lightweight noseclip, or use one provided by the lab, to be worn in order to prevent water from entering the nose during submersion. Despite jewelry's negligible weight, it should not be worn because of its high density (for example, gold has a density of 19.3 g·ml⁻¹, that is about 18 times heavier than an equivalent volume of muscle!). The subject should shower just prior to the test so that body oils or lotions are removed. The subject should be normally hydrated but should not be tested within 3 hours of eating (postprandial) or more than 12 hours after eating. The subject should urinate and defecate before arriving at the laboratory.

Many of the subject preparations attempt to avoid excess air trapped in the body. Trapped air results in a lower underwater weight, which converts to a higher percent fat. Persons with gastrointestinal (GI) disturbances should be rescheduled.

Anything that is apt to cause dehydration should be avoided, such as exercise under hot/humid conditions or sauna bathing. Due to higher estimates of percent fat from water retention, it may not be advisable to test females during the bloated period of the menstrual cycle[16] or within seven days on either side of the menstrual cycle.[30] Some investigators think that the fluid retention during normal menstruation may not be enough to affect the body density or percent fat.[20] However, a large hydration change equivalent to about 1–2 kg of body weight may increase the percent body fat estimation by hydrostatic weighing.[26]

Technician Preparations

The water in the tank should be clean, chlorinated, and at the proper temperature. For the comfort of the subjects, water temperatures should be above 33 °C, especially for lean persons, but probably no higher than 36 °C (91–97 °F). The technician should note the temperature of the water and consult Table 1 in order to find the water density for that temperature. The ability to float (buoyancy) improves with greater tank-water densities. Water densities increase with increased mineralization (hardness) or decreased temperatures, except near and at freezing when water turns into ice at 0 °C and then has the ability to float on water. Because warm water is lighter (less dense) than cold water, it is found above cold water. The standard density (1.000 g·ml^{-1}) is based on the heaviest density of pure water—that found at 4 °C.[21] In summary, the ability to float will be easier in harder and cooler waters, such as that typical of swimming pools between 25 and 27 °C (77–80 °F), than those typically found in laboratory underwater weighing tanks.

The technician should weigh the tare equipment at the water level likely to be encountered in the actual underwater weighing trials. If an electronic output from a load cell is used, it is likely that the weight (mass) monitor can be zeroed at the tare weight. In the latter case, there will be no need to subtract the tare weight from the subject's underwater weight in Equation 9. The position of the subject in the support device, whether it be sitting, semi-prone, or kneeling, should not affect the results of hydrostatic weighing.[29]

Procedures

Besides comforting and positioning the subject, three other concerns in the hydrostatic weighing procedures are to account for essential air, to eliminate excess air, and to read the underwater weight accurately.

Nonessential and Essential Air

In addition to fat, only two other parts of the body float: (1) the essential air compartments in the lungs and the gas-

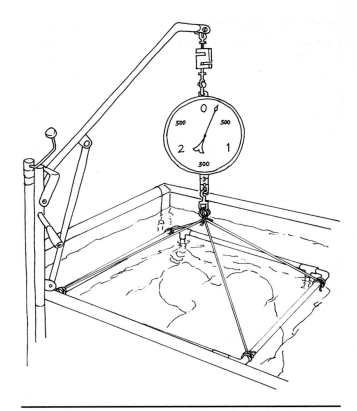

Figure 2 A subject being weighed under water in order to determine body density.

trointestinal (GI) tract, and (2) the nonessential air trapped in hair.

Nonessential Air. The first thing the subject should do upon entering the water is to dunk under the water, and then press the hands against the suit and body hairs in order to push the pockets of nonessential air from these sources. Nylon bathing suits trap air to a lesser extent than most conventional suits.

Essential GI Air. The GI air is a constant value of 100 ml assumed for all persons. Equation 10 accounts for this assumed constant value, but gas-producing foods or GI disturbances can increase this value to several hundred milliliters.[53]

Essential Lung Air. The lung volume, which is inserted into Equation 10, can be any known volume, such as total lung capacity (TLC), functional residual capacity (FRC), or residual volume (RV). The subject does not have to expel air during submersion, if the TLC, FRC, or partial expiration methods are used. These methods are more comfortable than the RV method, but less common.[42] The FRC,[57] TLC,[5,22,58,60] and partial expiration[34] methods appear to be as accurate as the RV method. The TLC or partial exhalation methods may be especially convenient for testing the elderly.[35,55]

The **RV method** of underwater weighing calls for the subject to rid the body of all lung air except the residual air by exhaling maximally. Usually the subject is in the seated position and forces the head towards the knees during the effort to expel the air. The technician can observe the formed bubbles of air as they escape from the subject's mouth to the top of the water. As long as there are noticeable bubbles, the subject still is not down to residual volume. The amount of time that subjects can remain under water while exhaling to residual volume is quite variable. Typically, it may be 5–10 s.[58]

Although a true research laboratory test of hydrostatic weighing would include the direct measurement of RV, it is possible to modify the hydrostatic test so that the RV is predicted by equations from either the vital capacity for men (Eq. 5) or women (Eq. 7)[62] or the age and height for men (Eq. 6)[10] or women (Eq. 8).[27] Sometimes the vital capacity is measured with the subject submerged to the neck.[55]

Men:

$$RV\ (L) = 24\%\ (or\ 0.24) \times VC_{BTPS} \qquad Eq.\ 5$$

$$RV\ (L) = (0.019 \times Ht) + (0.0115 \times Age) - 2.24 \quad Eq.\ 6$$

where: Ht = closest 0.5 cm; Age = closest y

For example, a 55-y-old man, who is 175 cm tall, has an estimated residual volume of 1.717 L based on Equation 6:

$$RV\ (L) = (0.019 \times 175\ cm) + (0.0115 \times 55\ y) - 2.24$$
$$= 3.325 + 0.632 - 2.24$$
$$= 1.717\ L$$

Women:

$$RV = 28\%\ (or\ 0.28) \times VC_{BTPS} \qquad Eq.\ 7$$

$$RV = (0.032 \times Ht) + (0.009 \times Age) - 3.90 \qquad Eq.\ 8$$

where: Ht = closest 0.5 cm; Age = closest y

Reading the Scale for Underwater Weight

The technician does not have much time to read the oscillating needle or digital display of the autopsy scale or force transducer, respectively. The time may be dependent upon the breath-holding ability of the subject and the degree of oscillation of the scale's indicating pointers or of the display. Force transducers reduce fluctuations compared to spring autopsy scales, but do not eliminate them.[48] The oscillations may be dependent upon the size of the tank, larger tanks requiring greater time. The oscillations should be small enough to be read to the nearest 20 g[31] or 25 g. However, it is not unusual to be able to read it only to the nearest 50 g. The technician reads the midpoint of the oscillations. The oscillations can be dampened if the technician loosely grasps the suspension hook of the autopsy scale with the fingers while the subject submerges.[a] Before reading the scale, the technician should check to be sure that all

---

[a]G. Rich, personal communication, May 1988

parts of the subject's body are submerged and that no air bubbles are visible. When the technician is satisfied with the reading, a prearranged signal (e.g., knocking on the tank) may be given to let the subject know it is time to surface. However, all subjects should feel free to ascend according to their own comfort.

The number of trials may vary according to the experience of the subjects. Usually, submerged subjects will reach their consistently highest expiratory capacities (hence heaviest weights), within 5 to 12 trials. Either the average of the last two or three trials or the average of the two heaviest weighings are chosen for insertion into the body density equation. Ideally, none of the readings used to calculate the average should differ by more than 100 g.[9,50]

Summary of Procedures

The following procedures are consistent with the RV method of hydrostatic weighing.

1. The technician measures and records the basic data and water-tank temperature onto Form HW 1.
2. The technician obtains one of the following lung volumes of choice:
   a. RV—directly measured or predicted from equations 5, 6, 7, or 8
   b. TLV (TLC)
   c. FRC
   d. Any partial volume
3. Being of normal hydration and after showering, the subject enters the water tank wearing, ideally, a nylon swimsuit and optional nose clip.
4. The technician records the tare weight and notes the depth of the chair at expected chin level of the subject.
5. The subject briefly submerges and then presses the air out of hair and swimsuit.
6. The subject sits in the chair or platform and, possibly, straps on a weighted belt to avoid floating when submerged.
7. Instructions for exhalation are given to the subject, and a signal is clarified by which to alert the subject that the technician is satisfied with the scale reading; the subject may ascend if becoming uncomfortable.
8. The subject begins to exhale while lowering head and shoulders under the water.
9. The technician may dampen the scale while observing the bubbles generated by the subject and the oscillations of the scale.
10. Usually near the 10th second, the technician gives the ascent signal and records the underwater weight to the nearest 20 to 50 g.
11. The procedure is repeated 5 to 12 times, depending on the consistency of the values.
12. The average of either the last two or three trials or of the two heaviest weighings are used in the body density equation.

Many modifications of the hydrostatic method have focused on ways to make the subject more comfortable in the water without losing any of the accuracy from the traditional technique. The FRC and TLC methods are two examples. Another example is one that permits the subject's head to remain above the water during the procedure.[24] Another modification eliminates the weight scale by having the subject grasp a 5.5 L plastic bottle to achieve neutral buoyancy in the measurement of body volume.[23] In general, it appears that modifications of the gold standard technique will continue to occur. Until valid electronic see-through techniques become practical and affordable to the exercise physiologist, the hydrostatic technique will continue to be a popular test.

Calculations

The density (D) of matter was shown to be a function of mass (M) per unit volume (V) in Equation 1 ($D = M/V$). This equation was the basis of Equation 2, which specifically related to hydrostatic weighing. However, the actual calculation of body density (D_b) from hydrostatic weighing data is slightly more complicated than Equation 2. The denominator—volume (V)—is found by using Equation 9.[64]

$$V = \left[\frac{(BM_a - BM_w)}{D_w} \right] - RV \qquad \text{Eq. 9}$$

where: BM_a = body mass (g) in air
BM_w = body wt in water (minus the tare wt if not zeroed electronically); net weight in water
D_w = density of water at given water temperature
RV = residual volume; other volumes could replace RV in Equation 9.

When Equations 2 and 9 are combined and modified from their original form[15] by accounting for the assumed 100 ml of air in the gastrointestinal (V_{GI}) tract, the complete equation (10) for body density is formed from the original density equation ($D = M/V$).

$$D_b = \frac{BM_a}{\left[\frac{BM_a - BM_w}{D_w} \right] - (RV + V_{GI})} \qquad \text{Eq. 10}$$

Because grams and milliliters are interconvertible, it does not matter which of these units is used in Equation 10; the resulting ratio is the same.

The body fat percentage is determined from body density based upon the two-compartment (FW and FFW) models of either the Siri[54] equation (Eq. 11) or the Brozek[14] equation (Eq. 12), which were developed from the chemical analysis of cadavers. Table 2 presents the body densities and equivalent body fat percentages based on the Brozek equation. The Brozek equation is preferred for elderly subjects.[55] Lohman and his colleagues feel that Equation 13 is preferable for young adult women.[37] Because indirect or non-vivo measurements have shown that Blacks have denser bones and muscles than Whites, the Schutte equation (Eq. 14) is recommended.[51]

$$\text{Siri } \%\text{Fat} = (495/D_b) - 450 \qquad \text{Eq. 11}$$

$$\text{Brozek (Older) } \%\text{Fat} = (457/D_b) - 414 \qquad \text{Eq. 12}$$

$$\text{Lohman (Young women) } \%\text{Fat} = (509/D_b) - 465 \qquad \text{Eq. 13}$$

$$\text{Schutte (Blacks) } \%\text{Fat} = (437.4/D_b) - 392.8 \qquad \text{Eq. 14}$$

Example of Calculating Body Density

A review of the respiratory volumes, such as vital capacity (VC), functional residual capacity (FRC), and residual volume (RV) is helpful prior to laboratory hydrodensitometry.[1]

Given the following conditions:

Male; Age = 27 y; BM_a = 83.62 kg or 83,620 g
VC_{BTPS} = 6.40 L or 6400 ml; the ATPS value can be multiplied by 1.063 to approximate the BTPS value.
Predicted RV = 1.536 L or 1536 ml (from Eq. 5)
Water Temperature (T_w) = 32 °C
Water Density (D_w) = 0.9950 (Table 1)
Underwater wt = 6.870 kg or 6870 g
Tare wt = 2500 g
Net BM_w = 6870 g − 2500 g = 4370 g

The calculation is performed as follows by using Equation 10:

$$D_b = \frac{83,620 \text{ g}}{\left[\frac{83,620 \text{ g} - 4370 \text{ g}}{0.9950} \right] - (1536 + 100 \text{ ml})}$$

$$= \frac{83,620}{\left(\frac{79,250}{0.9950} \right) - 1636}$$

$$= \frac{83,620}{79,648 - 1636}$$

$$= \frac{83,620}{78,012}$$

$$= 1.0719 \text{ g} \cdot \text{ml}^{-1}$$

The percentage of fat from the known body density of the man in our example can be found by using the Brozek equation (Eq. 12), Table 2, or the Siri equation (Eq. 11). The Brozek table gives a percent fat of 12.1% for a body density of 1.0720 (rounded). If we use the Siri equation (Eq. 11), which is not expected to differ by more than 1% body fat units from the Brozek-derived %Fat,[40] the percent fat is 11.7% based on the following calculation:

Given: D_b = 1.0720
then: %Fat = (495/D_b) − 450
= (495/1.0720) − 450
= 461.7 − 450
= 11.7%

Table 2 Body Densities (D_b) and Body Fat Percentages (%F) Based on the Brozek Equation

D_b (g·ml^{-1})	%F	D_b	%F	D_b	%F	D_b	%F
1.020	33.8	1.038	26.0	1.056	18.5	1.074	11.3
1.021	33.4	1.039	25.6	1.057	18.1	1.075	10.9
1.022	32.9	1.040	25.2	1.058	17.7	1.076	10.5
1.023	32.5	1.041	24.8	1.059	17.3	1.077	10.1
1.024	32.0	1.042	24.3	1.060	16.9	1.078	9.7
1.025	31.6	1.043	23.9	1.061	16.5	1.079	9.3
1.026	31.2	1.044	23.5	1.062	16.1	1.080	8.9
1.027	30.7	1.045	23.1	1.063	15.7	1.081	8.5
1.028	30.3	1.046	22.7	1.064	15.3	1.082	8.1
1.029	29.9	1.047	22.2	1.065	14.9	1.083	7.7
1.030	29.5	1.048	21.8	1.066	14.5	1.084	7.3
1.031	29.0	1.049	21.4	1.067	14.1	1.085	6.9
1.032	28.6	1.050	21.0	1.068	13.7	1.086	6.5
1.033	28.2	1.051	20.6	1.069	13.3	1.087	6.1
1.034	27.8	1.052	20.2	1.070	12.9	1.088	5.7
1.035	27.3	1.053	19.8	1.071	12.5	1.089	5.3
1.036	26.9	1.054	19.4	1.072	12.1	1.090	5.0
1.037	26.5	1.055	19.0	1.073	11.7		

Source: Data from Brozek & Keys.[15] Derived from Brozek Equation.

If the subjects were young adult women, then the Lohman equation (Eq. 13) is preferred. If the subjects were Black, then the Schutte equation (Eq. 14) is used.

Results and Discussion

Because the prediction of percent fat from body density values makes assumptions that probably are not totally valid, it may be advisable to rely on the body density values themselves for interpretive purposes.[40] Density values may range from a low of about 0.93 g·ml^{-1} in a very obese person to 1.10 g·ml^{-1} in a very lean man.[40] Most persons, however, will range from about 1.020 (~34% fat) to about 1.077 (~10% fat).

One authority feels that fat percentages between 10–22% for men and 20–32% for women are compatible with health.[36] Persons with percent body fat values at and above the 85th percentile (26% fat for men; 31.5% fat for women) may be considered obese.[44] Persons not satisfied with their body fat percentage will be more successful in altering it by combining diet and exercise rather than by modifying diet alone. It is not unusual for 35%–45% of the total weight loss to be lean body tissue when dieting and not exercising.[49] Many clinicians and researchers suggest a minimal fat percentage for men and women of 3–7% and 10–20%, respectively.[36] Persons known to have large muscle masses, such as body builders, power lifters, and Olympic lifters, have body fat percentages typically between 9–11%.[33]

References

1. Adams, G. M. (1994). *Exercise physiology laboratory manual.* Dubuque, IA: Brown & Benchmark.

2. Adams, J., Mottola, M., Bagnall, K. M., & McFadden, K. D. (1982). Total body fat content in a group of professional football players. *Canadian Journal of Applied Sport Science, 7,* 36–40.

3. Baker, P. T. & Angel, J. L. (1965). Old age changes in body density: Sex and race factors in the United States. *Human Biology, 37,* 104–119.

4. Bakker, H. K., & Struikenkamp, R. S. (1977). Biological variability and lean body mass estimates. *Human Biology, 49,* 187–202.

5. Ballard, T. (1984). *Hydrostatic weighing at total lung capacity versus residual volume.* Unpublished master's thesis, California State University, Fullerton.

6. Baumgartner, R. N., Heymsfield, S. B., Lichtman, S., Wang, J., & Pierson, R. N. (1991). Body composition in elderly people: Effect of criterion estimates on predictive equations. *American Journal of Clinical Nutrition, 53,* 1343–1353.

7. Behnke, A. R., Feen, B. G., & Welham, A. C. (1942). The specific gravity of healthy men: Body weight divided by volume as an index of obesity. *JAMA, 118,* 495–498.

8. Behnke, A. R., & Wilmore, J. H. (1974). *Evaluation and regulation of body build and composition.* Englewood Cliffs, NJ: Prentice-Hall.

9. Bonge, D., & Donnelly, J. E. (1989). Trials to criteria for hydrostatic weighing at residual volume. *Research Quarterly for Exercise and Sport, 60,* 176–179.

10. Boren, H. G., Kory, R. C., & Syner, J. C. (1966). The Veteran's Administration-Army cooperative study of pulmonary function. *American Journal of Medicine, 41,* 96–114.

11. Bosch, P. R., & Wells, C. L. (1991). Effect of immersion on residual volume of able-bodied and

spinal cord injured males. *Medicine and Science in Sports and Exercise, 23,* 384–388.

12. Brobek, J. R. (1968). Energy balance and food intake. In V. B. Mountcastle (Ed.), *Medical physiology* (pp. 498–519). St. Louis: C. V. Mosby.

13. Brooks, G. A., Fahey, T. D, & White, T. P. (1996). *Exercise physiology: Human bioenergetics and its application.* Mountain View, CA: Mayfield.

14. Brozek, J., Grande, F., Anderson, J., & Keys, A. (1963). Densitometric analysis of body composition: Revision of some quantitative assumptions. *Annals of New York Academy of Science, 110,* 113–140.

15. Brozek, J., & Keys, A. (1951). The evaluation of leanness-fatness in man: Norms and intercorrelations. *British Journal of Nutrition, 5,* 194–205.

16. Bunt, J. C., Lohman, T. G., & Boileau, R. A. (1989). Impact of total body water fluctuations on estimation of body fat from body density. *Medicine and Science in Sports and Exercise, 21,* 96–100.

17. Bunt, J. C., Lohman, T. G., Slaughter, M. H., Boileau, R. A., Lussier, L., & Van Loan, M. (1983). Bone mineral content as a source of variation in body density in children and youth [Abstract]. *Medicine and Science in Sports and Exercise, 15,* 172.

18. Buskirk, E., & Taylor, H. L. (1957). Maximal oxygen intake and its relation to body composition with special reference to chronic physical activity and obesity. *Journal of Applied Physiology, 11,* 72–78.

19. Buskirk, E. R., & Mendez, J. (1984). Sports science and body composition analysis: Emphasis on cell and muscle mass. *Medicine and Science in Sports and Exercise, 16,* 584–593.

20. Byrd, P. J., & Thomas, T. R. (1983). Hydrostatic weighing during different stages of the menstrual cycle. *Research Quarterly for Exercise and Sport, 54,* 296–298.

21. Clarke, G. L. (1954). *Elements of ecology.* New York: John Wiley & Sons.

22. Coffman, J. L., Timson, B. F., Beneke, W. M., & Paulsen, B. K. (1983). Measurement of body composition by hydrostatic weighing at residual volume and total lung capacity [Abstract]. From *Medicine and Science in Sports and Exercise, 15,* 172–173.

23. Denahan, T., Hortobagyl, T., & Katch, F. I. (1988). Validation of a new method of hydrostatic weighing. *Medicine and Science in Sports and Exercise, 20,* (2 Suppl.), Abstract #44, S8.

24. Donnelly, J. E., Brown, T. E., Israel, R. G., Smith-Sintek, S., O'Brien, K. F., & Caslavka, B. (1988). Hydrostatic weighing without head submersion: Description of a method. *Medicine and Science in Sports and Exercise, 20,* 66–69.

25. Freund, B. J., Wilmore, J. H., Boyden, T. W., Stimi, W. A., & Harrington, R. J. (1984). Relationships of aerobic fitness and body composition measurements to

bone density in post-menopausal women. *International Journal of Sports Medicine, 5,* 159.

26. Girandola, R. N., Wiswell, R. A., & Romero, G. T. (1977). Body composition changes resulting from fluid ingestion and dehydration. *Research Quarterly for Exercise and Sport, 48,* 299–303.

27. Goldman, H. I. & Becklake, M. R. (1959). Respiratory function tests. *American Review of Tuberculosis and Pulmonary Disease, 79,* 457–467.

28. Houtkooper, L. B., & Going, S. B. (1994). Body composition: How should it be measured? Does it affect sport performance? *Sports Science Exchange, 7*(5), 1–9.

29. Hsieh, S., Kline, G., Porcari, J., & Katch, F. I. (1985). Measurement of residual volume sitting and lying in air and water (and during underwater weighing) and its effects on computed body density [Abstract]. *Medicine and Science in Sports and Exercise, 17*(2), S204.

30. Jackson, A. S., Pollock, M. L., & Ward, A. (1980). Generalized equations for predicting body density of women. *Medicine and Science in Sports and Exercise, 12,* 175–182.

31. Jackson, A. S., & Pollock, M. L. (1985, May). Practical assessment of body composition. *The Physician and Sportsmedicine,* pp. 76–80, 82–90.

32. Katch, F. I., & Katch, V. L. (1980). Measurement and prediction errors in body composition assessment and the search for the perfect equation. *Research Quarterly for Exercise and Sport, 51,* 249–260.

33. Katch, V. L., Katch, F. I., Moffatt, R., & Gittleson, M. (1980). Muscular development and lean body weight in body builders and weight lifters. *Medicine and Science in Sports and Exercise, 12,* 340–344.

34. Kohrt, W. M., Malley, M. T., Dalsky, G. P., & Holloszy, J. O. (1992). Body composition of healthy sedentary and trained young and older men and women. *Medicine and Science in Sports and Exercise, 24,* 832–837.

35. Latin, R. W., & Ruhling, R. O. (1983). Comparison of hydrostatic weighing at total lung capacity, measured residual volume, and predicted residual volume in older men [Abstract]. *Medicine and Science in Sports and Exercise, 15,* 72–73.

36. Lohman, T. G. (1982, December). Body composition methodology in sports medicine. *The Physician and Sportsmedicine,* pp. 46–48, 51–53, 56–58.

37. Lohman, T. G., Slaughter, M. H., Boileau, R. A., Bunt, J., & Lussier, L. (1984). Bone mineral measurements and their relation to body density in children, youth, and adults. *Human Biology, 56,* 667.

38. Martin, A. D., Drinkwater, D. T., Clarys, J. P., & Ross, W. D. (1981). Estimation of body fat: A new look at some old assumptions. *The Physician and Sportsmedicine, 9,* 21–22.

39. Mathews, D. K., & Fox, E. L. (1976). *The physiological basis of physical education and athletics.* Philadelphia: W. B. Saunders.

40. McArdle, W. D., Katch, F. I., & Katch, V. L. (1996). *Exercise physiology: Energy, nutrition, and human performance.* Baltimore: Williams & Wilkins.

41. McClenaghan, B. A., & Rocchis, L. (1986). Design and validation of an automated hydrostatic weighing system. *Medicine and Science in Sports and Exercise, 18,* 479–484.

42. McGarty, J. M., Butts, N. K., Hall, L. K., & Fletcher, R. A. (1983). Comparison of three hydrostatic weighing methods [Abstract]. *Medicine and Science in Sports and Exercise, 15,* 181.

43. Morrow, J. R., Jackson, A. S., Bradley, P. W., & Hartung, G. H. (1986). Accuracy of measured and predicted residual lung volume on body density measurement. *Medicine and Science in Sports and Exercise, 18,* 647–652.

44. Mullins, N. M., & Sinning, W. E. (1996). Diagnostic utility of the body mass index as a measure of obesity in athletes and non-athletes. *Medicine and Science in Sports and Exercise, 28*(5), Abstract #1148, S193.

45. Nash, H. L. (1985, November). Body fat measurement: Weighing the pros and cons of electrical impedance. *The Physician and Sportsmedicine,* pp. 124–128.

46. Nieman, D. C. (1995). *Fitness and sports medicine: A health-related approach.* Palo Alto, CA: Bull Publishing.

47. Noble, B. J. (1986). *Physiology of exercise and sport.* St Louis: Times/Mirror College Publishers.

48. Organ, L. W., Eklund, A. D., & Ledbetter, J. D. (1994). An automated real time underwater weighing system. *Medicine and Science in Sports and Exercise, 26,* 383–391.

49. Oscai, L. B. (1973). The role of exercise in weight control. In J. H. Wilmore (Ed.), *Exercise and sport sciences reviews* (pp. 103–123). New York: Academic Press.

50. Quatrochi, J. A., Hicks, V. L., Heyward, V. H., Colville, B. C., Cook, K. L., Jenkins, K. A., & Wilson, W. L. (1992). Relationship of optical density and skinfold measurements: Effects of age and level of body fatness. *Research Quarterly for Exercise and Sport, 63,* 402–409.

51. Schutte, J. E. (1984). Density of lean body mass is greater in Blacks than Whites. *Journal of Applied Physiology, 56,* 1647.

52. Schutte, J. E., Longhurst, J. C., Gaffney, F. A., Bastian, B. C., & Blomqvist, C. G. (1981). Total plasma creatinine: An accurate measure of total striated muscle mass. *Journal of Applied Physiology, 51,* 762–766.

53. Siri, W. E. (1956). The gross composition of the body. *Adv. Biological Medical Physiology, 4,* 239–280.

54. Siri, W. E. (1961). *Body composition from fluid spaces and density: Analysis of methods in techniques for measuring body composition.* Washington, D.C.: National Academy of Science, National Research Council, 223–244.

55. Snead, D. B., Birge, S. J., & Kohrt, W. M. (1993). Age-related differences in body composition by hydrodensitometry and dual-energy X-ray absorptiometry. *Journal of Applied Physiology, 74,* 770–775.

56. Tanaka, K., Hijama, T., Watanabe, Y., Asano, K., Takedo, M., Hayakawa, Y., & Nakadomo, F. (1993). Assessment of exercise-induced alterations in body composition of patients with coronary heart disease. *European Journal of Applied Physiology, 66,* 321–327.

57. Thomas, T. R., & Etheridge, G. L. (1980). Hydrostatic weighing at residual volume and functional residual capacity. *Journal of Applied Physiology: Respiratory, Environmental and Exercise Physiology, 49,* 157–159.

58. Timson, B. F., & Coffman, J. L. (1984). Body composition by hydrostatic weighing at total lung capacity and residual volume. *Medicine and Science in Sports and Exercise, 16,* 411–414.

59. Trotter, M., Broman, G. E., & Peterson, R. R. (1959). Density of cervical vertebrae and comparison with densities of other bones. *American Journal of Physical Anthropology, 17,* 19–25.

60. Weltman, A., & Katch, V. (1981). Comparison of hydrostatic weighing at residual volume and total lung capacity. *Medicine and Science in Sports and Exercise, 13,* 210–213.

61. Williams, L., & Davis, J. A. (1987). Influence of functional residual capacity methodology on body fat determined by hydrostatic weighing [Abstract]. *International Journal of Sports Medicine, 8,* 243.

62. Wilmore, J. H. (1969). The use of actual, predicted, and constant residual volumes in the assessment of body composition by underwater weighing. *Medicine and Science in Sports and Exercise, 1,* 87–90.

63. Wilmore, J. H. (1980). A simplified method for determination of residual volume. *Journal of Applied Physiology, 27,* 96–100.

64. Wilmore, J. H., & Behnke, A. R. (1969). An anthropometric estimation of body density and lean body weight in young men. *Journal of Applied Physiology, 27,* 25–31.

Form *HW 1*

Individual Data for Hydrostatic Weighing

Basic Data

Name [   ] Date [   ] Time [   ] a.m. [   ] p.m. [   ]

Age [   ] y   Gender (M or F) [   ]   Ht [   ] in. = [   ] cm

Wt in air (BM_a) [   ] kg = [   ] g   Temperature (T_A) [   ] °C

Lung Volumes

VC (BTPS) [   ] L   In water: Yes [   ] No [   ] RV [   ] L   In water: Yes [   ] No [   ]

Estimated RV (L):

Men

1. $RV = 0.24 \times VC_{BTPS}$ [   ] L = [   ] L

2. or $RV = (0.019 \times Ht$ [   ] cm) $+ (0.0115 \times Age$ [   ] y) $- 2.24$

   $=$ [   ] $+$ [   ] $- 2.24 =$ [   ] L

Women

1. $RV = 0.28 \times VC_{BTPS}$ [   ] L = [   ] L

2. or $RV = (0.032 \times Ht$ [   ] cm) $+ (0.009 \times Age$ [   ] y) $- 3.90$

   $=$ [   ] $+$ [   ] $- 3.90 =$ [   ] L

Hydrostatic Weighing

Water T (T_w) [   ] °C D_w [   ]   Tare wt [   ] g

Body Wt in water (BM_w) to closest 25–50 g

Trial #1 [   ]   #2 [   ]   #3 [   ]   #4 [   ]   #5 [   ]   #6 [   ]

Trial #7 [   ]   #8 [   ]   #9 [   ]   #10 [   ]   #11 [   ]   #12 [   ]

[Circle two highest underwater weight (BM_w) values; average the two.]

Mean BM_w [   ] g $-$ Tare Wt [   ] g = Net BM_w [   ] g

Form *HW 2*

Hydrostatic Weighing Calculation Form

Body Density (Db) =

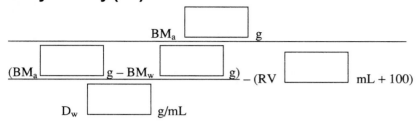

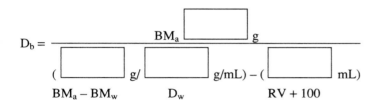

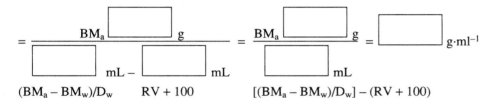

Percent Fat (%Fat):

(Siri equation: Men and Women)

%Fat = (495/D_b [____] $g \cdot mL^{-1}$) − 450 = [____] − 450 = [____] %Fat

(Lohman equation: Young Women)

%Fat = (509/D_b [____] $g \cdot mL^{-1}$) − 465 = [____] − 465 = [____] %Fat

(Schutte equation: Blacks)

%Fat = (437.4/D_b [____] $g \cdot ml^{-1}$) − 392.8 = [____] − 392.8 = [____] %Fat

(Brozek equation: Older Men and Women)

%Fat = (457/D_b) − 414 = [____] − 414 = [____] %Fat

Form HW 3

Group Data for Various Body Composition Methods

Men

Initials	Percent Fat				
	Girth		SF		Hydro
	1	2–3	AA[a]	JP	
1.					
2.					
3.					
4.					
5.					
6.					
7.					
8.					
9.					
10.					
11.					
12.					
13.					
14.					
15.					
16.					
17.					
18.					
19.					
20.					
Mean					

Women

Initials	Percent Fat				
	Girth		SF		Hydro
	1	2–3	AA[a]	JP	
1.					
2.					
3.					
4.					
5.					
6.					
7.					
8.					
9.					
10.					
11.					
12.					
13.					
14.					
15.					
16.					
17.					
18.					
19.					
20.					
Mean					

[a]AAHPERD

Appendix A

Cardiopulmonary Resuscitation (CPR)

Proper administration of CPR is essential for laboratory personnel who administer exercise stress tests. It appears that with proper screening, monitoring, and emergency procedures, the incidence of serious problems during exercise testing can be minimal. Successful treatment of a stricken victim often depends upon prompt treatment through basic life support (BLS) methods, followed shortly thereafter by advanced cardiac life support (ACLS) methods.

The following summary of basic life support represents a consensus of experts at the 1985 National Conference on Cardiopulmonary Resuscitation (CPR) and Emergency Cardiac Care (ECC).[8] The goal of BLS is to either (1) prevent circulatory or respiratory arrest or insufficiency or (2) externally support the victim via CPR techniques. The major objective is to promote the oxygenation of brain, heart, and other vital tissues. The key to success is prompt action. Success rates are best when CPR is initiated within 4 min of the time of arrest and when ACLS occurs within 8 min.[3]

Method

The acronym for remembering CPR techniques is ABC— Airway, Breathing, and Circulation. Each of these has an initial assessment phase to determine (1) unresponsiveness, (2) breathlessness, and (3) pulselessness. The assessment phase should not exceed several seconds. The one-rescuer method is outlined here in more detail than the two-rescuer method.

Airway

(1) Assessment—tap, gently shake, and shout, "Are you OK?"; (2) call for help; (3) position the victim supine on a firm surface; (4) open the airway by the head-tilt/chin-lift maneuver; (5) clear victim's mouth or throat if obstructed.

Breathing

(1) Assessment—look, feel, and listen for breath; (2) give two breaths, each lasting from 1 to 1.5 s, which are about 2 to 3 times greater (hence, 800–1200 ml) than a normal breath.

Circulation

(1) Assessment—feel carotid artery; (2) perform fifteen external chest compressions at a rate of 80–100 per min;

count one, two, etc. to fifteen; (3) open the airway (tilt) and administer two breaths as before; (4) repeat the fifteen chest compressions; (5) perform four complete cycles of fifteen compressions and two ventilations.

Reassessment

After the four cycles (15:2 ratio), reevaluate the victim. Check the carotid pulse (5 s); if it is absent resume the cycle, starting with two breaths. Check breathing (3–5 s). Do not interrupt CPR for more than 7 s.

Two-Rescuer Technique

Personnel should learn both the one-rescuer and the two-rescuer techniques. A compression rate of 80 to 100 per minute is used for both the one- and two-rescuer CPR method; however, the compression–ventilation ratio is 5:1 with a 1–1.5 s pause for ventilation in the two-rescuer technique.

Defibrillators

Only medical practitioners, or others specifically authorized by law, can legally use defibrillators.[1]

Discussion

Submaximal exercise tests are less risky than maximal tests—the maximal tests having percent death and myocardial infarction (MI) risks of $\leq 0.01\%$ and 0.04%, respectively, during or immediately after the test.[1] When exercise testing to the subjects' 85% predicted maximal heart rate, one group of investigators reported no deaths, nor cardiac arrests, nor ventricular fibrillation in more than five years involving more than 1000 tests.[9]

It appears that exercise testing is less risky in apparently healthy persons having preventive medicine exams than in symptomatic persons having diagnostic exams. In 1981, Dr. Ken Cooper said that their clinic had no deaths and only one resuscitation in more than 41,000 maximal Balke protocol tests in 20 years;[6] in that same preventive medicine clinic, as of 1989 there still had been no deaths in more than 70,000 maximal exercise tests.[4] When considering the non-eventful exercise tests administered at fitness clinics, Y's, corporations, safety and emergency facilities, and schools, it is clear that the risk of submaximal exercise testing is very low in the general population.

Only three fatalities in more than 100,000 exercise tests occurred on steps, cycle ergometers, and treadmills in apparently healthy subjects and heart disease patients.[5] Based upon a survey of over 500,000 exercise tests at over one thousand facilities, only 0.5 deaths occurred per 10,000 tests; about nine complications (total of MI, serious arrhythmias, and deaths) occurred per 10,000 tests.[10] No deaths were reported in 25,862 tests by Seattle-area physicians testing both symptomatic (63% with CHD) and asymptomatic persons in a nine-year period.[2]

The complication rates of tests supervised by certified clinical exercise physiologists are similar to physician-supervised rates; the non-physician-supervised tests having mortality, acute MI, and ventricular fibrillation rates of 0.0, 1.42, and 1.78, respectively, per 10,000 tests.[7] Low rates in a population that includes a high-risk sample is due to the constant monitoring of the exercising subject by trained personnel and to the proper application of emergency procedures.

References

1. American College of Sports Medicine (ACSM). (1995). *ACSM's guidelines for exercise testing and prescription.* Baltimore: Williams & Wilkins.
2. Bruce, R. A. (1981). Maximal exercise testing: Prognostic value for assessment of coronary heart disease risk. *Postgraduate Medicine, 70,* 161–168.
3. Eisenberg, M. S., Bergner, L., & Hallstrom, A. (1979). Cardiac resuscitation in the community. Importance of rapid provision and implications for program planning. *JAMA, 241,* 1905–1907.
4. Gibbons, L. W., Blair, S. N., Kohl, H. W., & Cooper, K. H. (1989). The safety of maximal exercise testing. *Circulation, 80,* 846–852.
5. Hornsten, T. R., & Bruce, R. A. (1968). Stress testing, safety precautions, and cardiovascular health. *Journal of Occupational Medicine, 10,* 640–648.
6. Jopke, T. (1981, March). Choosing an exercise testing protocol. *The Physician and Sportsmedicine,* pp. 141–146.
7. Knight, J. A., Laubach, C. A., Butcher, R. J., & Menapace, F. J. (1995). Supervision of clinical exercise testing by exercise physiologists. *American Journal of Cardiology, 75,* 390–391.
8. National Conference on Cardiopulmonary Resuscitation (CPR) and Emergency Cardiac Care (ECC). (1986). Standards and guidelines for cardiopulmonary resuscitation (CPR) and emergency cardiac care (ECC). *JAMA, 255,* 2905–2989.
9. Sheffield, L. T., Holt, J. H., & Reeves, T. J. (1965). Exercise graded by heart rate in electrocardiographic testing for angina pectoris. *Circulation 32,* 622–628.
10. Stuart, R. J., & Ellestad, M. H. 1980. National survey of exercise stress testing facilities. *Chest, 77*(1): 94–97.

Appendix B

Reporting Units and Symbols

In addition to those presented in Chapter UN, the following units and symbols are noted here along with some general comments.

1. The spelling of metric terms may vary with the country of the writer. For instance, an American may spell liter and meter as such, whereas a Briton may spell them as litre and metre, respectively.

2. The American Heart Association Task Force on Blood Pressure (1987) has not adopted the SI-approved kilopascals, thus retaining the mm Hg metric unit.[2] When referring to pressure inside the body, such as for blood pressure or dissolved gases, mm Hg units are acceptable. When referring to pressures outside the body, such as atmospheric pressures, torr is the preferred unit.

3. The symbol for the *micro* unit is not found on some computers; thus the symbol u is an acceptable replacement (e.g., uV = microvolt).

4. Time (t) symbols may be noted by the following:[3]

   s = seconds; h = hour; wk = week; mo = month;
   d = day; y = year

5. The following abbreviations are commonly used by scientists:

   $>$ = greater than; $<$ = less than;
   $\geq$ = equal to or greater than; $\leq$ = equal to or less than;
   $\sim$ = approximately

6. A number expressed by a negative exponent (e.g., $^{-1}$) is equal to the reciprocal of that number (e.g., 1/10) raised to the respective positive power.

   Examples:
   $10^{-1} = 1/10$; $10^{-2} = 1/100$;
   $ml \times kg^{-1} = ml \times 1/kg = ml/kg = ml \cdot kg^{-1}$
   $9.9 \times 10^{-9} = 0.0000000099$; decimal moved 9 places to left
   $1.2 \times 10^{6} = 1\ 200\ 000$; decimal moved 6 places to the right

7. Exponential Law of Half-life: This is defined as the time it takes for half of the substance to disintegrate, deplete, or decay.

8. A logarithm is related to exponential functions.

9. Avogadro's (1776 A.D.–1856 A.D.) number is the number of molecules in a mole of any substance: 6.02217×10^{23}. At standard temperature and pressure (STP) one mole of any gas occupies a volume of 22.414 L.

10. A kg·m is sometimes referred to as a kilopond meter (kp·m); theoretically, kp·m represents the force at normal acceleration of gravity that is dependent upon the global latitude (e.g., a person weighs more at the north pole than at the equator due to the greater pull of gravity at the pole); the difference between kg·m and kp·m has little practical significance for exercise laboratories.

11. International Unit (IU) is a measure of biological activity, not mass or volume. IU is often used for vitamins, but it is slowly disappearing in usage.

References

1. Astrand, I. (1988). *Work tests with the bicycle ergometer.* Varberg, Sweden: Monark Crescent AB.

2. Frohlich, E. D., Grim, C., Labarthe, D. R., Maxwell, M. H., Perloff, D., & Weidman, W. H. (1987). *Recommendations for human blood pressure determination by sphygmomanometers: Report of a special task force appointed by the steering committee, American Heart Association.* Dallas: National Center, American Heart Association.

3. Young, D. S. (1987). Implementation of SI units for clinical laboratory data. *Annals of Internal Medicine, 106,* 114–129.

Appendix C

Metric–American Conversions

Length Conversions

1 m = 39.370 in. = 3.281 ft = 1.0936 yd
1 cm = 0.3937 in.
1 mm = 0.03937 in.
1 km = 0.62137 mile

1 in. = 2.54 cm = 25.4 mm = 0.0254 m
1 ft = 0.3048 m
1 yd = 0.914 m = 91.44 cm
1 mile = 1609.35 m = 1.609 km

Mass (M) or Weight (Wt) Conversions

1 kg = 2.2046 lb
1 g = 0.0022 lb = 0.0352 oz

1 lb = 453.59 g = 0.454 kg
1 oz = 28.3495 g
1 grain = 65 mg

Force (F) Conversion

1 kg = 9.80665 N
1 N = 0.10197 kg = 0.2248 lb

Volume (V) Conversions

1 L = 1.0567 US qt (1 US qt and 1 US gal are
    > 1 Imperial qt and gal)
1 ml = 1 cm^3 = 0.03381 fluid oz = 0.061 cu in.

1 US qt = 0.9464 L
1 US gal = 3.785 L
1 cup liquid = 250 ml
1 tablespoon = 15 ml

Work (w) and Energy (E) Conversions

1 N·m = 1 J = 0.7375 ft-lb
1 kg·m = 9.80665 J = 7.2307 ft-lb
1 ft-lb = 0.1383 kg·m = 1.3560 N·m
1 kJ = 0.239 kcal
1 kcal = 4186 J = 4.186 kJ
1 kcal = 426.85 kg·m at 100% efficiency

1 J = 1 N·m = 0.10197 kg·m
1 L VO$_2$ ~ 21 kJ at R of 1.0

Velocity (v) Conversions

1 m·s^{-1} = 2.2371 miles per hour (mph)
1 m·min^{-1} = 0.03728 mph
1 km·h^{-1} = 0.6215 mph

1 mph = 26.822 m·min^{-1} = 1.6093 km·h^{-1}
    = 0.4470 m·s^{-1} = 1.4667 ft·s^{-1}

Radial Velocity Conversions

1 rad·s^{-1} = 57.3°·s^{-1}
rad = radian = 0.5 Π = radius of circle = 57.3°
1° = 0.01745 radian
Π = 3.1416 = ratio of the circumference of a circle to
    its diameter.

Power (P) Conversions

1 W = 1 J·s^{-1} = 60 J·min^{-1} = 0.060 kJ·min^{-1}
    = 6.12 kg·m min^{-1} = 0.1019 kg·m·s^{-1}
1 kW = 1000 W = 1.34 horsepower (hp)
1 kg·m min^{-1} = 0.1635 W = 0.000219 hp

1 hp = 745.7 W = 745.7 J·s^{-1} = 75 kg·m·s^{-1}
    = 4562 kg·m min^{-1} = 10.688 kcal·min^{-1}

Acceleration (a) Conversion

a of gravity = 9.81 m·s^{-2} = 32.2 ft·s^{-2}

Temperature (T) Conversions

each °C = 1 °K = 1.8 °F
each °F = 0.56 °C = 0.56 °K

Pressure Units, Symbols, and Conversions

1 pascal (Pa) = 1 N·m^{-2}
Barometric Pressure (P$_B$): 1 in. = 25.4 torr
29.92 in. Hg = 760 torr = 1 atmosphere (atm) = 14.7 lb/in.^{2}
1 mbar = 0.750 mm Hg = 0.750 torr

Appendix D

Sample Problems and Solutions

Most of the problems presented here may be solved in more than one way. These different approaches to the same problem may sometimes produce small differences in the answers. Also, differences may be produced due to rounding off of the various conversion factors. These differences are small enough to be of little practical significance in most exercise physiology laboratory classes.

Before starting any calculations, students are encouraged to "guesstimate" the answer. Guessing will prevent making obvious errors such as in the placing of the decimal point and also will force metric thinking and visualization.

1. How tall in centimeters and meters is a six-footer?

   $6 \text{ ft} \times 12 \text{ in.} = 72 \text{ in.}$
   $2.54 \text{ cm} = 1 \text{ in.}$
   Therefore: $2.54 \text{ cm} \times 72 \text{ in.} = 182.88 \text{ cm} = 182.9 \text{ cm}$
   $= 1.83 \text{ meters}$
   Optional solutions:
   (a) $1 \text{ ft} = 0.3048 \text{ m}; 0.3048 \text{ m} \times 6 = 1.83 \text{ m}$ (183 cm)
   (b) $72 \div 0.3937 = 182.9 \text{ cm}$

2. Which is longer—250 yd or 240 m?

   Answer: 240 m; optional solutions:
   (a) $1.09 \text{ yd} = 1 \text{ m}$; thus $250 \text{ yd} \div 1.09 = 229 \text{ m}$
   (b) $1.09 \times 240 = 261.6 \text{ yd}$

3. A ski length of 68.9 in. is how many centimeters?

   $1 \text{ in.} = 2.54 \text{ cm}$; thus, $68.9 \text{ in.} \times 2.54 = 175 \text{ cm}$
   Option: $1 \text{ cm} = 0.3937 \text{ in.}$; thus $68.9 \div 0.3937$
   $= 175 \text{ cm}$

4. $35 \text{ mph} = ? \text{ km·h}^{-1}$

   $1 \text{ mile} = 1.6 \text{ km}$
   Therefore: $1.6 \text{ km} \times 35 = 56 \text{ km·h}^{-1}$
   Option: $1 \text{ km} = 0.62 \text{ mile}$; thus, $35 \div 0.62$
   $= 56.5 \text{ km·h}^{-1}$

5. $160 \text{ lb} = ? \text{ kg}$

   $\text{lb} = 1 \text{ kg}$; therefore: $160 \div 2.2 = 72.7 \text{ kg}$
   Option: $1 \text{ lb} = 0.454 \text{ kg}$; thus $0.454 \times 160 = 72.6 \text{ kg}$

6. Most distance racing shoes weigh less than 10 oz. How many grams is this?

   $1 \text{ oz} = 28.3 \text{ g}$; thus, $28.3 \times 10 = 283 \text{ g}$
   Option: $1 \text{ g} = 0.0352 \text{ oz}$; thus, $10 \div 0.0352 = 284 \text{ g}$

7. $2.5 \text{ gallons} = ? \text{ L and ml}$

   $2.5 \text{ gal} = 10 \text{ qt}$ ($1 \text{ gal} = 4 \text{ qt}$)
   $1 \text{ qt} = 0.9464 \text{ L}$
   Therefore: $10 \text{ qt} \times 0.9464 \text{ L} = 9.464 \text{ L} = 9464 \text{ ml}$
   Option: $1 \text{ L} = 1.0567 \text{ qt}$; thus, $10 \div 1.0567 = 9.463 \text{ L}$
   $= 9463 \text{ ml}$

8. True or False: 12.5 quarts is > 13 liters

   $12.5 \text{ qt} \times 0.9464 \text{ L} = 11.83 \text{ L}$
   Thus, the answer is False because $11.8 \text{ L is} < 13 \text{ L}$
   Option: $1 \text{ liter} = 1.0567 \text{ qt}$; thus, $12.5 \div 1.0567$
   $= 11.8 \text{ L}$

9. $28 \text{ miles per gallon} = ? \text{ km per liter}$

   $1 \text{ mile} = 1.6 \text{ km}$; thus, $28 \times 1.6 \text{ km} = 45 \text{ km}$
   $1 \text{ qt} = 0.9464 \text{ L}$; thus, $4 \times 0.9464 \text{ L} = 3.78 \text{ L}$
   Therefore, $45 \text{ km per } 3.78 \text{ L} = 11.9 \text{ km per L}$
   Option: $1 \text{ km} = 0.62 \text{ mile}$; thus $28 \div 0.62 = 45.2 \text{ km}$
   $1 \text{ L} = 1.0567 \text{ qt}$; thus $4 \div 1.0567 = 3.78 \text{ L}$
   $45.2 \text{ km} \div 3.78 \text{ L} = 11.96 \text{ km per liter}$

10. A person loads 200 crates weighing 30 lb each into a truck bed that is 3 feet above the location of the crates. What is the total positive work in N·m and joules?

    $+w = F \times D; F = 30 \text{ lb} \div 2.2 = 13.6 \text{ kg} = 136 \text{ N}$
    $D \text{ in meters} = (200 \text{ lifts} \times 3 \text{ ft} \times 0.3048) = 183 \text{ m};$
    $+w = 183 \text{ m} \times 136 \text{ N} = 24\,888 \text{ N·m} = 24\,888 \text{ J or}$
    24.89 kJ

11. Suppose the above task takes 20 minutes. What is the rate of the work (power) in N·m·min^{-1} and watts?

    $P = w/t = 24\,888 \text{ N·m·min}^{-1} \div 20 \text{ min}$
    $= 1244 \text{ N·m·min}^{-1} = 20.7 \text{ N·m·s}^{-1} = 20.7 \text{ W}$

12. A person weighing 120 lb walks from an elevation of 900 ft to 3400 ft. How much positive work was accomplished in this ascent?

    $+w = F \times D; D = 3400 \text{ ft} - 900 \text{ ft} = 2500 \text{ ft}$
    $1 \text{ meter} = 3.28 \text{ ft}$; thus, $2500 \text{ ft} \div 3.28 = 762 \text{ m}$
    $120 \text{ lb} \div 2.2 = 54.5 \text{ kg} = 545 \text{ N}$
    $545 \text{ N} \times 762 \text{ m} = 415\,290 \text{ N·m or } 415\,290 \text{ J}$
    or 415.3 kJ
    Option: $1 \text{ ft} = 0.3048 \text{ m}$; thus, $0.3048 \times 2500 \text{ ft}$
    $= 762 \text{ m}$
    Option: $1 \text{ lb} = 0.454 \text{ kg}$; thus, $0.454 \times 120 = 54.5 \text{ kg}$
    $= 545 \text{ N}$

13. The return descent resulted in how much negative (eccentric) work?

   [assumes negative work $(-w) = 1/3$ positive work (^+w)]
   $^-w = 415\,290\ \text{N·m} \div 3 = 138\,430\ \text{N·m} = 138\,430\ \text{J}$
   $= 138.4\ \text{kJ}$

14. During the 1.5 mile run test, a person consumes 35 liters of oxygen. How many kcal were burned?

   L $VO_2 = 5$ kcal; thus, $35\ \text{L} \times 5 = 175$ kcal

15. True or False: 82 °F is < 30 °C?

   $°C = (°F - 32) \times 0.56;\ (82 - 32) \times 0.56 = 50 \times 0.56$
   $= 28\ °C$

Option: $°C = (°F - 32) \div 1.8 = 50 \div 1.8 = 27.8\ °C$
Option: $°F = (1.8 \times °C) + 32 = (1.8 \times 30) + 32$
$= 54 + 32 = 86\ °F$
Answer: True, because 27.8 °C (or 28) is < 30 °C; or 82 °F is < 86 °F; also, mnemonic- 28 is reverse of 82

16. A barometric pressure equal to 29.92 in. of Hg is equal to how many torr (or mm) of Hg?

   1 mm = 0.03937 in.; thus, $29.92 \div 0.03937$
   $= 760$ torr (mm)
   Option: 1 in. = 25.4 mm; thus, 29.92×25.4
   $= 760$ torr (mm)

Appendix E

Informed Consent for Participating in Lab

Explanation of the Graded (Progressive) Exercise Tests

You will perform several different graded exercise tests on a cycle ergometer and/or treadmill. The exercise intensity will increase each 2–4 minutes. Depending on your heart rate or other symptoms and variables, you may continue to work harder or the test will end. We may stop the test at any time because of signs of fatigue or discomfort. Also you may stop any time you feel the test is becoming too strenuous. You may also perform a very strenuous test of anaerobic power with slightly more risk of cardiovascular complications.

Explanation of Other Tests

You will also perform several other tests including evaluations of your body composition, pulmonary function, blood pressure, flexibility, and muscular strength. All of these tests involve minimal risk of injury.

Risks and Discomforts

The possibility does exist that certain changes could occur during the graded exercise test. They include abnormal blood pressure, fainting, disorders of heart beat, and in very rare instances, heart attack or death. Every effort will be made to minimize the risk of these changes through preliminary screening and by observation during the testing. Emergency procedures and trained lab personnel are available to deal with any unusual situations that may arise. All of the other tests involve minimal risk but could result in overstretching muscles, respiratory difficulties, muscle cramps, and light headedness.

Benefits to be Expected

The results obtained from the graded exercise test and related tests will assist in the assessment of your current level of physical fitness. You will learn how it feels to perform these tests and how to administer them, in addition to learning how to interpret them.

Inquiries

Any questions about the procedures used in the exercise tests are encouraged. If you have any doubts or questions, please ask us for further explanations.

Freedom of Consent

Your permission to perform the tests is voluntary. We will work together toward making an effort to find a substitute assignment for any of the tests in which you do not feel comfortable in performing.

"I have read this form and I understand the test procedures that I will perform. I freely consent to participate voluntarily in all of the described laboratory tests."

_____   _____
(Signature of Participant)   (Date)

Source: Courtesy of Dr. William Beam, CSUF.

Index